Communicable Diseases

A Global Perspective

4th Edition

*This book is dedicated to Michael Colbourne (1919–1993),
malariologist, teacher and previous Dean in the Universities of Hong Kong and
Singapore, who while at the London School of Hygiene and Tropical Medicine
gave me considerable help in its preparation.*

And also to

*Brian Southgate (1930–2011) teacher, mentor and an authority
in many fields who has been a constant support and helper
in the development of this book.*

Communicable Diseases

A Global Perspective

4th Edition

Roger Webber

Watermell, Ardfern, Lochgilphead, Argyll PA31 8QN, UK
r-webber@live.co.uk
Formerly of London School of Hygiene and Tropical Medicine

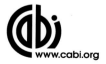
www.cabi.org

CABI is a trading name of CAB International

CABI
Nosworthy Way
Wallingford
Oxfordshire OX10 8DE
UK

CABI
875 Massachusetts Avenue
7th Floor
Cambridge, MA 02139
USA

Tel: +44 (0)1491 832111
Fax: +44 (0)1491 833508
E-mail: cabi@cabi.org
Website: www.cabi.org

Tel: +1 617 395 4056
Fax: +1 617 354 6875
E-mail: cabi-nao@cabi.org

A catalogue record for this book is available from the British Library, London, UK.

Library of Congress Cataloging-in-Publication Data

Webber, Roger.
  Communicable diseases : a global perspective / Roger Webber. -- 4th ed.
    p.; cm.
  Rev. ed. of: Communicable disease epidemiology and control / Roger Webber. 3rd ed. c2009.
  Includes bibliographical references and index.
    ISBN 978-1-84593-938-0 (pbk. : alk. paper) -- ISBN 978-1-84593-939-7 (hbk. : alk. paper)
I. Webber, Roger. Communicable disease epidemiology and control. II. Title.
[DNLM: 1. Communicable Disease Control. 2. Communicable Diseases--epidemiology. WA 110]

614.4--dc23

2012004198

First edition 1996 ISBN 978 0 85199 138 2
Second edition 2005 ISBN 978 0 85199 902 9
Third edition 2009 ISBN 978 1 84593 504 7 (pbk) 978 1 84593 505 5 (hbk)

ISBN: 978 1 84593 938 0 (pbk)
     978 1 84593 939 7 (hbk)

Commissioning editor: Rachel Cutts
Editorial assistant: Alexandra Lainsbury
Production editor: Tracy Head

Typeset by SPi, Pondicherry, India
Printed and bound by Gutenberg Press Limited, Tarxien, Malta

Contents

Introduction

Since the last edition of this book – *Communicable Disease Epidemiology and Control* – communicable diseases have again been at the forefront of concern, not only by the medical fraternity but by the population at large with the steady progress of A(H1N1) influenza, so-called swine flu. This was declared a pandemic in 2010, the first pandemic of influenza since 1977. Fortunately, the last major scare of an epidemic disease, severe acute respiratory syndrome (SARS), was completely contained, with no further cases since July 2003, while the steady decline of variant Creutzfeldt–Jakob disease (vCJD) gives hope that this awful condition is coming to an end. On the negative side has been the increase in food-borne transmitted infections due to international trade in poultry and meat produce and the alarming appearance of multi-drug-resistant organisms in many infections. This has caused considerable problems in the treatment of tuberculosis, while some hospital infections are now resistant to every known antibiotic. There has also been the appearance of artemesinin-resistant malaria and the realization that human immunodeficiency virus (HIV) infection potentiates the spread and severity of malaria.

Communicable diseases are still the major killers in the world, with tuberculosis, malaria and HIV taking a huge annual toll (approximately 4–5 million deaths). In the developing world, just to survive childhood is the major challenge to life as acute respiratory infections (ARIs) and diarrhoeal diseases account for some 6 million young lives every year.

The news is not all bad though. Since the first edition was published poliomyelitis has been eradicated from Europe, the Americas and the Western Pacific, and although there have been setbacks, continued good progress is being made towards the goal of global eradication. Guinea worm has been cleared from most of the endemic area by simple improvements in water supply, a tribute to rudimentary health measures. Leprosy, the disease of antiquity has, owing to an active search and find programme, decreased by such a degree that it is no longer a health problem in many countries. Chagas' disease, the awful debilitating condition that has troubled South and Central America for such a long time, has been eradicated from Uruguay, Chile, Brazil and Argentina, with good progress continuing to be made in Bolivia and Paraguay. This has been by simple control of the vector and improvement in standards of housing – attention to detail rather than some newly discovered invention.

The development of new vaccines has been a tribute to the research and development sector, with the general availability of vaccines against meningitis, pneumococcal infection, rotavirus and human papilloma virus now added to the routine vaccination programmes in many countries. As well as the polio eradication campaign, there is the real possibility of eliminating measles as a public health problem; between 2000 and 2008 it is estimated that 4.3 million deaths due to measles were prevented.

The appearance of new diseases and the persistence of infections that have always been with us means that a knowledge of communicable diseases is still necessary. This is even more so in the developing world where the burden of communicable diseases is the major health problem.

While individuals fall sick and require the expertise of the medical profession, it is the overall assessment of the cause of diseases and how to control them that will most rapidly solve the problem in the community. Indeed, communicable diseases are community problems and need to be looked at in this way. Epidemiology is the science of communities: looking at many individuals to try and discover common features. From this analysis, the cause and characteristics of a disease can be worked out. However, this is not an epidemiology book and it appears that the previous title might have suggested this, so the present title has been shortened to remove this confusion.

Learning about these diseases one by one is a long and complicated process, yet it is the method of transmission that is the key to control, with several diseases sharing the same method of transmission.

This allows diseases to be grouped together so that knowing the characteristics of one means that any of the diseases in the group can probably be controlled in a similar way. While there are always exceptions, grouping communicable diseases makes this easier and is one of the intentions of the book. This approach seems to have been borne out as the previous editions have been used as course books for several teaching programmes and it is hoped that changes made in this edition will make it even more suitable.

Communicable diseases tend to behave in a similar pattern. Such generalizations determine the first chapters, which look at communicable disease theory, formulating common principles in both epidemiology and control. Entomology and parasitology are often taught as separate disciplines, but because they form such an integral part of many communicable diseases the essentials have been included. A knowledge of the various vectors needs to be known for those diseases in which vectors are involved and the life cycles of parasites determine the clinical signs as well as indicating the best places to aim control programmes.

The range of communicable diseases occurring throughout the world is considerable. A comprehensive list is given in Chapter 20, but only those of importance are covered in detail in the main part of the book. Emphasis is placed on developing countries, as this is where most communicable diseases are found. It is hoped this selection of diseases provides a representative perspective of the world situation (Table I.1).

While the emphasis of this book is on diseases found in tropical and developing countries, several diseases more common in developed countries, have also been included. A balance had to be achieved though between attempting to cover everything superficially or concentrating on certain diseases in more depth, and within the constraints of trying to keep this book to a manageable size, it is hoped the right balance has been achieved. The main addition in this edition is a new chapter on infection and pregnancy, a more important subject than it at first seems. By bringing together all the infections that can afflict the pregnant woman the full magnitude of the problem is shown.

Many of the examples are taken from the author's personal experience of working in Solomon Islands and Tanzania, with shorter periods in South America and various Asian countries. Much of what I have learnt has come from the large number of people who have helped and worked with me in these countries. I owe them a considerable debt for their wisdom and assistance, help that I hope I pass on in the following pages.

Experience is invaluable, but organizing one's thoughts and developing a critical judgement comes from working in an academic environment and many people in the London School of Hygiene and Tropical Medicine (LSHTM) helped me in the previous editions. David Bradley provided the inspiration for the system of classification. I have borrowed heavily from the classification he developed for the water- and excreta-related diseases, continuing with these principles for the other communicable diseases. I also owe a special thanks to Brian Southgate, who sadly died in May 2011 after a long illness. He introduced me to many original concepts and has been a kindly guide to being more scientific.

In this edition, I particularly wish to thank Deborah Bateson, Director of Family Planning, New South Wales, Australia, John Walley and Kirstie Graham of the Nuffield Centre for International Health and Development, Leeds and Sandy Cairncross of the LSHTM. Rupert Gude, while working in Tanzania, kindly supplied me with useful information on the management of the pregnant woman with HIV. Other material I found on the helpful web sites mounted by the World Health Organization (WHO) and the UK Health Protection Agency. The Internet has changed the whole way of researching for a book, and to the many unknown writers who have contributed to the various sites I have used I give my thanks. Many of these sites, particularly that of WHO, allow you to download their publications free of charge, making a very useful source of reference for the reader who requires more information.

Many organizations assisted me, and I am especially grateful to WHO for allowing me to use copies of its many figures. The Department for International Development (DFID) was my employer while I worked in Solomon Islands and Tanzania, and as a member of the Tropical Diseases Control Programme at LSHTM. It has given me considerable assistance in this entire endeavour and I would particularly like to thank the Health and Population Division Low Cost Book Programme for a generous grant towards the publishing costs of the first edition. I have had a very happy working relationship with CABI, the book's publisher, ever since 1995 when my manuscript for the first edition was accepted. CABI has given me considerable support, and as a non-profit organization renders a most valuable service to the developing world.

In these days of rising prices and commercial competition it is becoming increasingly difficult to produce books that are affordable in developing countries. Every effort has been made to produce this volume as cheaply as possible, without sacrificing quality, but even so the copy price is higher than I would like it to have been. This is mainly to allow production at a lower cost for developing countries, so every copy bought is helping more copies to be made available where they are most needed.

Table I.1. The burden of communicable diseases in the world 2004. Data from the World Health Organization, Geneva.

Disease	DALYs[a] ('000)	%	Deaths ('000)	%
Lower respiratory infections	94,511	25.42	4109	32.9
Diarrhoeal disease	72,777	19.57	2127	17.03
HIV/AIDS	58,513	15.74	2040	16.33
Tuberculosis	34,217	9.20	1464	11.72
Malaria	33,976	9.14	1021	8.17
Measles	14,853	3.99	424	3.39
Meningitis	11,426	3.07	340	2.72
Pertussis	9882	2.66	254	2.03
Lymphatic filariasis	5941	1.60	0	0
Tetanus	5283	1.42	163	1.30
Chlamydia	3748	1.01	9	0.07
Gonorrhoea	3550	0.95	1	0.008
Syphilis	2846	0.76	99	0.79
Hepatitis B	2068	0.56	105	0.84
Leishmaniasis	1974	0.53	47	0.38
Hookworm	1851	0.50	2	0.02
Ascariasis	1851	0.50	2	0.02
Upper respiratory infections	1787	0.48	77	0.62
Schistosomiasis	1707	0.46	41	0.33
Trypanosomiasis (African)	1673	0.45	52	0.42
Otitis media	1488	0.40	5	0.04
Trachoma	1334	0.36	0	0
Trichuriasis	1012	0.27	2	0.02
Hepatitis C	955	0.26	54	0.43
Japanese encephalitis	681	0.18	11	0.09
Dengue	670	0.18	18	0.14
Chagas' disease	430	0.12	11	0.09
Onchocerciasis	389	0.10	0	0
Leprosy	194	0.05	5	0.04
Diphtheria	174	0.05	5	0.04
Poliomyelitis	34	0.01	1	0.008
Total	371,795	100.00	12,489	100.00

[a]Disability-adjusted life years. The DALY is a calculation of the morbidity and mortality of the particular disease averaged out over the expected life of a person, so it reflects the prevalence of the disease and the disability it produces. For example, a common disease such as lymphatic filariasis will have a high DALY because of the large number of people infected and the disability caused, although nobody dies from the disease.

1 Elements of Communicable Diseases

1.1 What Are Communicable Diseases?

A *communicable disease* is an illness that is transmitted from a person, animal, or inanimate source to another person either directly, with the assistance of an intermediate host or by a vector. Communicable diseases cover a wider range than the person-to-person transmission of infectious diseases; they include the parasitic diseases, infections transmitted by a vector, the zoonoses and all the transmissible diseases.

Communicable diseases present in an epidemic or endemic form. An *epidemic* is the introduction of a new infection or the presence of an illness in excess of normal expectancy. This can be seasonal such as, with influenza or when the number of susceptible persons is sufficient for a new epidemic to take place, e.g. measles. Any unknown infection will be epidemic when first introduced. An *endemic* disease is constantly present in a geographical area or population group, e.g. malaria is found in tropical countries and endemic in the adult population.

Communicable diseases are dependent on the person being susceptible to infection, so children meeting an infection for the first time or communities that have been isolated from the infection are more liable to become infected. They are found particularly in conditions that encourage transmission such as overcrowding or poor hygiene so are more common in developing countries. They are invariably associated with poverty.

Epidemic diseases devastate whole populations, as when measles ravaged Fiji, killing adults as well as children. Populations then have to start again from the survivors to recover their former strength. These are essentially young and growing populations.

With endemic diseases it is children that are particularly vulnerable, so there is a high birth rate to compensate. With so many young people in the population, non-communicable diseases are uncommon, but as people live longer then they become more frequent. Non-communicable diseases such as coronary heart disease (CHD) are the main problem of older aged populations as seen in the Western world.

This division between the developed and developing world is purely artificial where diseases are concerned. When the plague, or 'Black Death' as it was known, spread across Europe it caused as much devastation as when communicable diseases were introduced to newly found nations by Western explorers. The population started again from the survivors as it has had to do in developing countries. Just over 100 years ago measles was as serious a cause of childhood death in large European cities as it is today in developing countries without well-organized vaccination programmes. A tropical environment is more favourable to many diseases than the cooler temperate regions, but even here such tropical diseases as malaria were once common in Europe. There is nothing new or different about these artificially divided parts of the world except for the resources that each is able to devote to the improvement of their health. Communicable diseases could be reduced to manageable problems if enough resources, both in financial and educational terms, could be spent on them.

The difference between communicable and non-communicable diseases used to be quite clear cut. Where there was an organism that was transmitted it was communicable; otherwise the disease was classified as non-communicable. However, this strict boundary is becoming less well defined as new suspect organisms are discovered, or diseases, by their very nature, suggest a communicable origin. Various cancers are good examples; the link between hepatitis B virus (HBV, Section 14.11) and hepatocellular cancer is well established, and is now being prevented by routine vaccination. Epstein–Barr virus (EBV) seems to be a pathogenic factor in Burkitt's lymphoma, but there is also a causal relationship with malaria, so controlling malaria (Section 15.6) in Africa and Papua New Guinea, where this tumour is found, could have a double benefit. EBV might also have a causal effect in non-Hodgkin's lymphoma and nasopharyngeal cancer. Kaposi's sarcoma may well be transmitted by the sexual route as shown by the number of people with it who acquire human immunodeficiency virus (HIV) infection via sexual transmission as compared with those becoming infected from blood transmission, in which the tumour occurs only rarely. The trematode worms *Schistosoma haematobium* (Section 11.1) and *Clonorchis sinensis* (Section 9.5) are causative factors in bladder cancer and cholangiocarcinoma, respectively, so their control as communicable diseases will also reduce cancer incidence. *Helicobacter pylori*, an organism that thrives in gastric secretions, is probably a causative factor in gastric cancer. The commonest cancer with a communicable cause is cancer of the cervix, due to infection with the human papilloma virus (HPV, Section 14.9). Prevention of this infection by vaccination offers the greatest hope of reducing this important cause of female mortality.

Equally intriguing is the possibility that atheroma has an infective cause or association. With arteriosclerosis being largely responsible for CHD and the major killer in Western countries the possibility of preventing it by finding the infective causal agent is attractive. *Chlamydia pneumoniae* has been found within atheroma lesions, but not normal arteries, while cytomegalovirus (CMV) is able to infect the smooth muscle cells of arterial walls. The association of *H. pylori* and CHD now seems unlikely, but herpesvirus 1 could induce an endothelial cell response. The cause will probably be found to be multifactorial, but perhaps in time nearly all diseases will be shown to have a transmissible factor in their causation. Even road accidents – for which there seems no need to look for a predisposing cause in a communicable disease – might be made more likely to occur as a result of infection with toxoplasmosis (Section 17.5). *Toxoplasma gondii*, the causative organism, is also thought to be a causal factor in neurosis and schizophrenia, and recent work also suggests a correlation with brain cancer.

While avoiding infection is normally the best strategy, our obsession with cleanliness might be responsible for the increase in allergies, type 1 diabetes, inflammatory bowel disorders and multiple sclerosis in developed countries. These are found less commonly in developing countries where conditions of hygiene are poor and were rare in developed countries in the early part of the last century. It is thought that our obsession with cleanliness and using antibacterial products prevents minor infections that stimulate the immune system. A little bit of dirt is good for us, and especially for young children when they are developing their immune response.

The key to any communicable disease is to think of it in terms of *agent, transmission, host* and *environment*. These components are illustrated in Fig. 1.1, which will be used as a framework in the description of this section. There needs to be a causative agent, which requires a means of transmission from one host to another, but the outcome of infection will be influenced by the environment in which the disease is transmitted and the response of the host.

1.2   The Agent

The agent can be an organism (virus, prion, bacteria, rickettsia, protozoa, helminth, fungus or arthropod) or a physical or chemical agent (toxin or poison). If it is an organism, the agent needs to *multiply*, find a means of *transmission* and *survive*.

1.2.1   Multiplication

Two methods of multiplication occur, *sexual* and *asexual* reproduction, which have different advantages. In asexual reproduction a succession of exact or almost exact replicas are produced, so that any natural selection will act on batches or strains, rather than on individuals. By contrast, sexual reproduction offers great scope for variety, both within the cells of the single organism and from one organism to another. This means that natural selection acts on individuals, and variations of vigour and adaptability occur.

There are different consequences of these two methods of reproduction. With asexual organisms the strain of the organism is either successful or unsuccessful in invading the host, whereas in sexually reproducing organisms certain individuals will succeed while others will not. In continuing its existence, only one organism of the asexual parasite requires to be transmitted, whereas with the sexually reproducing parasite, both male and female adults must meet before reproduction can take place. Some parasites seem to be at a tremendous disadvantage, e.g. the filarial worm *Wuchereria bancrofti*, in which both male and female individuals go through long migrations in

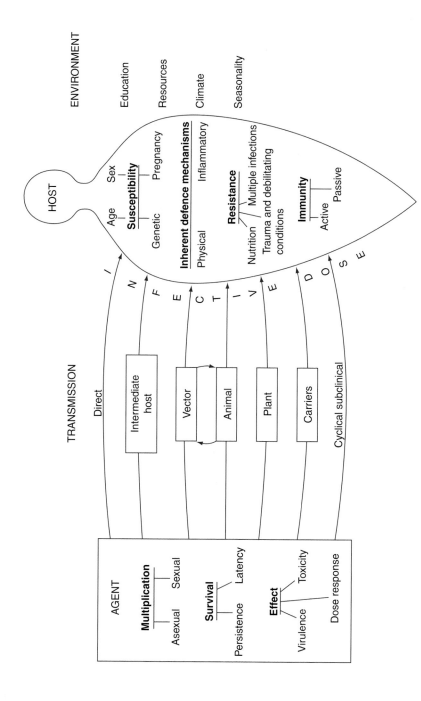

Fig. 1.1. The interrelationship of the agent, transmission, host and environment.

the body to find an individual of the opposite sex, but despite all these problems this is one of the most successful of all parasites.

Whether the organism reproduces sexually or asexually is relevant in treatment and control. If a treatment is successful at destroying an asexually reproducing organism then it will be successful against all the other individuals of that strain of the organism – unless a mutation occurs which renders the individual resistant to treatment, when this resistance will be conferred on all other organisms developing from this strain. In contrast, sexual reproduction produces individuals of different vigour, meaning that some individuals will succumb to treatment, while others will not. However, having two sexes can be a disadvantage for the organism in that methods of control can be devised which attack only one of the sexes, or designed to reduce the chance of individuals of each sex from meeting.

1.2.2 Survival

Parasitic agents survive by finding a suitable host within a certain period of time. They have been able to improve their chances of finding a new host or surviving in the environment by a number of different methods.

Reservoirs and parasite adaptability

A reservoir is a storage place for water but also serves as an appropriate term to describe a suitable place for storing agents of infection. Once an agent invades a host there is normally a latent or waiting period while sufficient organisms are produced before the main attack is mounted. If the host survives but is not able to eliminate the invading organism, then the organism can continue to live and reproduce in the host.

The relationship between the parasite and host is one of continual challenge, what has been termed a biological arms race. When the parasite first attacks a new species the host attempts to eliminate it, resulting in a severe reaction. In time, adaptation can occur so that the reaction of the host diminishes and the adaptability of the parasite increases. The parasite is then able to live in the host with few ill effects (e.g. *Trichuris trichiura*), forming an established population, and continuing with minimal reaction from the host. The host then acts as a reservoir from which parasites attack new hosts of the same species or attempt to colonize different species. Reservoirs can be humans, animals, vectors or the inanimate environment (e.g. soil, water). Intermediaries may be required before the final reservoir host is colonized. However, it is always within the parasite's interest to improve its reproductive capability, so if a new mutation arises which is beneficial to this end then this will be selected, generally to the host's disadvantage.

The adaptability of parasites to their human hosts might even have advantages for us. *Ascaris*, *Trichuris* and the hookworms (particularly *Necator americanus*) secrete substances to reduce the host immune response, which inadvertently are absorbed by the gut lining. These have been found to help reduce allergic reactions such as hay fever. Our more hygienic surroundings, by decreasing these parasites, may be responsible for the increase in allergic diseases such as asthma in developed countries. It is a strange irony that it may be preferable to actually introduce (rather than control) these parasites to combat some allergic reactions.

Persistence

Another mechanism used by parasites to survive is the development of special stages that resist destruction in an adverse environment. Examples are the cysts of protozoa, e.g. *Entamoeba histolytica*, and the eggs of nematodes, e.g. *Ascaris*. Bacteria can persist in the environment by the development of spores, as with anthrax and tetanus bacilli. Destruction of persistent organisms requires the use of antiseptics or sufficient heat for a prolonged period of time, as shown in Fig 1.2.

Latency

The production by the organism of a developmental stage in the environment that is not infective to a new host is called latency. This allows the parasite to wait until suitable conditions develop before changing into the infective form. *Ascaris*, the hookworms and *Strongyloides* exhibit latency.

1.2.3 The effect of the agent

If enough agents survive to infect a new host, they will produce illness, the severity of which is determined by their toxicity and virulence.

Infectious agents produce a toxic reaction due to the foreign proteins they consist of or

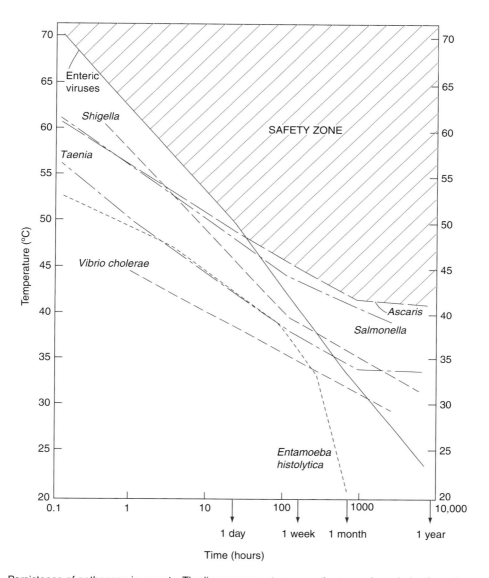

Fig. 1.2. Persistence of pathogens in excreta. The lines represent conservative upper boundaries for pathogen death – that is, estimates of the time–temperature combinations required for pathogen inactivation. Organisms can survive for long periods at low temperatures, so a composting process must be maintained at a temperature above 43°C for at least a month to effectively kill all pathogens likely to be found in human excreta. (From Feachem, R.G, Bradley, D.J., Garelick, H. and Mara, D.D. (1983) *Sanitation and Disease: Health Aspects of Excreta and Wastewater Management*. The World Bank, Washington, DC, p. 79. Reprinted by permission of John Wiley & Sons Ltd.)

produce in their respiratory or reproductive processes (e.g. malaria). Sometimes the organism produces very little toxicity or, conversely, this can be out of all proportion to the insignificant primary infection, as for example with tetanus.

Some organisms produce toxins when they grow in food, causing illness at a distance. An example is *Clostridium botulinum*. Toxic chemicals can also contaminate food, e.g. adulterated cooking oil, and produce an illness that has all the appearances of an epidemic produced by a living organism.

Some agents have a very marked effect on their host, while others have a mild one. A good example is influenza. In the so-called Spanish flu of 1918–1920, it is estimated that 70 million people were killed worldwide, while subsequent epidemics of influenza have caused mainly mild infections, with mortality only in the young or aged. As an infection progresses in a community, virulence can increase or decrease owing to its passage through several individuals. Generally virulence decreases, and passage through many experimental animals is a method used in developing vaccines.

1.2.4   Excreted load and infective dose

The number of organisms excreted can vary considerably according to the type of infection or the stage of the disease. In diseases such as cholera there may be vast numbers of organisms excreted (10^6–10^{12} vibrios/g of faeces), whereas in hookworm infection the number of eggs may be comparatively few. In *Schistosoma mansoni* asymptomatic children excrete the largest number of eggs, whereas adults exhibiting severe manifestations may be almost non-infectious. In the otherwise harmless typhoid carrier, a bout of diarrhoea can cause the passage of a sufficient number of organisms to initiate an epidemic.

For each infectious agent, a minimum number of organisms, the infective dose, is required to overcome the defences of the host and cause the disease. A large dose of organisms may be required, such as with *Vibrio cholerae*, or very few, as in *Entamoeba histolytica*. In most infections, once this number is surpassed, the severity of the disease is the same whether a few or large number of organisms are introduced, while in others there is a correlation between dose and severity of illness. Estimates of doses have been attempted in cholera and typhoid using healthy volunteers, but variables such as host susceptibility prevent any degree of precision in such estimations. A more precise example is found in food poisoning, where the severity of the illness is determined by the quantity of the infected food item that is consumed. On the beneficial side, a low dose of organisms may produce no symptoms of disease, but be sufficient to induce immunity. Poliomyelitis is one of many such examples.

Infections with a low infective dose (such as enteric viruses and *E. histolytica*) can spread by person-to-person contact. This means that the provision of a safe water supply or sanitation will have little or no effect. At the other extreme are organisms like typhoid and cholera, for which a high infective dose (of the order of 10^6 organisms/ml of water) is required to produce the disease. Improving water quality and the reduction of pathogens in the sewage will be beneficial to the community.

1.3   Transmission

Communicable diseases fall into a number of transmission patterns, as illustrated in Figs 1.1 and 1.3.

1.3.1   Direct

Direct transmission includes person-to-person contact, as from dirty fingers, or via food and water as in the diarrhoeal diseases. Direct transmission also occurs through droplet infection in the respiratory diseases. Auto-infection can occur where humans contaminate themselves directly from their external orifices. Examples are the transmission of *Enterobius* from anal scratching or the infection of skin abrasions with bacteria from nose picking.

1.3.2   Human reservoir with intermediate host

The adults of the schistosomiasis parasite live in humans but for transmission to another human the parasite must undergo developmental stages in a snail intermediate host. In the flukes *Clonorchis*, *Opisthorchis* and *Paragonimus*, and the fish tapeworm *Diphyllobothrium*, more than one kind of non-mammalian intermediate host is required.

1.3.3   Animals as intermediate host or reservoir

Animals can either be intermediate hosts, as with *Taenia saginata* and *T. solium* (the beef and pork tapeworms) where cysticerci must develop in the animal muscle before they infect humans, or they can be reservoirs as in Chagas' disease (caused by *Trypanosoma cruzi*). In the latter, the infection is maintained in a wild rodent reservoir, from which the foraging dog becomes infected, bringing infection into the home of a vulnerable human.

1.3.4   Vectors

A vector carries the infection from one host to another either as part of the transmission process, as in the mosquito, or mechanically, as in the house fly,

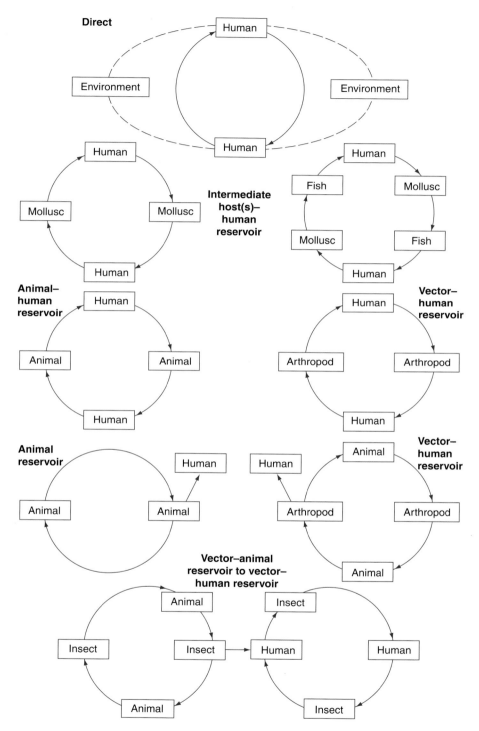

Fig. 1.3. Transmission cycles.

which inadvertently transmits organisms to the host on its feet and mouthparts. All vectors of importance are either insects; mosquitoes, flies, fleas, lice, etc., or arachnids; ticks and mites. Infection may occur as a result of either the feeding of the arthropod or its habits. The cycles of transmission are:

- direct insect to human as in malaria;
- insect to animal with humans entering the cycle as an abnormal host, e.g. bubonic plague;
- insect to animal, including humans, from which it is transmitted to other humans by the same or another insect vector. Examples are yellow fever and East African sleeping sickness.

(Snails, especially in descriptions of schistosomiasis, are often called vectors, but they do not carry the infection from one host to the other so are intermediate hosts not vectors.)

1.3.5   Zoonosis

In their classification by transmission cycle, communicable diseases fall into two main groups, the diseases where only humans are involved, and those in which there is an animal reservoir or intermediate host. The latter include the *zoonoses*, which are infections that are naturally transmitted between vertebrate animals and humans. These can be grouped according to the intimacy of the animal to the human being:

- *Domestic*: those invited animals that live in close proximity to man, e.g. pets and farm animals.
- *Synanthropic*: animals that live in close association with man, but are not invited, e.g. rats.
- *Exoanthropic*: animals that are not in close association with man, e.g. monkeys.

The importance of this type of classification is that it indicates the *focality* of the disease. As domestic animals are universally distributed then domestic zoonotic diseases are cosmopolitan, whereas at the other extreme, in an exoanthropic zoonosis such as scrub typhus or jungle yellow fever it is quite possible for humans to live in the same locality but separate from the disease area. Humans have no part in the disease cycle, but come into contact with it only when they accidentally enter the affected place (focus).

In zoonoses, the animal is all important in control. In some diseases, such as beef and pork tapeworm infections, good hygiene practice and inspection of the animal carcass may be all that is required to interrupt transmission. At the opposite extreme, a disease such as yellow fever can never be eradicated from the population even if every man, woman and child were immunized because the reservoir of disease remains in the monkey population. In a zoonosis the animal reservoir is of prime importance, and only by studying the ecology of the animal population can any rational attempt be made to control it.

1.3.6   Plants

Vegetable material that is eaten by the host can serve as a method of transmission. This can either be a specific plant, such as water calthrop on which the cercariae of the fluke *Fasciolopsis buski* encyst, or non-specific, such as any salad vegetable that might be carrying cysts of *E. histolytica*.

1.3.7   Carriers and subclinical transmission

Diseases in which there is an animal reservoir, intermediate host or vector are complex and difficult to control, but even in the simplified transmission cycle of direct spread from human to human, complications occur with the *carrier* state. A carrier is a person that can transmit the infective agent but is not manifesting the disease. There are several types of carriers:

- Incubating or prodromal carriers who are infectious but unaware that they are in the early stages of the disease.
- Asymptomatic carriers who remain well throughout the infection.
- Convalescent carriers who continue to be infectious after the clinical disease has passed.

The carrier state can either be *transient* or *chronic*. The important features of carriers are:

- The number of carriers may be far greater than the number of those who are sick.
- Carriers are not manifest so they and others are unaware that they can transmit the disease.
- As carriers are not sick they are not restricted and therefore disseminate the disease widely.
- Chronic carriers may produce repeated outbreaks over a considerable period of time.

Identification of carriers is a singularly difficult and generally unsuccessful exercise. If the carrier is asymptomatic the organism is often in such reduced numbers, or excreted at such infrequent intervals, that routine culture techniques will not detect it. The investigation has to be repeated many times and is probably only successful at specific instances, e.g. during a minor diarrhoeal episode in a suspected typhoid carrier. A further difficulty is that clinically well people object to having investigations performed on them, so coverage is incomplete. Examples of diseases in which the carrier state is important are typhoid, amoebiasis, poliomyelitis, meningococcal meningitis, diphtheria and hepatitis B. More on carriers will be found in the sections dealing with each of these diseases.

In some diseases, the carrier state appears to be prolonged, or is perpetuated when there are in fact no carriers. This may be due to *cyclical subclinical transmission* when infection is transmitted within a family or throughout a community that is tolerant or has a high level of immunity, without the subjects being aware of any particular symptoms. One member of a family passes on the infection to another, a process which is continued, producing asymptomatic infection. When someone who is susceptible to the disease accidentally enters this cycle, or the organism is more widely disseminated, then a clinical outbreak occurs. This is a mechanism by which poliomyelitis is maintained in the community. Most subclinical transmissions result from infection acquired in childhood.

1.4 Host Factors

If the agent is transmitted to a new host its successful invasion and continuation will depend upon a number of host factors.

1.4.1 Susceptibility

Genetic

Certain diseases can only affect animals, and when they are transmitted to humans they are not able to establish themselves. An example is *Plasmodium berghei*, the rodent malaria parasite, which cannot produce disease in man although it is closely related to the human malaria parasites. However, some newly emergent diseases have succeeded in crossing this genetic barrier, such as HIV and new variant Creutzfeldt-Jakob disease (vCJD).

The heterozygous (the union of two unlike gametes) genetic make-up of animals, including humans, gives added protection from infection in that some individuals will be highly susceptible to a certain

disease whereas others might be quite resistant. This is well shown in tuberculosis and leprosy where the mycobacterium is common in the environment but only certain people develop tuberculosis or leprosy. The type of disease, e.g. tuberculoid or lepromatous leprosy, is also determined by the genetic make-up of the individual. Particular genetic traits, such as sickle-cell anaemia, give protection against infection, in this case malaria. Certain individuals have been found to be resistant to HIV infection even in high-risk situations such as prostitution.

The wider the heterozygote separation the greater is the possibility of producing offspring resistant to some infections, and it has been the introduction of genetically diverse people into some populations that has increased their resistance to disease. Widely diverse heterozygotes are at least 20% better at resisting infection than related heterozygotes.

Age

During the course of life different diseases affect particular age groups. The childhood diseases of measles, chickenpox and diphtheria are found at one end of the lifespan, with the degenerative diseases and neoplasms predominating at the other.

Sex

The same advantages as parasites derive from having two sexes, producing many individuals of different vigour also benefit humans, and it is thought that evading parasites might be one of the main reasons why mammals evolved with two sexes. However one or other sex might more commonly succumb to illness, such as in poliomyelitis which is more common in females, and in mumps which is a more serious condition in males. Occupation can determine which sex is more likely to be involved, such as in East Africa where males who hunt and collect honey in tsetse fly infested forest are more likely to contract *Trypanasoma brucei rhodesiense* sleeping sickness. Social habits may also be determinant, such as the custom of the Fore people in Papua New Guinea, where the women eat the brains of the recently dead, making kuru predominantly a disease of women.

Pregnancy

When a woman is pregnant, her physiological mechanisms are altered and she becomes more susceptible to infections. Chickenpox is a severe disease in pregnancy and malaria attacks the pregnant woman as though she had little acquired immunity. The pregnant woman that contracts Lassa fever is more likely to die from the illness. More on pregnancy and infection can be found in Chapter 18.

1.4.2 Inherent defence mechanisms

Any infecting organism must be able to overcome the body's *inherent defence mechanisms*. These can either be:

- *physical*, such as the skin, mucous-secreting membranes or acidity of the stomach; or
- *inflammatory*, the localized reaction of increased blood flow, the isolation of the site of inoculation, the attraction of white blood cells and the increased lymph cell activity (often resulting in lymphadenopathy). The range of white blood cells includes macrophages, granulocytes, natural killer cells and dendritic cells, which produce an array of armaments that passively engulf organisms to secreting substances that immobilize them. These cells also process the foreign material of the invading organism to initiate the immune response.

1.4.3 Immunity

Experience of previous infection by a host can lead to the development of immunity. This consists of two parts: a cellular and a humoral response. In the *cellular* response, the material processed by white blood cells is served in a histocompatibility complex to T-lymphocytes which then destroy host cells exhibiting this foreign material. In the *humoral* response, B-lymphocytes which have pre-formed antibodies on their surfaces are stimulated by the foreign material of an infection to synthesize specific antibodies, tailor-made to the antigen. These antibodies can either be antigen specific or able to act on a wider range of antigenic structures. In addition, B-cell activation will stimulate memory cells which reside in the bone marrow to produce long-term protection. Immunity can be either *active* or *passive*.

Active

Active immunity follows an infection (with or without symptoms) or vaccination with attenuated (live or dead) organisms. This will induce the body to develop an immune response in a number of diseases. Immunity is most completely developed against the viral infections and may be permanent. With protozoal infections, e.g. malaria, it is only maintained by repeated attacks of the organism.

Passive

Passive immunity is the transfer of antibodies from a mother to her child via the placenta. Passive immunity is short lived, as in the protection of the young infant against measles for the first 6 months of life. Passive immunity can also be introduced by the transfer of antibodies from animals or convalescent human serum, e.g. in rabies immune serum.

1.4.4 Resistance

The person's resistance to infection may be lowered by the following:

- *Nutrition.* Where the nutritional status is decreased the susceptibility to a disease is increased, or the clinical illness is more severe.
- *Trauma and debilitating conditions.* Poliomyelitis may be a mild or inapparent infection, but if associated with trauma, such as an intramuscular injection, then paralytic disease can result. The appearance of shingles or fungal infections in debilitated people is often seen.
- *Multiple infections.* The presence of one disease may make it easier for other infecting organisms. Secondary respiratory infections commonly occur in measles. Yaws has been noticed to increase and spread more rapidly following an outbreak of chickenpox.
- *Immunodeficiency.* This can rarely be present at birth but is more commonly the result of certain infections such as HIV, which interferes with the host immune response.

1.5 The Environment

The transmission cycle used by the agent to reach the host takes place within an environment which determines the success and severity of the infection. Environmental factors are subtle, diffuse and wide ranging. A few of the more important ones are mentioned in this section. These will be divided into the social environment and the physical environment.

1.5.1 The social environment

Education

Sufficient is known about most of the communicable diseases for them to be prevented, if only people were taught how. Education is a complex process, it is not just teaching people; they must be able to understand to such an extent that they are able to modify their lives. This is not a sudden process; changes made by one generation are used as the starting place for improvements or modifications in the following one. Change is always opposed, and steps that seem easy to the educated are mountains for the uneducated to climb.

It is not the tropical climate that determines much of the disease found in developing countries but poverty and lack of education. Parts of Australia and South America lie in the tropics but a high standard of living prevents potential diseases from being a problem. This is even more finely divided in the great conurbations of Asia where the educated rich live in a good state of health, while their less fortunate neighbours residing in slum conditions suffer from a range of preventable diseases. Indeed, countries in Western Europe have suffered from epidemic diseases that devastated the population. In the time of Shakespeare, England was struggling to maintain its population after plague had reduced it by 6% in the previous decade. Another great killer was smallpox, which was no respecter of privilege, almost carrying off Queen Elizabeth I. Measles, rickets, dysentery and every kind of fever were problems of the time. While many of these diseases can be identified as typhus, malaria or scarlet fever, there are others which seem to be new diseases that subsequently died out. The most notorious was the 'English sweat', where people developed fever and died on the same day, although acquired immunity drove the disease to extinction by the 1550s. Another was the 'New sickness', which killed thousands in a series of epidemics between 1556 and 1559.

An improvement in the level of education and understanding was probably the most important reason that endemic communicable diseases largely disappeared from the developed world. As education improved there was a demand for improved living standards. Good water and proper sewage disposal were provided, personal hygiene became a normal rather than abnormal practice, and cleanliness was sanctioned as a desirable attribute. These changes all occurred before the advent of antibiotics.

The decline of tuberculosis in England and Wales (Fig. 13.3) is a classic example of how a major communicable disease decreased as living standards rose.

Resources and economics

The lack of resources leads to poverty, which reduces the ability to combat disease. By resources are meant everything that people have to carry out their livelihood. Perhaps the most important resource is land, which is used by the family for living on and growing crops. Alternatively, this land can be used to produce commodities that can be sold as part of a manufacturing process. As the society develops, then education, or the ability to perform a service, becomes a resource.

Resources are required to enact the preventive methods or raise standards that have come to be demanded by education. At its simplest, food is required to build up body processes and prevent malnutrition. But with a little extra money a water supply can be built or a better house constructed.

Resources, education and disease are inextricably linked. Diseases are best prevented by educating people to overcome them, but resources are required to achieve this. Greater resources allow increased education and improved education the greater utilization of resources. These both act in reducing communicable diseases.

Making the most use of resources and balancing what is needed with what is available is the province of health economics. When someone is ill they need treatment, but there may be several alternatives available so the cheapest producing the desired effect will be the most appropriate for the health service of the country. A good example is the World Health Organization (WHO) essential drugs programme, which recommends the pharmacological component of the medicine rather than generic alternatives, so limiting unnecessary expenditure on treatment.

A community will express its needs on what it perceives is the best requirement to solve its problems, but financial restriction will limit what can be supplied. Health services will need to make choices between one implementation and another, such as a mass drug administration programme or improved curative services, basing their choices on cost-effectiveness and cost–benefit analysis.

With *cost-effectiveness*, programmes that yield the greatest health improvement for the available resources, such as a vaccination programme, are chosen, whereas with *cost–benefit* the outputs of different projects are measured and emphasis given to the one producing the greatest benefit per unit of cost. Although cost–benefit analysis is the more desirable for long-term planning, measuring the benefit of a health intervention is difficult to do.

A development of these methods is the concept of *marginal costs*, as seen in the three different strategies of a vaccination programme: fixed units, mobile clinics and outreach programmes. Using fixed units (clinics and hospitals), the greatest number of children will be reached for the least cost, but to obtain higher coverage it will cost more per child by this method (building more clinics) than adding an outreach programme to the existing clinics. To contact the last remaining children (at the margin of an outreach programme) it will be cheaper to use mobile clinics. So each strategy has its value and it is more cost-effective to use them in this stratified fashion. The same principle can be applied to disease control, as illustrated in Fig 1.4 for dengue. The cheapest method is to get people to remove all collections of water (in tin cans, coconut shells, etc.), whereas the longer term more permanent control will be to cover all water containers near people's houses, which will be more expensive to do. Where there are collections of people, such as a refugee camp, then costly ULV (ultra-low volume) fogging or aerial spraying might be required to prevent an impending epidemic. The most economic strategy will be to use a mix of methods. (More details on dengue will be found in Section 15.4.)

The cost of disease can be considerable as witnessed by many developing countries. It was the success of developed countries to overcome diseases that helped them to become more affluent. However, this can easily be brought down by new and epidemic diseases which can strain the resources of a country just when they are least expected. The SARS (severe acute respiratory syndrome) epidemic of 2002–2003 was estimated to cost US$11 billion.

Communities and movements

People gather together into communities and construct some form of habitation in which to live. The type of structure they live in can play an important part in the diseases they succumb to. In South America the Reduviidae bugs that transmit Chagas' disease live in the mud walls of houses, so replacing these with more permanent materials can prevent the disease. Conversely, if a fire is lit within the house for cooking and heating, the smoke-filled interior leads to an increase in acute respiratory infections, one of the most common of all health problems.

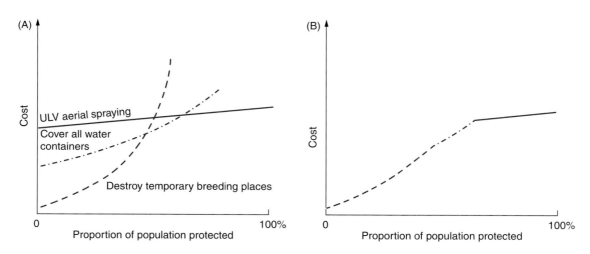

Fig. 1.4. (A) The relative costs of alternative methods of dengue control. (B) The optimum mix of methods.

The attraction of cities has resulted in one of the largest demographic changes in recent times; whereas before the majority of the population lived in rural areas, urban areas have now become the commonest place of residence in tropical countries. Slums have developed in which the diseases of poverty thrive and the imbalance of the sexes has led to an increase in sexually transmitted diseases. At the other extreme is the nomad continually moving from place to place, making it difficult to provide maternal and child health services, with the result that children are not vaccinated, making them vulnerable to many childhood infections.

People have to move to get to their place of work, attend school, visit the clinic, or for many other reasons, but all movements incur a health risk. The woman collecting water may make herself more vulnerable to contracting a diarrhoeal disease by drinking from a polluted source, while the tsetse fly vectors of Gambiense sleeping sickness favour biting people at water-gathering places. The mother carrying her baby to market with her makes it more liable to contract measles and whooping cough at a younger and more vulnerable age. Fishermen, with their greater contact with water, are more likely to contract schistosomiasis.

Local migrations from one country to a neighbouring country for trade or to visit relatives can risk the health of individuals or families. In much of South-east Asia borders generally follow ridges of high ground, which by their nature are inaccessible and generally contain remnants of forest. Mosquitoes inhabit these forests, where there are the right conditions in which to breed. As a consequence, malaria is more intense along these borders so that crossing to the next country and staying for a few days has been found to increase the chance of contracting malaria by as much as six times. This is a complex process (designated 'forest fringe malaria') involving forests and the illegal cutting of timber, which is well illustrated in Fig. 1.5. Insurgents and traffic in narcotics often complicate the picture. Illegal loggers set up camps to exploit the remaining forest, and these are also likely to be the areas in which people spend the night when crossing from one country to another, increasing the likelihood of them contracting malaria.

Following trading routes was the manner in which classical cholera was taken to East Africa in the 19th century and repeated with El Tor cholera in the 20th century. Schistosomiasis was carried to the Americas and Arabia along with the slaves

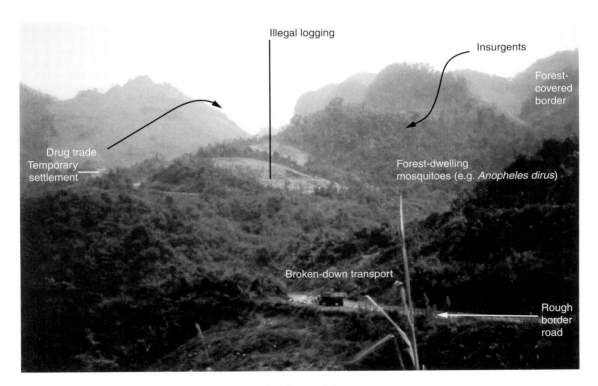

Fig. 1.5. The complexity of forest/border malaria in South-east Asia.

that were forcibly taken to these parts of the world; a continuing vengeance for the evils inflicted on them.

The intriguing story of the jigger flea (*Tunga penetrans*), which burrows into the foot causing painful swellings and a passage for bacterial infection, tells how it was carried the other way round. First described in 1525 by the Spanish in South America, it was brought to Angola in South-west Africa by the British ship *Thomas Mitchell* in 1872. Originating from Rio de Janeiro, the *Thomas Mitchell* was carrying sand ballast on its return voyage (probably from transporting slaves), the perfect soil type for the development of *Tunga* larvae. When this was offloaded the jigger found a ready host in the barefoot African and travelled with the slave caravans to reach Zanzibar, on the other side of Africa, only 25 years later. It is now endemic in the continent producing much misery, especially in poverty-ridden children.

Travel to another country permanently to seek employment or escape from civil conflict is a particularly vulnerable time for the individual and family. Refugees in particular need extra help, but sometimes this can be misplaced and the situation made worse. During the Cambodian crisis, water containers were provided to households in refugee camps along the Thai border, but these proved excellent breeding places for *Aedes* mosquitoes, with the result that there were large outbreaks of dengue. In Tanzania, refugees were settled in a large uninhabited forest area, but it was uninhabited because it was infested with tsetse flies, so soon cases of sleeping sickness began to appear. *Refugee health* has become a subject in its own right and communicable diseases are one of the many troubles that these unfortunate people suffer from.

As with refugee health, a new speciality has developed around the *health of travellers*. The phenomenal increase in air travel has brought the risk of contracting a communicable disease in a foreign country to all kinds of people. Several thousand cases of malaria are imported to England and Wales every year, making it more important than many of the indigenous health problems. HIV infection in European countries has changed from being predominantly in the homosexual community to an increasing problem in the heterosexual, mainly due to infections contracted overseas. Problems also travel in the other direction as when students from malarious areas come to temperate countries to study, so losing their acquired immunity and rendering them liable to contract serious malaria when they return home. Influenza generally arises in the northern hemisphere and is carried to the south by air travel.

1.5.2 The physical environment

Topography

The nature of the physical surroundings can influence the diseases that are found there. In much of Asia a complex interaction termed 'forest fringe malaria', described above, increases the likelihood of developing malaria at the forest margin. A similar cycle of transmission occurs with yellow fever, illustrated in Fig. 15.4. Destruction of primary forest, to be replaced by secondary growth, also makes ideal conditions for the development of the 'mite islands' that are important in scrub typhus (see Section 16.2).

Human activity not only destroys the natural balance of nature but often changes the landscape to make it more suitable for the transmission of communicable diseases. The growing of rice in paddy fields provides suitable conditions for the *Culex* mosquitoes that transmit Japanese encephalitis (JE) and for *Anopheles sinensis*, the vector of malaria in much of China. The construction of dams and irrigation canals has encouraged the proliferation of intermediate host snails of schistosomiasis. However, the *Simulium* fly that transmits onchocerciasis breeds in fast-flowing oxygenated streams that are often destroyed when dams are built, depriving them of their breeding place. All major construction projects should therefore have a health evaluation to determine how the health risk can be minimized.

Climate

Climate can be divided into different components of *temperature*, *rainfall* (humidity) and, less importantly, *wind*. These attributes of the climate have a marked influence on where diseases are found and the ways in which they are to be controlled.

Temperature

Temperature varies by distance from the equator, altitude, prevailing winds and the size of land masses. A number of diseases are found only in the tropics, which is the main area for communicable diseases. Temperature decreases with altitude, so that malaria will be found at the lower hot altitude, while respiratory diseases are commoner in the colder hills. At the fringe of the mosquito range, exceptional conditions of temperature and humidity can produce epidemic malaria.

Temperature not only affects the presence or absence of disease, but often regulates the amount. The malaria parasite has a shorter developmental cycle as the temperature rises and so permits an increased rate of transmission. Many insect vectors have a more rapid development in the tropics, making them difficult to control. The life cycles of a number of parasites are directly related to the temperature.

Rainfall

Rainfall is perhaps the most essential element in human livelihood. Rainfall must be sufficient and regular (Fig. 1.6) allowing people to plant crops and ensure they come to fruition. An irregular rainfall can be as disastrous as a low rainfall, leading to failed crops, malnutrition and a reduction of resistance to infection.

Rainfall also has a direct effect on certain diseases. Moderate rainfall creates fresh breeding sites for *Anopheles* mosquitoes, but excessive rain can wash out larvae and cause a reduction in the number of mosquitoes. Some diseases, such as trachoma, favour dry arid regions.

Wind

Winds produce local alterations to the weather. A major wind system is the monsoon, which brings rainfall to the Indian subcontinent and South-east Asia. In West Africa, the hot dry Harmattan blows down from the Sahara reducing humidity and increasing dust. It is these secondary effects on rainfall and temperature that determine the disease patterns.

The winds are appreciated by man to improve living conditions in the warm moist areas of the world but are avoided in the hot dry zones. However, excess wind in hurricane areas or localized tornadoes cause destruction and loss of life (Fig. 1.7). Natural disasters disrupt the normal pattern of life, destroy water supplies and provide ideal conditions for epidemics to occur.

Seasonality

Temperature and rainfall together determine the seasons. This will have a major influence on the best time to grow crops and produce a seasonal pattern of a number of diseases. In areas of almost constant rain there is very little seasonal variation, but in the drier regions, seasonality can be quite marked. These areas are illustrated in Fig. 1.6.

The pattern of life determined by seasonality can be generalized as follows:

- Food stores are low or absent during the rains as it is the longest time since the harvest.
- When the rains come people are required to work their hardest when they have the least amount of food.
- The rains bring seasonal illnesses, especially diarrhoea and malaria, which debilitate just when complete fitness is required.
- The time of the rains often coincides with late pregnancy for the woman, conception having taken place during harvest. As all members of the family are required to work in the fields and much of the burden of cultivating falls on the woman, the increased strain threatens her pregnancy, while her physical reserves are stretched even further.
- Once harvest comes, then body weight is restored, excess crops are stored or sold, and some respite taken before the cycle repeats itself.

This pattern leads to the following observations:

1. Attendance for treatment at medical institutions and admission to hospital often follow a cyclical pattern. This is illustrated in Fig. 1.8, where it will be seen that the reporting of ill health is least during the dry months and increases with the rains.
2. Knowledge of the seasonality of disease can be used in health planning, the deployment of manpower, the ordering of supplies, the best time to take preventive action, etc.
3. Many illnesses show a marked seasonal pattern. Mosquitoes require water to breed so rainfall will determine a seasonal pattern for many of the vector-borne diseases. The massive contamination of rivers caused by the first rains washing in accumulated pollutants from the many dry months makes this a period of diarrhoeal diseases. The seasonality of cholera allows a warning system to be implemented and prevention initiated (see Section 8.4, especially Fig. 8.2.)

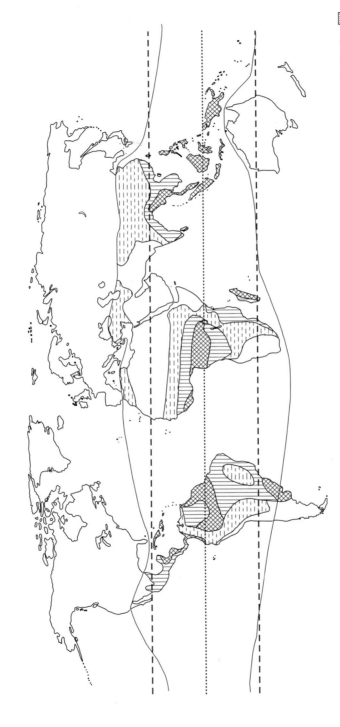

Fig. 1.6. The tropics, rainfall and seasonality. – – –, The tropics, Cancer to Capricorn; – –, developing country zone. Seasonality within the tropical region: ▨, rainfall in every season; ▦, heavy seasonal rainfall; ▦, variable seasonal rainfall; ☐, arid.

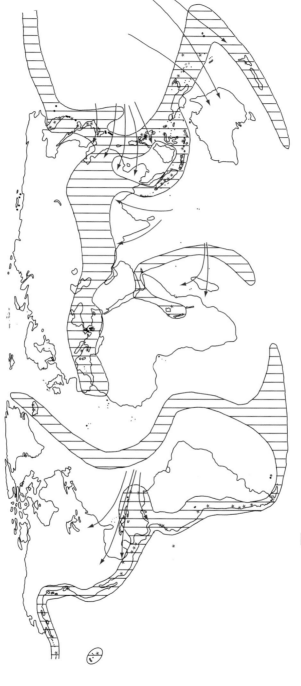

Fig. 1.7. Natural disaster zones. ▦, earthquake areas; *, active volcanoes; ←, revolving tropical storms (tornadoes, hurricanes, cyclones).

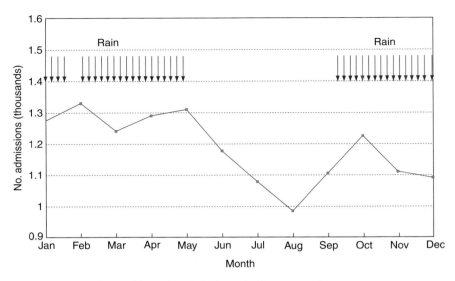

Fig. 1.8. Seasonality of admissions to Mbeya hospital, Tanzania (3 year mean).

4. A different pattern of seasonal diseases occurs with the viral infections, measles (see Figs 1.9 and 12.2) being a good example. As measles confers lifelong immunity then the only way that sufficient susceptibles can accumulate for another epidemic to occur is by immigration or reproduction. If the birth rate is high a critical number of susceptibles will soon be produced and annual epidemics will occur. If the birth rate is low then the interval may be every 2–3 years.

5. Knowledge of the seasonality of disease allows planned preventive services. If a mobile or mass vaccination campaign is used to combat measles, then timing it in the few months before an expected epidemic is the most cost-effective action. In Tanzania, measles outbreaks often occur in the rainy season (Fig. 1.9), a time of shortages, malnutrition and difficult communications; the worst possible time to have to do emergency vaccination to contain the epidemic. Just a few months before, there was little ill health, nutritional status was high, road conditions good and medical staff were at their slackest. This would have been the best time to ensure that every child was vaccinated.

1.5.3 Climate change due to global warming

The increase in carbon dioxide (CO_2) and other pollutants in the atmosphere due to the burning of fossil fuels (coal, petrol, etc.) has led to an increase in global temperature. While only a comparatively small increase, this has begun to have a major effect on the climate, with a disruption of weather systems and a raising of the sea level. This has been most marked on a system of currents off the west coast of South America known as the El Niño Southern Oscillation. Climatic systems are reversed or severely disrupted, with heavy rains and flooding when no rain is normally expected and drought conditions when there should normally be rain. Countries in South America, South-east Asia and Oceania are mostly affected, but effects are felt all over the world. While these effects will be more general in the diseases they affect, such as the association of illness with the rains (see Fig. 1.6), outbreaks of plague in Ecuador have been shown to have a possible connection with the appearance of El Niño. An association has also been shown between influenza pandemics and La Niña events as the last four pandemics were preceded by cooling of ocean surface temperatures, which occur with the La Niña phase of the El Niño Southern Oscillation. This alters the migration of birds, possibly favouring gene swapping among them and also contacts with domestic birds and animals. (See further in Section 19.2.)

As well as major climatic disruption, there has also been an increase in the severity and frequency of storms leading to flooding and destruction by

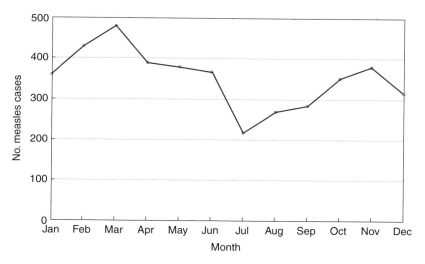

Fig. 1.9. Mean monthly measles cases over a 5 year period, Mbeya region, Tanzania.

winds. Flooding will make diarrhoeal diseases more likely and extend the range of diseases such as leptospirosis, which favour a watery environment.

Increase in temperature has the potential to expand the range of infections that are normally constrained by temperature, such as malaria. This has led to speculation that malaria could become a problem in the developed countries of Europe and North America where it occurred in former times. However, this is unlikely as good preventive measures are able to keep the disease from spreading even if the malarial mosquito re-establishes itself. A good example is Australia, where much of the county lies within the tropical region, the main malaria vector *Anopheles farauti* (the same as in Papua New Guinea and the Solomon Islands) is present, yet control methods have eradicated the parasite and continued surveillance has prevented it from being reintroduced.

A more serious problem is in areas of highlands within tropical countries such as East Africa and South America. At a certain level of altitude, where the lower temperature prevents the mosquito vector and parasite from developing, malaria is not found, but evidence from Ethiopia and Kenya has shown that this level is already rising. Malaria is now found at higher altitudes, with the rate of ascent linked to the rise in temperature. There is also a wider fluctuation of temperature, resulting in a greater risk of epidemic malaria in

people who have no immunity. Other diseases transmitted by mosquitoes – dengue, JE and other arboviruses, such as Rift Valley Fever, are likely to increase.

Leishmaniasis is an established disease in southern Europe and with the changing climate, conditions might well become favourable for the vector sandfly to extend its range further north. However, the *Phlebotamus* species already have a wider range than the pathogen (*Leishmania infantum*) and reservoir dogs are common in central and northern Europe, so there are no compelling reasons to suggest that this disease will increase its range. In contrast, *Ixodes ricinus*, the main vector of Lyme disease, and tick-borne encephalitis (TBE) in Europe, has been found to have already extended its range into higher latitudes (Scandinavia) and higher altitudes (the mountainous area of the Czech Republic) so there is likely to be an increase in spread of these two diseases. Also, the prolonged season could intensify transmission in areas where these infections are already prevalent. A similar scenario is likely to have taken place with the vector ticks of Lyme disease in North America.

If ocean levels rise then small island nations will be threatened by a reduction in land area on which to live and grow their crops, and by salt water intrusion into freshwater aquifers. Thirteen of the 20 major conurbations are at sea level and the population at risk from storm surges could rise from 45 to 90 million people. Countries at greatest risk are Bangladesh, China, Egypt and the small island nations of the Pacific, Caribbean and Indian Oceans.

Climate change will be most felt at the extremes of the world, the Arctic and Antarctic regions. A rise in temperature could damage the permafrost, upsetting the balance of nature and the livelihood of indigenous people who live in the colder parts of the world. The increase in CO_2 will result in preferential conditions for tree growth and the development of forests, which would be beneficial in the long run, but the animals that live in these lands might not be able to adjust to the rate of change and might become extinct.

While most of the concern on increase in disease due to global warming has been expressed in the Western world it is more likely that most of the effects will be concentrated in the poorer regions of the world, with an increase in vector-borne and diarrhoeal diseases, malnutrition and natural disasters.

1.5.4 Geographical information systems (GIS) and remote sensing

Such features as topography, climate and altitude are more commonly the province of geography than of medicine, but epidemiologists are making more use of geographical tools to help them understand the distribution and spread of disease. The classic tool is the map and many examples of this will be found in several sections of this book where maps are used. A development of mapping is geographical information systems (GIS) using complex computer software packages to analyse a range of coordinates to identify links between them. The power of GIS is its ability to integrate and manipulate multiple layers of spatial data that can then be applied to larger areas. Also, data can be continually updated to incorporate seasonal changes or long-term alterations in the topography, such as forest clearance. As well as its facility to map diseases, GIS can also be used to quantify risk and create databases for further analysis.

GIS are particularly useful in vector-borne diseases and has been used to good effect in mapping the risk areas for Lyme disease in Europe and North America. In Mexico, villages with high levels of *Anopheles albimanus* were identified and multivariate analysis indicated that transitional swamps and unmanaged pastures were the most important landscape features in vector abundance. Looking for these particular landscape features could then be used to estimate malaria risk. Measures of malaria incidence can also be directly applied to geographical features, as was done in the Red River Basin in Yunnan Province in China. This showed that the more paddy fields around the household and the closer people lived to areas of forest, the higher was the risk of contracting malaria.

While GIS collect information in detail for a small area, particular features identified as risk factors can be looked for by remote sensing over larger areas. Remote sensing initially used aerial photographs, but the advent of orbiting satellites such as Landsat and SPOT has considerably extended the use of geographical data. These map the surface of the world at frequent intervals, allowing detailed features identified by GIS to be applied to areas, and comparisons made over time. For example, in the study in China mentioned above, paddy fields and forest can be identified on satellite images for a much larger area and the malaria risk predicted (Fig 1.10). Both of these features will change as forest is cut down and new paddy fields created, so continued monitoring of malaria risk can be visualized without having to make detailed surveys.

A malaria risk map for Africa (MARA) has been developed for the whole continent using GIS and remote sensing. Remote sensing has also been used to identify new settlements in the Amazon forest where yellow fever is endemic. Remote sensing is at the forefront of identifying alterations that are resulting from global climate change.

Summary

- A communicable disease requires an agent and a means of transmitting the infection to a susceptible host within an amenable environment.
- The agent needs to be able to multiply and survive if it is to have an effect on the host.
- Transmission can be direct, via an intermediate host or by a vector.
- The host's susceptibility is influenced by age, sex, defence mechanisms and immunity.
- The social environment is modified by education and resources and altered by movements of communities or individuals.

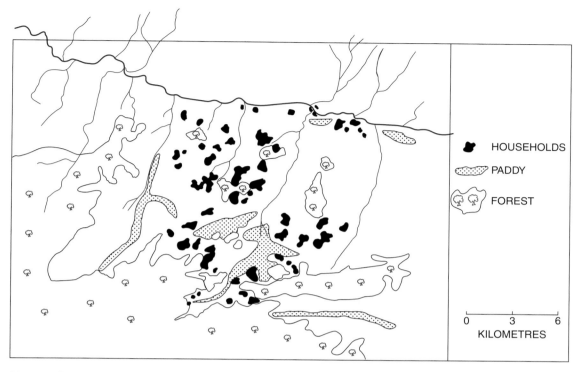

Fig 1.10. Simplified satellite image to show forest, rice paddy and people's households in part of Yunnan, China. (Modified from Luo Da-Peng (2000) Spatial prediction of malaria in the Red River Basin, Yunnan, China, using geographical information systems and remote sensing. PhD thesis, University of London. Reproduced with permission.)

- The physical environment is affected by the nature of the surroundings, seasonality and climate change.

Further Reading

Abramson, J.H. and Abramson, Z.H. (2008) *Research Methods in Community Public Health: Surveys, Epidemiological Research, Programme Evaluation, Clinical Trials*, 6th edn. John Wiley and Sons, Chichester, UK.

Githeko, A.K., Lindsay, S.W., Confalonieri, U.E. and Patz, J.A. (2000) Climate change and vector-borne diseases: a regional analysis. *Bulletin of the World Health Organization* 78, 1136–1147.

Available at: www.who.int/bulletin/archives/78(9)1136.pdf (accessed 22 February 2012).

Thompson, R., Jowett, M., Witter, S. and Ensor, T. (2000) *Health Economics in Developing Countries: A Practical Guide*. Macmillan, Basingstoke, UK.

Vaughan, J.P. and Morrow, R.H. (2011) *Manual of Epidemiology for District Health Management*, 2nd edn. World Health Organization, Geneva.

Walley, J., Wright, J. and Hubley, J. (2009) Public Health, 2nd edn. Oxford University Press, Oxford, UK.

World Health Organization (2003) *The World Health Report 2002: Reducing Risks, Promoting Healthy Life*. WHO, Geneva. Available at: http://www.who.int/whr/2002/en/index.html (accessed 22 February 2012).

Wright, J. (1998) *Health Needs Assessment in Practice*. BMJ Books, London.

2 Communicable Disease Theory

The previous chapter attempted to unify communicable diseases into basic units, the *agent*, a route of *transmission* to a *host*, and the way the *environment* influenced the outcome. Generalizations were made in an attempt to limit all the alternatives and variations that are possible, developing principles rather than discovering exceptions. This chapter looks at interactions between these various elements in an analytical way.

2.1 Force of Infection

In a communicable disease, the number of new cases occurring in a period of time is dependent on the number of infectious persons within a susceptible population and the degree of contact between them. Persons, whether infectious or susceptible, and a period of time, are all quantifiable factors, but the degree of contact can depend upon very many variables. Such things as proximity (density) of populations, carriers, reservoirs, climate and seasonality will all have separate effects. To single these out and ascribe values to them will involve considerable, and generally unnecessary, complexity. In some disease patterns, certain factors have sufficient influence that they require to be given values, but for the time being these will all be considered together as a *force of infection*. This can be summarized as:

The force of infection
  = Number of infectious individuals
  × Transmission rate

Therefore:

Number of newly infected individuals
  = Force of infection
  × Number of susceptible individuals in the
    population

If the susceptible population is sufficiently large to maintain a permanent pool of susceptibles (as would happen in a disease where there is little or no immunity) and the force of infection is constant, then newly infected individuals will continue to be produced while infectious individuals remain in the population. One healthy carrier might continue to infect a large number of individuals over a long period of time, or a brief devastating epidemic, with a short period of infectiousness, may infect a large number of people over a short period of time. Parasitic infections such as the hookworm would be an example of the former, and measles of the latter. Of course, measles produces immunity which will alter the size of the susceptible population.

The proportion of susceptible individuals can either be reduced by mortality, immunity or emigration, or increased by birth or immigration. After a certain period of time a sufficient number of non-immune persons will have entered the population for a new *epidemic* of the disease to occur.

2.2 Epidemic Theory

Epidemics can occur unexpectedly, as when a new disease enters a community, or can occur regularly at certain times of the year, as in epidemics of measles. Epidemic contrasts with *endemic*, which means the continuous presence of an infection in the community and is described by *incidence* and *prevalence* measurements. This section will cover epidemics and how they are measured.

Epidemic means an excess of cases in the community from that normally expected, or the appearance of a new infection. The point at which an endemic disease becomes epidemic depends on the usual presence of the disease and its rate. With an unusual disease, a few cases could be an epidemic, whereas with a common disease (such as gastroenteritis) an epidemic is when the usual rate of the disease is substantially exceeded. Criteria can be set so that when the number of cases exceeds this level the *epidemic threshold* is crossed. The epidemic threshold can either be the upper limit of cases expected at that particular time, an excess mortality, or a combination of both the number of cases and the mortality.

Characteristics of an epidemic (Fig. 2.1) are as follows:

- *Latent period*, the time interval from initial infection until the start of infectiousness.
- *Incubation period*, the time interval from initial infection until the onset of clinical disease. The incubation period varies from disease to disease and for a particular disease has a *range*. This range extends from a *minimum* incubation period to a *maximum* incubation period (for incubation periods see Chapter 20).
- *Period of communicability*, the period during which an individual is infectious. The infectious period can start before the disease process commences (e.g. hepatitis) or after (e.g. sleeping sickness). In some diseases, such as diphtheria and streptococcal infections, infectiousness starts from the date of first exposure.

Various factors modify the incubation period so that if it is plotted on a time-based graph, it is found to rise rapidly to a peak and then tail off over a longer period (Fig. 2.2). The infecting dose, portal of entry, immune response of the host and a number of other factors modify the normal distribution to extend the tail of the graph. By using a log timescale this skewed curve can be converted to a normal distribution and the mean incubation period measured.

An epidemic can be either a *common-source* epidemic or *propagated-source* epidemic (Fig. 2.3).

- Common-source epidemics can further be divided into a *point-source* epidemic resulting from a single exposure, such as a food poisoning episode, or an *extended* epidemic resulting from repeated multiple exposures over a period of time (e.g. a contaminated well).
- In a propagated-source epidemic the agent is spread through serial transfer from host to host. With a disease having a reasonably long incubation period, the initial peaks will be separated by the median incubation periods. Chickenpox (varicella) can start as an epidemic in one school; then mingling children will lead to transfer to another school, leading to a series of propagated epidemics.

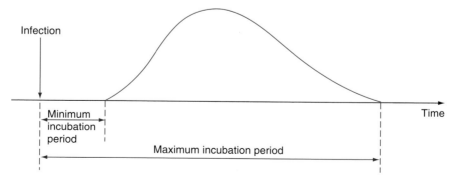

Fig. 2.1. Parameters of an infection (see text for definitions).

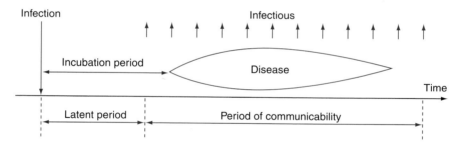

Fig. 2.2. Distribution curve of incubation times (the epidemic curve).

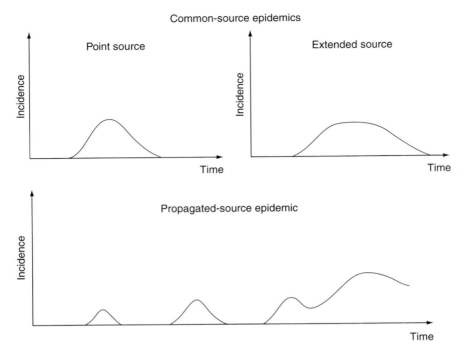

Fig. 2.3. Epidemic types.

2.2.1 Investigation of an epidemic

In the investigation of any outbreak of a disease the basic approach is to gather information on the following.

1. *Persons*: age, sex, occupation, ethnic group, etc., comparing the number infected with the population at risk.
2. *Place*: country, district, town, village, household and relationship to geographical features such as roads, rivers, forests, etc., conveniently marked on a map.
3. *Time*: annual, monthly (seasonal), day and hour (nocturnal/diurnal). The number of cases occurring within each time period is viewed as a graph.

To instil conformity on what is regarded as a case of the particular disease a *case definition* is developed. This needs to be tried out as an over-complex case definition will exclude a number of cases while too simple a definition will include cases that might not be of the infection in question. Fever could be used as a presumptive diagnosis for malaria to inform the health worker to take a blood slide, so the case definition for malaria would be fever with a positive blood slide. A case definition for measles could be fever with the characteristic rash, but this

could either be defined more specifically or health workers given a course of training so that they all know what the characteristic rash looks like. Where a specific epidemic is being investigated then time and/or place can be added. For example, if it is an epidemic of measles, then it would be all cases of fever with the characteristic rash between say January and February in village X.

In a *point-source* epidemic the number of cases of the disease occurring each day is plotted on a graph to produce an epidemic curve. The earliest cases will be those with the minimum incubation period and the last those with the maximum incubation period if all were infected at a single point in time, as illustrated in Fig. 2.4.

Three factors describe a point-source epidemic:

- the epidemic curve;
- the incubation period of the disease; and
- the time of infection.

If only two of these factors are known then the third can be deduced. From the epidemic curve, the median (or geometric mean) of the incubation periods is determined. If the disease is known from its clinical features, then the incubation period will

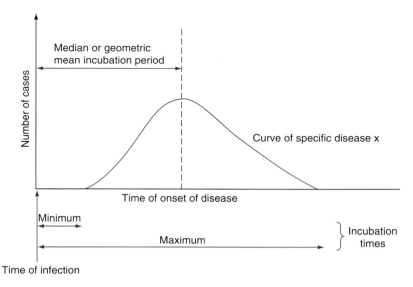

Fig. 2.4. Investigation of a point-source epidemic.

also be known (Chapter 20). So measuring this known incubation period back in time from the median incubation period on the curve, or the minimum incubation period from the beginning of the curve, the time of infection can be calculated. The source, now localized to a restricted period of time, can more easily be investigated.

If the disease is unknown, but there is evidence of the time of infection (e.g. a particular event in time that brought all the cases together or linked them by a common phenomenon), then the incubation period can be calculated and a disease (or aetiological agent producing a disease) with this incubation period suspected. This method was used to work out the incubation period for the first epidemic of Ebola haemorrhagic fever, as there were a large number of fatal cases that occurred in one hospital at the same time.

In an *extended-source* epidemic, the time of infection can be deduced by measuring back in time from the first case on the rising epidemic curve to the maximum and minimum incubation periods of the diagnosed disease. Search within this defined period of time can elucidate the source.

With a *propagated-source epidemic*, phases of infection occur at regular intervals. The time period between these phases is called the *serial* interval (Fig. 2.5). Features of the epidemic are measured in the same way as a common-source epidemic, while an estimate of time of recurrence is given by the serial interval.

After several propagated epidemics, cases remaining from the previous epidemic will merge with the next so that the regular serial pattern will be lost.

2.2.2 Attack rates

Epidemics are suitably described by expressing them in *attack rates*. In a common-source epidemic, the *overall attack rate* is used.

$$\text{Overall attack rate} = \frac{\text{Number of individuals affected during an epidemic}}{\text{Number (of susceptibles) exposed to the risk}}$$

In a new infection, everyone will be at risk (e.g. with the SARS virus), but as the infection proceeds, persons will become immune and are therefore no longer at risk. Where an epidemic occurs at regular intervals (e.g. measles) only those people who have not met the infection before or have not been vaccinated will be at risk.

Contagiousness or the probability that an exposure will lead to a transmission is measured by:

$$\text{Secondary attack rate} = \frac{\text{Number of cases within the period of one minimum and one maximum incubation period (secondary cases) from the primary case}}{\text{Number (of susceptibles) exposed to the risk}}$$

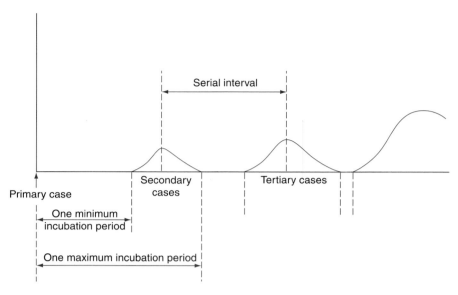

Fig. 2.5. Investigation of a propagated-source epidemic.

An example is smallpox, which had a high secondary attack rate and was therefore very contagious. Since smallpox was eradicated and people are no longer vaccinated the level of immunity has waned and there is the fear that a very similar disease, monkeypox, could now increase and be a threat. However, it has a lower secondary attack rate so we can rest assured that this is unlikely to happen (see also Section 19.3).

2.2.3 Dynamics of epidemics

The increase in cases in an epidemic has given rise to a measure called the *basic reproductive rate*. This measures the average number of subsequent cases of an infection from a single case in an unlimited, wholly susceptible population. For example, if one case gave rise to two and these two to four, etc., as illustrated in Fig. 2.6, the basic reproductive rate would be 2. This is the most extreme situation. In reality the epidemic is modified by immunity or the population limited by people having already become infected, so such a rapid increase does not occur. If the basic reproductive rate is less than 1, as illustrated in Fig 2.7, the epidemic will not take off. The importance of this concept is in control, whereby, if the basic reproductive rate can be reduced below 1, then the disease will die out.

By giving values to parameters that influence the outcome of the infection a mathematical formula can be developed to hypothesize the likely outcome of different control strategies. The basic reproductive rate has been used in this way to develop mathematical models of disease, particularly for malaria (Section 15.6) and filariasis (Fig. 15.11).

2.2.4 Population size and characteristics

As already mentioned, the continuation of an epidemic is determined by the number of susceptibles remaining in the population. Once an individual has experienced an episode of the disease (whether manifest or not) they will develop immunity (either temporary or permanent) and recover. When a certain number of individuals have developed immunity then there are insufficient susceptibles and the infection dies out. This collective permanent immunity (as occurs in viral infections) is called the *herd immunity*. After a period of time, depending on the size of the population, this herd immunity becomes diluted by new individuals born (or by immigration), and a new epidemic can take place. This is called the *critical population* (the theoretical minimum host population size required to maintain an infecting agent). It depends upon the infectious agent, the demographic structure and the conditions (hygiene, etc.) of the host population. In developing countries with their high birth rates the critical population is less than in developed countries. Examples of the critical human population size are 500,000 for measles and 10,000 for varicella.

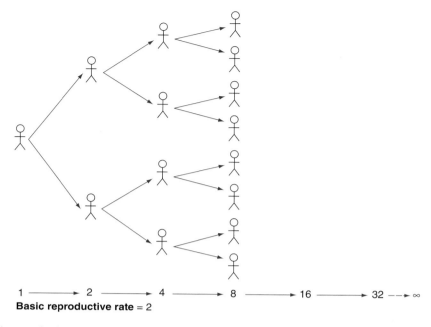

Fig. 2.6. Basic reproductive rate increasing, i.e. >1. Maximal transmission: every infection produces a new case.

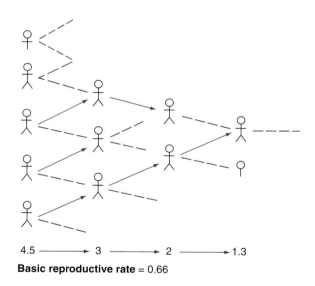

Fig. 2.7. Basic reproductive rate decreasing, i.e. <1. Unsustained transmission: each transmission gives rise to less than one new case and the infection dies out.

If the population is less than the critical size, then regular epidemics will occur at intervals related to the population size. An example is given in Fig. 12.2 of a measles epidemic which occurred regularly every 3 years in a well-defined community. These regular epidemics can be analysed in the same way as a propagated-source epidemic, from which it can be deduced that the smaller the community, the longer the interval between epidemics.

An extension of the concept of herd immunity shows that not everyone in a population needs to be vaccinated to prevent an epidemic. On the same principle as calculating the critical population, the *critical rate of vaccination coverage* can also be worked out – in other words, the population that will need to be successfully vaccinated to reduce the population at risk below the epidemic threshold. It can similarly be seen that even if this target is not reached, then the epidemic will be put off until a future date when the susceptible unvaccinated children will have grown older and therefore be able to cope with the infection better. This is illustrated in Fig. 12.2.

In a serious epidemic there will be a high death rate which is generally expressed as the *case fatality rate*. This is the number of people with the disease that die from it within a defined period of time. The time period will have to be stated, for example for measles it could be children dying within 4–6 weeks of developing the rash. A decreasing case fatality rate could indicate improvement of treatment, the result of a preventive vaccination programme or decreasing virulence of the infection.

The mortality rate is the number of people dying out of the population at risk. The population at risk will need to be defined if it is a localized epidemic, such as the population in region A. Mortality rates are often measured sequentially (generally monthly) during the course of an epidemic to judge whether the epidemic is declining or its severity decreasing.

Epidemics often start from a small group of people, spread to other related groups and then become more widely dispersed. These small groups of people are called *clusters*. A good example of clustering has been with bird flu and is well illustrated in Fig. 19.1. Clusters can be defined by place or time, while in this particular case there was also an occupational grouping with people who had close contact with poultry.

2.2.5 Investigating food-borne and waterborne epidemics

Other epidemiological techniques are useful for investigating food-borne and waterborne epidemics, particularly case-control and cohort study methods.

Case-control studies

The importance of a suspected aetiological item, in this case fish, can be measured using a case-control study in a cholera investigation. In the community being investigated the people preferred to eat fish

marinated, but uncooked, and it was suspected that this might have been the cause of the disease. Cases were interviewed as to whether they ate raw fish and compared with a similar group who had not had the disease. The results were set out in a two-by-two table and calculation showed a significant finding with a χ^2 of 50.47, $p < 0.001$.

	Cases	Controls	Total
Ate raw fish	31	8	39
Did not eat raw fish	3	60	63
Total	34	68	102

A reasonable estimate of the *relative risk* can be arrived at (as the incidence rates are not known) from the two-by-two table, using the odds ratio: *ad/cb*.

Suspected cause	Cases	Controls
Present	*a*	*b*
Absent	*c*	*d*

In the example above, the relative risk of contracting cholera after eating raw fish is:

$$\frac{31 \times 60}{3 \times 8} = 77.5.$$

Cohort studies

A cohort is a group of people all exposed to the same aetiological agent. By following this group over time the risk of developing disease can be measured. A modification of the technique can be used in outbreak investigation, particularly food poisoning. This compares the attack rate in the persons exposed to the factor with the attack rate in those not exposed to the factor. In a food poisoning outbreak where various foods are suspected then the attack rates in those eating and not eating the range of foods can be compared. This is best illustrated by using an example, as shown in Table 2.1. The relative risk for each food item is calculated as above and the results set down in a table. Most of the relative risk values are about one, but there is over four times the risk of becoming ill if you ate fish, so the investigator would suspect fish as being the most likely cause.

2.3 Endemicity

An endemic disease implies that there is a constant rate of infection occurring in the community.

As new individuals are born, they become infected, are cured (including self-cure), retain the infection for life, or become immune. Prevalence rates will measure the level of endemicity as it applies to the community. Incidence rates will measure change in the level of infection over a period of time.

While it is useful to compare prevalence from one community to another, on more careful investigation it will be found that within a community, prevalence rates can also vary. These areas of increased prevalence within a community are called foci. Two types of foci occur:

- *Host focality*, where some individuals have more severe infection than others, e.g. worm load in schistosomiasis.
- *Geographical focality*, where certain localities have a higher prevalence rate than others. Malaria exhibits geographical focality.

These concepts are important in control strategy. When a control method is applied equally to a community then the overall decrease in disease will leave the foci to maintain infection. However, if the foci are identified and treated then the infectious source is contained (Fig. 2.8).

Incidence rates show change in the endemicity, either upwards, downwards or remaining the same. A decreasing incidence will indicate that the disease may be dying out, especially if control measures have been used. Incidence rates often show a seasonal pattern (Fig. 1.8) and threshold levels that take into account this seasonal variation can be set to give early warning of the disease becoming epidemic.

2.4 Quantitative Dynamics

The concept of a force of infection was introduced earlier as a general term to incorporate all the

Table 2.1. Food-specific attack rates and the relative risks of eating different foods. Meal eaten by 152 persons.

	Ate			Did not eat			
Food item	Sick	Well	Attack rate (%)	Sick	Well	Attack rate (%)	Relative risk
Rice	115	28	80.4	45	4	55.5	1.4
Potatoes	111	31	78.2	9	1	90.0	0.9
Fish	93	22	80.9	17	30	18.9	4.3
Beans	101	29	77.7	16	6	72.7	1.1
Coconut	86	22	79.6	24	20	54.5	1.5
Bananas	109	32	77.3	10	1	90.9	0.8

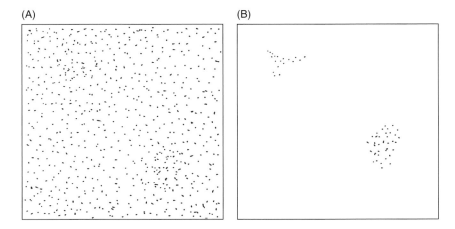

(A)   (B)

Fig. 2.8. The focality of endemic disease. (A) A universally homogenous prevalence rate is measured in an area. (B) Once control measures have been implemented, foci of persistent transmission are revealed.

variable components that could alter the outcome of an infection. Parasite infections in particular are markedly influenced by alterations in some of these variables, e.g. the length of life of the vector mosquito in its ability to transmit malaria. Identifying the important variables and quantifying them can give an estimate of the magnitude of the infectious process, and so enable calculations of the degree of control necessary. As an introduction to quantitative dynamics, examples of helminth infections are used.

2.4.1   Hookworm infection

If we take as an example a family of five people with four out of the five infected with hookworms, producing on average some 4000 eggs/g of faeces. Approximately 200 g of faeces are voided by the average person each day so the four people are excreting $4 \times 4000 \times 200 = 3.2 \times 10^6$ eggs/day. If each of these eggs results in a viable larva then the potential for infection would be astronomical.

If the head of the household is now persuaded to install a latrine and he encourages his family to use it, then hopefully there should be no further contamination of the surroundings and infection will decrease as the worms die off. Unfortunately, his youngest child does not understand how to use a latrine and despite being taken to it by his mother, half of the stools are still deposited indiscriminately around the neighbourhood. This results in 100 (g) $\times$ 4000 (eggs) $= 4 \times 10^5$ eggs deposited, which means that the potential for infecting the rest of the family

has hardly altered. (This is a simplistic example implying that the eggs will still be concentrated where infection is most likely to occur.)

2.4.2   Schistosomiasis

An idealized situation is illustrated in Fig. 2.9. Ten people with schistosomiasis are all potential polluters of a body of water. Each gram of faeces might contain 80 eggs, but if only half of them reach the water then there are still 40×200 (an average stool specimen is 200 g) $= 8 \times 10^3$ eggs per person or 8×10^4 eggs from all ten people reaching the water every day. The miracidium that hatches from the egg needs to find a host snail to complete its development. Snails can reproduce rapidly so that one snail can produce a colony in 40 days and be infective in 60. The numbers of cercariae liberated from a snail are immense, but because they need to find a human host within 24 h (generally less) few are successful. The ten people entering the water at the other side of the picture could all become infected, but in reality only a proportion are likely to be so.

When control is considered, there is the choice of preventing pollution of the water, destroying the snails or preventing water contact. (There is also mass treatment of the population which will reduce the total egg load, but for the present argument it will not be discussed here.) If latrines are provided and nine out of the ten people used them, there would still be 8×10^3 eggs from the tenth person going into the water, sufficient to maintain almost

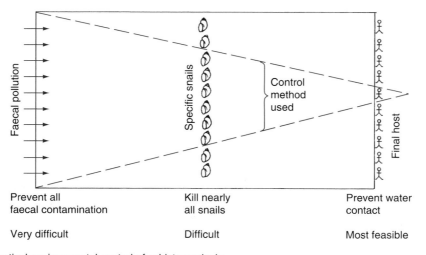

Fig. 2.9. Theoretical environmental control of schistosomiasis.

the same level of snail infections. If all the snails were destroyed except a few, then within 60 days the situation would return to what it was before. However, if any one of the ten people could be prevented from making contact with the water then his/her freedom from infection would be absolute.

Of course, the situation is never as clear cut as this, but the illustration is made to show that a sanitation or molluscicide programme needs to be virtually perfect, whereas prevention of water contact can provide complete protection to the individual. This is a simplified example, but a more realistic situation can be simulated by the use of mathematical models.

Mathematical models will not be covered in any more detail here, but examples will be found in measles (Fig. 12.1), malaria (Section 15.6 and Fig. 15.8) and lymphatic filariasis (Fig. 15.11). They are especially useful in determining control strategy, which is the subject of the next few chapters.

Summary

- A disease can either be epidemic or endemic.
- Epidemic diseases can be common source or propagated but by measuring the minimal and maximum incubation period from the first case the time of infection can be determined.
- The size of the population will determine the frequency of epidemics and the number that need to be vaccinated to produce herd immunity.
- An endemic disease is described by its incidence and prevalence, but foci of infection can also occur.
- Mathematical models can look at different parameters of a disease and determine the best strategy for control.

Further Reading

Bonita, R. (2006) *Basic Epidemiology*, 2nd edn. World Health Organization, Geneva.

Cooper, C., Rose, G. and Barker, D.J.P. (1998) *Epidemiology in Medical Practice*. Churchill Livingstone, London.

Giesecke, J. (2001) *Modern Infectious Disease Epidemiology*, 2nd edn. Hodder Arnold, London.

Kirkwood, B.R. and Sterne, J. (2003) *Essentials of Medical Statistics*, 2nd edn. Blackwell Scientific Publications, Oxford, UK.

Last, J.M. (2001) *A Dictionary of Epidemiology*, 4th edn. Oxford University Press, New York.

Stolley, P.D., Lilienfield, A.M. and Lilienfield, D.E. (2001) *Foundations of Epidemiology*. Oxford University Press, New York.

3 Control Principles and Methods

3.1 Control Principles

Control can be directed at either the agent, the route of transmission, the host, or the environment. Sometimes it is necessary to use several control strategies. The general methods of control are summarized in Fig. 3.1.

3.1.1 The agent

Destruction of the agent can be by specific treatment, using drugs that kill the agent *in vivo*, or if it is outside the body, by the use of antiseptics, sterilization, incineration or radiation.

3.1.2 Transmission

When the agent is attempting to travel to a host it is at its most vulnerable so many methods of control have been developed to interrupt transmission.

Quarantine or isolation

Keeping the agent at a sufficient distance and for a sufficient length of time away from the host until it dies or becomes inactive can be effective in preventing transmission. Quarantine or isolation can be used for animals as well as humans, but is more effective in the former because they can be forcibly restrained. Because it is difficult to quarantine people it is not widely practised as a method of control, except where the disease is very infectious or the patient can be restrained easily, e.g. in hospital (Lassa fever).

Contacts

People who might have become infected because of their close proximity to a case are called contacts. They can be isolated, given prophylactic treatment or kept under surveillance.

Environmental health

Methods of personal hygiene, water supplies and sanitation are particularly effective against all agents transmitted by the faecal-oral route, whether by direct transmission or complex parasitic cycles involving intermediate hosts.

Animals

Whether they act as reservoirs or intermediate hosts animals can be controlled by *destruction* or *vaccination* (e.g. against rabies). If animals are to be eaten, their carcasses can be *inspected* to make sure they are free of parasitic stages. The excretions or tissues of an animal can be infectious so protective clothing and gloves should be worn when handling animals.

Cooking

Proper cooking renders plant and animal produce safe for consumption, although some toxins are heat-resistant. Food should be prepared hygienically before cooking and stored properly afterwards.

Vector

Vector control is one of the most highly developed methods of interrupting transmission because the parasite utilizes a vulnerable stage for development and transport. Attack on vectors can either be on their larval stage by using *larvicides* and methods of biological control, or while they are adults with *adulticides*.

3.1.3 Host

The host can be protected by physical methods (mosquito nets, clothing, housing, etc.), by vaccination against specific diseases, or by taking regular prophylaxis.

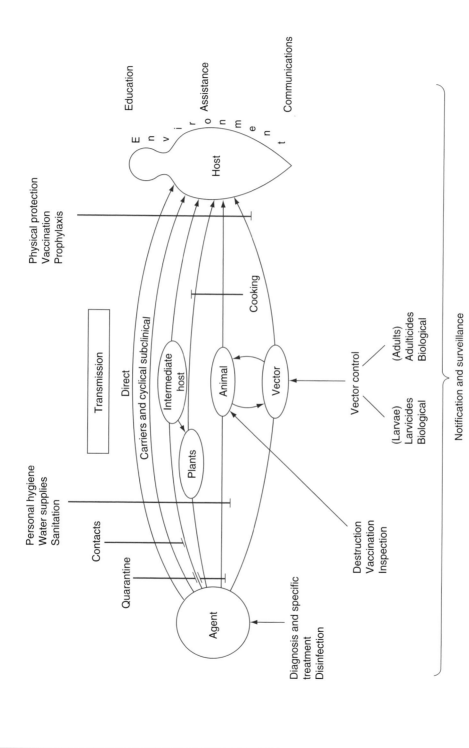

Fig. 3.1. Control principles.

3.1.4 Environment

The physical environment can be modified to reduce breeding places for vectors and warning systems set up to advise people on destructive storms and other natural hazards.

The social environment of the host can be improved, by education, assistance (agricultural advice, house building, subsidies, loans, etc.), and improvement of communications (to market produce, reach health facilities, attend school, etc.). In time these will be the most effective methods of preventing continuation of the transmission cycle.

3.2 Control Methods – Vaccination

3.2.1 Vaccines

The newborn baby carries antibodies transmitted from its mother across the placenta and from early breastfeeding, so protecting it at a very vulnerable stage in life. The effects of these antibodies wear off after 6 weeks to 6 months so the baby starts making its own antibodies from natural or artificial infections that it acquires.

Artificial infection is given by vaccination, or rather the objective is to administer the antigenic substances produced by the disease organisms in a vaccine without the host developing the disease. Vaccine can be given but immunity does not always result, owing to poor administration, the vaccine no longer being potent, or the host not developing an immune response. Therefore the term vaccination is mostly used in this book to indicate the giving of the vaccine rather than immunization, which can be misunderstood as immunity having been given.

The immune system of the full-term newborn is capable of producing antibodies and mobilizing cellular defences. Bacillus Calmette–Guérin (BCG) and polio vaccines can be given shortly after birth and killed antigen vaccines are also effective from the first month of life. Some live vaccines – like measles – do not provide protection if given early because of circulating maternal antibodies.

Vaccines are of four main kinds:

- *Live attenuated organisms* give the body an actual infection, inducing antibody production. This is the best kind of vaccine as it generates maximal response from a single dose and as a consequence immunity is long lasting. The danger with live attenuated vaccines is that the organisms could revert to the virulent strain.

Examples are measles and oral polio, which are attenuated virus infections, and BCG, which is an attenuated bacterium.

- *Killed organisms* are used when it is not possible to produce a live attenuated strain. Immunity does not develop so well and the vaccine has to be repeated to induce the body defence mechanisms to increase their response. An example is pertussis (whooping cough).
- *Active components* can be separated from organisms and conjugate vaccines made from these. Good immunity is produced, but they are expensive to manufacture. An example is hepatitis B vaccine, which is a recombinant DNA or plasma-derived vaccine.
- *Toxoids* are detoxified bacterial exotoxins and are an important way of producing antibodies to bacterial toxins. They do not prevent the infection, but counteract the dangerous effects of the toxin. Like killed organisms, several doses have to be given to induce a sufficient antibody response and booster doses repeated from time to time to maintain the level. Diphtheria and tetanus toxoid are two vaccines in this category.

3.2.2 Vaccine schedules

The type of vaccine and the age of risk of developing the target disease determine the optimum time and schedule for giving each vaccine. The characteristics of the principal vaccine preventable diseases (included in the EPI (Expanded Programme of Immunization) programme in most developing countries) are as follows:

Tetanus

Tetanus can enter the neonate through an infected umbilical cord, producing a high mortality. Protection is by immunizing pregnant women with tetanus toxoid. This protection is short lived and the child should be given tetanus toxoid early in infancy. Vaccination is started at 6 weeks minimum, and is combined with diphtheria and pertussis as DTP, given in three doses, followed later in life with a booster. Toxoid (Ta) is also given to adults as a course of three vaccinations to prevent tetanus, or prophylactically if they have a cut or wound and did not have a full course. Booster doses should be given, after which long-lasting protection is achieved. The World Health Organization (WHO) policy is to vaccinate all women of childbearing age with a lifetime total of five doses of tetanus toxoid.

Whooping cough (pertussis)

Whooping cough is a serious disease of young children, often with a fatal outcome in infants less than 6 months old. Vaccination must start before this time, so is given from 6 weeks with diphtheria and tetanus as DTP. Immunity wanes so a booster dose between 1 and 6 years is recommended.

Diphtheria

Diphtheria is a dangerous disease at any age, so it is preferable to start protection early. Vaccination is with the combined DTP in childhood and a booster dose at 1–6 years of age. Adults should have booster doses of tetanus and diphtheria vaccine (Td) depending on the level of risk in the community. This particularly applies to travellers visiting high-risk areas.

Poliomyelitis

Poliomyelitis infection is by three different strains of virus. The oral polio vaccine (OPV) contains all three attenuated strains of the virus, but the gut may not be infected by three strains at the same time and so three doses are required to ensure protection. In developing countries where wild poliovirus is circulating a first dose is given as soon after birth as possible, followed by three other doses at the same time as DTP. Endemic polio is now only found in Africa and Asia. Inactivated polio vaccine (IPV) is favoured in many developed countries, but is more expensive and produces less herd immunity. As the reservoir of wild virus is being eliminated IPV is the preferred vaccine as there is no risk of reversion of the vaccine to a pathogenic form.

Hepatitis B

Hepatitis B leads to chronic liver disease, especially cirrhosis, which is a predisposing cause of primary liver cell cancer. The prevalence of hepatitis B is as high as 8% in many parts of the world, but if the vaccine is administered before infection the disease and carrier state are prevented. Hepatitis B vaccine should be given as soon after birth as possible and then either by three doses at the same time as DTP, or the second dose with the first DTP and the third dose with the third DTP. It should also be given to adults at risk who have not been vaccinated in childhood, e.g. drug users and those coming into frequent contact with blood.

Haemophillus influenzae *type b*

H. influenzae is an important cause of meningitis and pneumonia in children under 6 years, particularly those 4–18 months old, and a vaccine given before this age gives a high degree of protection. The vaccine is a conjugate known as Hib and has the advantage of inducing antibody response and immunological memory in infants as well as reducing nasopharyngeal carriage of the organism, thereby reducing transmission. It is given at the same time as DTP.

Pneumococcal vaccine

The pneumococcus is the cause of a range of illnesses, including milder respiratory infection right up to life-threatening pneumonia. It also causes meningitis and otitis media, a common ear infection in childhood. The conjugate pneumococcal vaccine (PCV) is included in the routine vaccination schedule at the same time as DTP, but given at a different site.

Rotavirus

Rotavirus is a common cause of diarrhoea in young children and the vaccine (RV) can be given at the same time as DTP/OPV vaccination. It can either be given as a three-dose schedule (Rota Teq) with each DTP or as a two dose (Rotarix) with the first and second DTP.

Measles

Measles is one of the most important causes of childhood death and disability in the tropics. It reaches maximal prevalence by the end of the first year of life, but many children will already have been infected by 6–12 months. Maternal antibodies do not diminish sufficiently until 6 months for the attenuated virus to be effective, so the optimal time for vaccination is 9 months in developing countries. Prolonged immunity is obtained if the vaccine is given later (at 12–13 months) so this is a preferable time for developed countries or those in which there is a low disease prevalence. A second dose should be administered at 12–18 months (see Section 12.2), depending on when the first dose was given. In areas with a high level of human immunodeficiency virus (HIV) and measles the first dose can be given at 6 months followed by two further doses.

Rubella

The objective of giving rubella vaccination is to reduce congenital rubella syndrome (CRS), which occurs if a woman becomes infected just before or in the first 20 weeks of pregnancy. If the vaccination programme is efficient (over 80% coverage) then a strategy to eliminate rubella is by giving a combined measles and rubella (MR) or measles, mumps and rubella (MMR) vaccine at the same time as the measles vaccination programme. If the objective is to reduce CRS then all adolescent girls and women of childbearing age should be vaccinated (see Section 12.3).

Mumps

An infection of the salivary glands, mumps can cause orchitis and meningitis and, more rarely, encephalitis. Vaccination is conveniently combined with measles and rubella vaccines (see Section 12.4).

Tuberculosis

The maximum age risk of tuberculosis depends on the prevalence of active infection in the community. Where there are many open cases even small children are at risk, but in a society where most cases are in older people and individuals do not contact many others until they start work in young adulthood, the period of greatest risk is adolescence. In developing countries vaccination is given at birth, whereas in developed countries BCG is given when the child starts school, or selectively to risk groups such as immigrants from high-risk countries. BCG should not be given to pregnant women or those with symptomatic HIV infection. However, even in countries where there is a high level of HIV and tuberculosis, BCG should be given to all infants at birth unless they are known to be infected with HIV.

Human papilloma vaccine

Infection with the human papilloma virus (HPV) can lead to cancer of the cervix so giving the vaccine (HPV vaccine) to girls before they become sexually active is recommended. Initially it will also need to be given to older and 'catch-up' popula-

tions. The age of vaccination varies from country to country within a range of 9–13 years. Where possible it should be included in the school vaccination programme.

Meningitis

Meningitis due to *Neisseria meningitidis* (meningococcal) occurs in epidemics in a belt across tropical Africa and is a risk factor in collections of people such as in schools. Several vaccines are now available containing groups A, C, Y and W-135 meningococcal polysaccharides. Children over 2 years of age can be given any of these vaccines or combinations in mass campaigns and emergencies when in a high-risk situation, such as collections of people, or travel to an epidemic area. Group C conjugate vaccine (MenC) is safe in young children and is often incorporated into the routine childhood vaccination programme in countries that can afford it, given at 3 months, 4 months and 12 months of age. A booster dose may be required in adolescence.

Yellow fever

In endemic areas of Africa and South America yellow fever is a serious disease with high mortality so vaccination should be given to all children of 9 months or older. Many countries carry out mass campaigns to immunize the adult population, whereas in South America vaccination stations are situated at important road junctions to make sure anyone entering an infected area is vaccinated. Yellow fever vaccine is an international requirement for travellers entering infected areas. It is an extremely effective vaccine and provides immunity for at least 10 years.

Japanese encephalitis

Japanese encephalitis (JE) is a cause of severe neurological symptoms and can be an important cause of death in parts of Asia. Where there is a public health problem then vaccination can be added to the routine schedule, given as a single dose at 1 year of age.

Combinations and schedules

Different vaccines can be combined, as in DTP, or can be given together, e.g. DTP and polio.

A sufficient interval must be left between doses to allow time for the antibody response to take place, 1 month normally being sufficient. All these factors and the national characteristics of a country will determine the vaccination schedule to be followed. A suggested regime is as follows:

Before birth	Tetanus toxoid to all women of childbearing age with at least two doses in the first pregnancy and one in the second
Birth	BCG. Hepatitis B vaccine and oral polio vaccine (OPV) in endemic areas
6–8 weeks	DTP plus OPV plus Hepatitis B vaccine plus Hib plus PCV plus RV
10–12 weeks	DTP plus OPV plus Hepatitis B plus Hib plus PCV plus RV
14–16 weeks	DTP plus OPV plus Hepatitis B plus Hib plus PCV plus RV
9–15 months	Measles vaccine (see Section 12.2). Yellow fever vaccine in yellow fever endemic areas of Africa and South America. Japanese encephalitis vaccine in problem areas
12–18 months	Measles booster dose
1–6 years	DTP booster dose
9–13 years	HPV vaccine to all girls
13–18 years	Tetanus and diphtheria booster (Td)

DTP (diphtheria tetanus pertussis) and OPV can be given even if the child has a mild illness. Measles vaccine can also be given if the child is having a mild illness, as it does not have any effect for several days, by which time the minor illness will have finished. Vaccination should always be given to the malnourished child who is at particular risk from infection. Protective response is good except in cases of severe kwashiorkor. In high-risk populations the following vaccines can be included: meningococcal vaccine, and vaccines for rabies, typhoid, cholera and hepatitis A. (See further under the respective diseases, Sections 13.6, 17.1, 8.8, 8.4 and 8.9.) See text for other definitions.

The routine childhood vaccination programme used in the UK National Health Service is:

Age	Vaccination
2 months	DTP/IPV/Hib/PCV
3 months	DTP/IPV/Hib/MenC
4 months	DTP/IPV/Hib/MenC/PCV
12–13 months	Hib/MenC, PCV, MMR
3 years 4 months to 5 years	DTaP/IPV/MMR
Girls 12–13 years	HPV vaccine
13–18 years	Td/IPV

See text for definitions.

Other vaccines specific to particular diseases, e.g. influenza, will be discussed in the relevant disease sections of the book.

3.2.3 Operational factors

In planning vaccination programmes cultural, logistic and other operational factors largely determine the coverage. Some of these are:

- The strongest motivation to attend Maternal and Child Health (MCH) clinics is immediately after the child has been born, so the shorter the interval between birth and vaccination, the more likely is the child to be brought by its mother.
- A range of ages, days and combinations should be available so that the time of attendance is always the right time for vaccination. If a mother is told to bring her child back at a set time or age of the child, then she probably will not bother.
- Admission to hospital is an ideal opportunity to check that the vaccination schedule is up to date. Measles vaccination is particularly important as many children contract serious measles when admitted to hospital for another complaint.
- A primary course need never be repeated, even if the booster dose is long delayed.
- An interrupted course can be resumed whenever feasible without starting from the beginning again.
- If the interval between doses ends up as being longer than planned, the immunological effect will not be reduced. The only disadvantage to long, drawn-out schedules is that the individual is not rapidly protected.

3.2.4 The cold chain

The cold chain is a descriptive term for the whole sequence of links that must be maintained in transporting the vaccine in a viable condition from the manufacturer to the person to be vaccinated. Vaccines will only survive when they are maintained at the correct temperature. There are certain limits when the vaccine can be allowed to depart from the optimal temperature, but the range and time are very short and vaccines rapidly lose their potency. To vaccinate with non-potent vaccine is not only a waste of time and money but brings discredit to the vaccination programme.

Some vaccines are stored at freezing temperature (poliomyelitis, BCG and measles), while others are kept at the standard refrigerator temperature of 4–8°C (DTP and tetanus). If stored at the wrong temperature the vaccine will be destroyed. The two elements of the cold chain are speed of transport and maintenance of a steady temperature, so the fastest means of getting a vaccine from one place to another is used. A temperature-sensitive strip that changes colour if the batch becomes too warm during the period of transport accompanies most vaccines. The viability of the vaccine can then be checked and the problem link in the cold chain detected.

Cold boxes are well-insulated containers lined with freezer packs in which vaccines can be transported or stored for up to 7 days. They are valuable for mobile vaccination teams, but for the individual vaccinator, a hand-held vacuum flask will store vaccines for 1–2 days, depending on the outside temperature.

Certain vaccines, such as the measles vaccine and BCG, are sensitive to light and need to be protected while they are being diluted, stored and given to the person. Special dark glass syringes can be obtained, but covering with a cloth is just as efficient. Many potent vaccines are destroyed by being drawn up into syringes that are still warm from the sterilizing process, a sad end to a long cold chain.

3.2.5 Mobile and static clinics

Vaccination can be from static and/or mobile clinics. Their various advantages and disadvantages are:

	Static	Mobile
Coverage	Limited to 10 km radius	Large areas
Availability	Always	Occasional
Transport	Not required	Required
Costs	High capital, low recurrent	Moderate capital, high recurrent
Vaccine supplies	Often erratic	Good

A static clinic responsible for providing primary care services (including delivery) for both the mother and child is the most effective. A child stands a greater chance of receiving all its vaccines from a static health unit. However, as the distance from a clinic increases, the probability of a mother bringing her child to the clinic decreases for every kilometre to be walked. Coverage is best closest to the clinic and decreases further away, with often large gaps between clinics, as shown in Fig. 3.2. It is the inadequately covered areas between the static clinics where an epidemic is likely to occur. Outreach services or mobile clinics then become valuable in vaccinating the in-between areas.

Mobile clinics are easier to organize where only one dose of vaccine is required (e.g. yellow fever), and have a special place in mass campaigns.

3.2.6 Seasonality and vaccination campaigns

Many infections follow a seasonal pattern with sufficient regularity for peaks of incidence to be forecast. If known, the epidemic can be averted by carrying out mass vaccination before it is expected (see Fig. 1.8).

3.2.7 Ring vaccination

If an epidemic is spreading it can be contained by vaccinating everyone in a ring round the site of the epidemic. Villages should be chosen where cases have not yet been reported and an attempt made to vaccinate as many people as possible. If the ring is too close to the epidemic, then the disease may already have affected some people outside the defensive ring and then another will need to be started even further away.

3.2.8 Economies of vaccination

Vaccination coverage is often poor because of constraints put on staff about the cost of vaccines. Vaccines should be supplied in small dose quantities so that a vial can be opened even if there is only one child to be vaccinated. Spare vaccine can often be used up on other children attending the health centre for other reasons. The cost of vaccination is not just the price of the actual vial of vaccine but includes the whole cold chain and the salary of the vaccinator. To have a vaccinator sitting around not vaccinating because there are not enough children to warrant opening a vial is a false economy. Proportional costs have been calculated as follows:

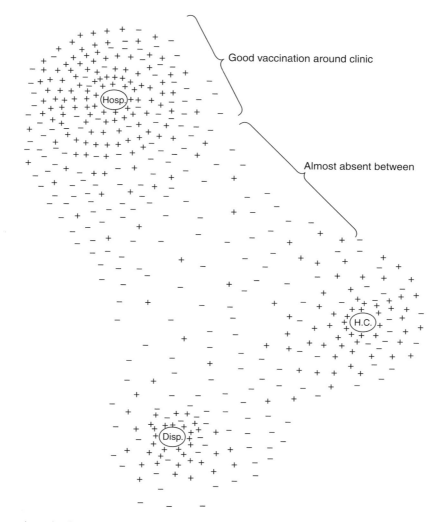

Fig. 3.2. Unequal vaccination coverage from static clinics. +, vaccinated child; –, non-vaccinated child; Hosp., hospital; H.C., health centre; Disp., dispensary.

Capital	12–15%	Transport	20%
Salaries	45%	Vaccine	5%
Training	2–3%	Other	12–16%

3.2.9 Vaccine efficacy

Vaccine efficacy (VE) is calculated by:

$$VE = \frac{(AR\ in\ unvaccinated - AR\ in\ vaccinated)}{AR\ in\ unvaccinated} \times 100\%$$

where AR is the attack rate (discussed in Section 2.2.2).

The VE indicates the maximum achievable level, but poor vaccination technique or storage can reduce this. Also, the more people that are vaccinated the greater the number of apparent vaccine failures, as shown in Fig. 3.3. If the above equation is rewritten to express the percentage of cases vaccinated (PCV) in terms of the percentage of the population vaccinated (PPV) and VE then:

$$PCV = \frac{PPV - (PPV \times VE)}{1 - (PPV \times VE)}$$

By knowing two of these variables, the third can be calculated. Figure 3.3 shows three curves

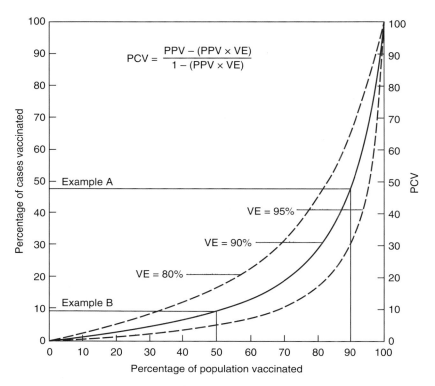

$$PCV = \frac{PPV - (PPV \times VE)}{1 - (PPV \times VE)}$$

Fig. 3.3. Percentage of cases vaccinated (PCV) per percentage of population vaccinated (PPV) for three values of vaccine efficacy (VE). (Reproduced by permission from *Weekly Epidemiological Record* 7, 20 February 1981. World Health Organization, Geneva.)

generated from the equation, each for a different vaccine efficacy. These curves predict the theoretical proportion of cases with a vaccine history. For example, if a measles epidemic is observed in a population with homogeneous measles exposure where 90% of the individuals are vaccinated (PPV = 90%) with a 90% effective vaccine (VE = 90%), the expected percentage of measles cases with a history of being vaccinated would be 47% (PCV = 47%: Example A). However, if only 50% were vaccinated, then 9% of the cases would be found to have been vaccinated (Example B). This is not to say that there is anything wrong with the vaccination programme, but explains why there may appear to be an unexpected number of vaccinated individuals among the cases.

3.3 Environmental Control Methods

Many diseases result from contamination of the environment by faecal matter with transmission by the direct route (e.g. by fingers), or via food and water. The mechanisms are schematically illustrated in Fig. 3.4. The various control methods available are as follows:

- personal and domestic hygiene;
- the proper preparation, cooking and storage of food;
- use of water supplies;
- proper disposal of excreta and waste; and
- miscellaneous methods including meat inspection and hygiene.

Classifying the water- and sanitation-related diseases into well-defined categories allows rational control methods to be applied (Table 3.1). The potential impact of these control methods is seen in Table 3.2.

3.3.1 Personal hygiene

Personal hygiene is the understanding by the individual of how infections can be transmitted to

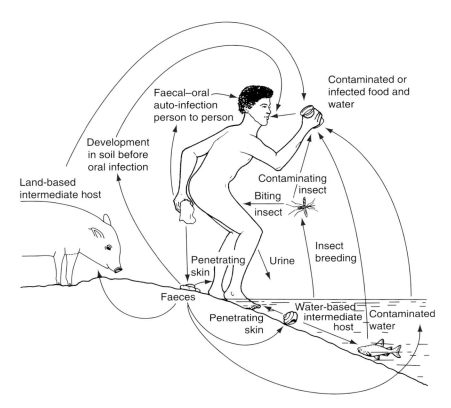

Fig. 3.4. Routes of transmission of the water- and sanitation-related diseases.

them or others by unclean habits, and using appropriate methods to avoid them. Infection can be avoided by preventing bad habits, e.g. promiscuous defecation, or introducing good habits, e.g. hand washing before eating. Teaching of personal hygiene is best started at an early age and reinforced when the child goes to school. The main infections that can be reduced by personal hygiene are shown in Table 3.3, but see also Chapters 6 and 20.

Category 1 diseases are reduced by washing of the body and clothing with water and soap (water-washed diseases). Categories 2 and 3 diseases are reduced by rigorous hand washing after defecation and before eating.

Personal hygiene is closely related to the availability of water in sufficient quantity. Water quality is of less importance. Washing is improved by using soap, which reduces surface tension and emulsifies oils, allowing bacteria to be more easily removed. Where soap is not available then mud or ash can be used.

3.3.2 Protection of foods

Food-transmitted infections can spread either through contamination or by a specific intermediate host. Flies indirectly contaminate food.

Protection of the food we eat can be by the following methods:

- inspection of raw produce;
- packaging and avoiding contamination;
- suitable storage conditions and time limits;
- washing and correct preparation;
- adequate and even cooking;
- preventing contamination of cooked foods; and
- eating cooked foods immediately.

Infections that can be reduced by the proper protection of food are shown in Table 3.4.

Category 2 infections contaminate food before or after cooking. Flies are often involved. Even if contamination has occurred, correct storage and the disposal of cooked foods after a limited time

Table 3.1. A classification of water- and excreta-related diseases. (Modified from Bradley, D.J. (1978), in Feachem, R.G. et al. (eds) *Water Wastes and Health in Hot Climates*. Reprinted by permission of John Wiley & Sons Ltd, Chichester, UK.)

Category	Characteristics	Examples	Transmission	Control measures
1. Water-washed diseases	Diseases of poor hygiene	Skin diseases, eye diseases, louse-borne typhus	Person to person (and autoinfection)	Personal hygiene Increase water quantity
2. Faecal–oral diseases	a. Low infective dose	*Enterobius*, amoebiasis, enteric viruses	Person to person (and autoinfection)	Personal hygiene Increase water quantity
	b. High infective dose. Able to multiply outside host	Diarrhoeal diseases, cholera, typhoid, hepatitis A	Contamination of food or water	Excreta disposal Cook food Improve water quality
3. Soil-mediated diseases (helminths)	a. Development in soil	*Ascaris*, hookworms, *Strongyloides*	Larvae penetrate skin or swallowed	Personal hygiene Excreta disposal
	b. Development in animal (cow or pig) intermediate host	*Taenia* spp.	Cysts in meat	Meat inspection Cooked food
4. Water-based diseases	Helminths requiring intermediate hosts			
	a. Copepods	Guinea worm	Ingested in water	Improve water quality
	b. Snails only	Schistosomiasis	Penetrates skin	Reduce water contact
	c. Two intermediate hosts	*Fasciolopsis*, *Clonorchis*, *Paragonimus*, *Diphyllobothrium*	Eating uncooked specific foods	Excreta disposal Cook food
5. Water and excreta-related insect vectors	a. Breeding in water or sewage	Malaria, filariasis, arboviruses	Mosquitoes	Drain breeding sites Maintain water supplies and sanitation
	b. Breeding or biting near water	Onchocerciasis Trypanosomiasis	*Simulium* Tsetse fly	Water supply at site of use
	c. Breeding in excreta	Diarrhoeal diseases	Housefly	Excreta disposal

Table 3.2. The potential impact of environmental control methods (compare with Table 3.1).

Disease category	Personal hygiene	Cooking of foods	Water supplies	Sanitation	Miscellaneous
1. Water-washed diseases	+++	–	++	+	–
2. Faecal–oral diseases	+++	+	++	+	–
3. Soil-mediated diseases	++	+++	–	+++	Meat inspection
4. Water-based diseases	–	+++	++	+	Reduce water contact
5. Water- and excreta-related insect vectors	–	–	±±	±±	Protection from insects

+++, Very effective; ++, moderately effective; +, effective; –, not effective; ±, can be either effective or not effective.

can prevent sufficient multiplication of bacteria to reach an infective dose. Where food has been stored it can be reheated to render it safe in most circumstances, but precautions need to be taken against food poisoning, especially that produced by staphylococci (see Section 9.1.1).

Categories 3b and 4c infections require specific intermediate hosts in their transmission so

Table 3.3. Infections that can be reduced by personal hygiene.

Category	Infection
1	Skin sepsis and ulcers
1	Conjunctivitis
1	Trachoma
1	Scabies
1	Yaws
1	Leprosy
1	*Tinea*
1	Louse-borne fevers
1	Flea-borne infections (including plague)
2	Enteric viruses (including hepatitis A and polio)
2	*Enterobius*
2	Amoebiasis
2	*Trichuris*
2	*Giardia*
2	*Shigella*
2	Typhoid
2	Other salmonellae
2	*Campylobacter*
2	Non-specific diarrhoeal diseases
2	Cholera
2	Leptospirosis
3a	Ascaris

their destruction or proper cooking is an effective means of control. Cooking needs to be at a sufficiently high temperature to kill off the intermediate stages and procedures such as roasting on a spit or cooking meat 'underdone' do not provide high enough temperatures inside the meat. Meat inspection can be effective in *Taenia* infection (3b).

3.3.3 Water supplies

Contaminated water can be the vehicle of transmission of a number of disease-producing organisms. Water is also important in diseases of poor hygiene, as a medium for intermediate hosts, and as a breeding place for vectors of disease.

The infections and possible improvements that may occur from installing a water supply are shown in Table 3.5.

The provision of water

There are four aspects of water supply which can help to control disease transmission.

- improve water quantity;
- improve water quality;
- reduce water contact by bringing water to site of use; and
- prevent spillage by proper maintenance of supplies and drainage.

It will be noticed how this is the normal process in the supply of water. The first objective is to provide water in sufficient quantity, which is followed by improving its quality, and finally a piped system is made. If this is the pattern followed, then similarly it can be anticipated that the first group of diseases to be reduced will be the water-washed and faecal–oral, then the waterborne, etc. However, water supplies need to be maintained and when they break down disease can be expected to return.

In rural water supplies where chlorine treatment of the water is costly, difficult to maintain or inappropriate, then a different standard to that in large centralized supplies may be acceptable. This should not be considered to be unsatisfactory as the provision of a properly constructed water supply is an improvement on what was used before. Also, quality is closely related to quantity. By providing a greater volume of water at a more accessible site, quality will usually be improved.

Health aspects are the concern of the medical worker, whereas the villager looks upon water as a basic necessity. His, or rather her (as women are nearly always the carriers of water) major concerns will be quite different, as follows:

- availability of water at a more convenient place (preferably in the village);
- a continuous and reliable supply; and
- additional water for crops and domestic animals.

It is a combination of these health and social factors that needs to be used in deciding the appropriateness and benefits of water supplies.

Economic and planning criteria

Everybody wants the best possible water supply they can get, but resources are limited so it will be many years before everyone has the supply they desire. Decisions have to be made as to which sections of the community should be served, when they should receive their supply and the level of

Table 3.4. Reduction of infection by food protection.

Category	Infection	Type of food	Possible reduction
2	Enteric viruses (including hepatitis A and polio)	All	+
2	*Hymenolepis*	All	+
2	Amoebiasis	All	+
2	*Trichuris*	All	+
2	*Giardia*	All	+
2	*Shigella*	All, especially dairy produce	++
2	Typhoid	All, especially dairy produce	++
2	Salmonellae	All, especially dairy produce	++
2	*Campylobacter*	All, especially dairy produce	++
2	Non-specific diarrhoeal diseases	All, plus fly contamination	++
2	Cholera	Marine animals, salad	++
2	Leptospirosis	Rat-contaminated foods	++
2	Brucellosis	Milk produce	++
3a	*Ascaris*	All	+
3b	*Taenia*	Cow or pig meat	+++
4b	*Trichinella*	Pig	+++
4c	*Fasciolopsis*	Salad	+++
4c	*Opisthorchis*	Fish (freshwater)	+++
4c	*Paragonimus*	Crustacea (freshwater)	+++
4c	*Diphyllobothrium*	Fish (freshwater)	+++

availability. There are many alternative strategies that may be, or inadvertently will be, used. They might include the following:

- priority of an area on health grounds;
- priority to an area of water scarcity;
- encouragement of development to an area of high potential;
- priority to communities that can contribute in money and labour;
- first come, first served; and
- political favouritism.

Other alternatives in the nature of the supply can also be considered:

- supplying a large number of people with the simplest of supplies;
- restricting supplies to certain demonstration areas with a high standard;
- starting with the most available natural water sources; and
- planning a major project, such as a dam, followed by extensions in subsequent years.

The strategy adopted will depend on how much the country, region, district or village is prepared to pay for the price of water. Savings can be made by the following means:

- economies of scale;
- standardizing the equipment; and
- self-help labour.

The initial water master plan is best formulated by skilled engineers, but its execution can be carried out by a purpose trained technician, utilizing community effort. The plan needs to take account of health, engineering, political and community demands.

Water capacity and use

In selecting a suitable source, the amount of water it produces and its regularity needs to be known. If a spring or stream does not flow all the year round, then it is not suitable, unless a dam is also built. Measurements of water flow should be made at the end of the dry season and the people asked if the source has ever dried up. A temporary dam can be made, and the rate of filling a measured bucket estimates the flow. Wells can be mechanically pumped out and the fall noted for a given flow of water. Rainwater catchment is derived from the simple formula:

1 mm of rainfall on $1\,m^2$ of roof in plan will give 0.8 l of water

Table 3.5. Expected improvements when installing a water supply. (From Bradley, D.J. (1978) in Feachem, R.G. *et al.* (eds) *Water, Wastes and Health in Hot Climates.* Reprinted by permission of John Wiley & Sons. Ltd, Chichester, UK.)

Category	Infection	Water improvement required	Possible reduction (%)
1	Skin sepsis and ulcers	Increase water quantity	50
1	Conjunctivitis	Increase water quantity	70
1	Trachoma	Increase water quantity	60
1	Scabies	Increase water quantity	80
1	Yaws	Increase water quantity	70
1	Leprosy	Increase water quantity	50
1	*Tinea*	Increase water quantity	50
1	Louse-borne fevers	Increase water quantity	40
1	Flea-borne diseases (including plague)	Increase water quantity	40
2	Enteric viruses (including hepatitis A and polio)	Increase water quantity	10?
2	*Enterobius*	Increase water quantity	20
2	*Hymenolepis*	Increase water quantity	20
2	Amoebiasis	Increase water quantity	50
2	*Trichuris*	Increase water quantity	20
2	*Giardia*	Increase water quantity	30
2	*Shigella*	Improve water quality	50
2	Typhoid	Improve water quality	80
2	Other salmonellae	Improve water quality	50
2	*Campylobacter*	Improve water quality	50
2	Non-specific diarrhoeal diseases	Improve water quality	50
2	Cholera	Improve water quality	90
2	Leptospirosis	Improve water quality	80
3a	*Ascaris*	Increase water quantity	40
3a	Hydatids	Increase water quantity	40
3a	*Toxocara*	Increase water quantity	40
3a	Toxoplasmosis	Increase water quantity	40
4a	Guinea worm	Reduce water contact	100
4b	Schistosomiasis	Reduce water contact	60
5a	Malaria	Water piped to site of use and maintenance of water supplies	10
5a	Filariasis	Water piped to site of use and maintenance of water supplies	10
5a	Arboviruses	Water piped to site of use and maintenance of water supplies	10?
5b	Onchocerciasis	Water piped to site of use	20?
5b	Gambian trypanosomiasis	Water piped to site of use	80

As an example, if the roof plan area is 10×5 m and the average annual rainfall is 650 mm, then $10 \times 5 \times 650 \times 0.8 = 26,000$ l/year or 71 l/day, on average.

The demand for water will be determined by the availability, the number of people and the use to which it is put. The availability is the most crucial factor as water that has to be carried some distance will be used much more sparingly than when there is a tap inside the house. Average figures taken from a number of studies are as follows:

Rural supply	20 l/person/day
Standpipe	40 l/person/day
Single tap in the home	80 l/person/day
Multiple taps with bath, WC, etc.	200–300 l/person/day

At least 50% extra capacity is allowed for future growth of the community and expansion of the supply. A water source is chosen where the expected demand on the supply will never be exceeded, even in the driest time of the year. If this is not possible then some form of storage will be required. Water use during the night is far less than in the day, so a poor supply can be boosted by providing a storage tank that fills at night. In areas of wide seasonal variation, more extensive storage facilities may be required to save the rain falling in the few wet months, such as a dam.

Choice of water supply

Choosing a water source will depend upon the following:

- proximity to user;
- reliability;
- quantity of water;
- quality of water;
- technical feasibility;
- resources available;
- social desirability or taboo; and
- maintenance.

The alternative choices are illustrated in Figs 3.5 and 3.6. Rainwater naturally seeps through the earth until it finds an impervious layer (such as clay) on which it collects. Where this impervious layer comes to the surface the water runs out of the ground as a spring. It can also form the bed of a river or, in an enclosed area, a lake. This groundwater can be tapped by a shallow well. At a much deeper level, a second impervious layer can trap a large quantity of water. A deep well or borehole is required to reach this source of water. Island populations (Fig. 3.6) have particular problems in obtaining water and are generally left with only two alternatives. Providing they have suitable roofing material (e.g. corrugated iron), rainwater can be collected and stored in a tank. The alternative is to sink a well to tap the freshwater lens. Due to a fortunate quality of coral rock it acts like a large sponge holding freshwater that has percolated through, floating on the denser sea water. Providing the well is sunk just far enough and not pumped out too hard, then freshwater can be obtained. The different water sources are summarized in Table 3.6.

Wells are often a good supply, as long as contamination can be prevented, and have the advantage that they can be sited close to houses. This can be achieved by sealing them and fitting a pump, but this will require maintenance. Deep wells and boreholes need special equipment for their construction and complex pumps to lift water from these depths. They are mainly applicable in areas of severe water shortage, such as deserts. Lakes and rivers provide convenient, but poor, quality water. Other sources should be used if possible, but if there is no alternative, then some form of water treatment, such as filtration and storage, should be incorporated. A constant spring that never dries up is a very suitable source, as it is comparatively free from contamination and can normally be led to an outlet without requiring pumping.

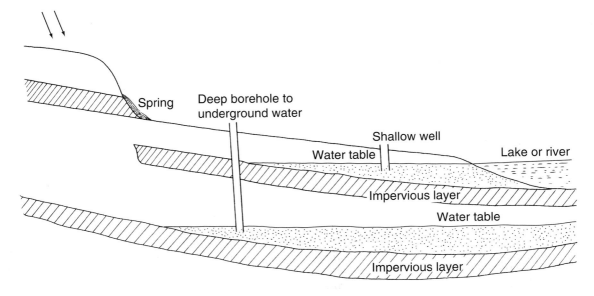

Fig. 3.5. Sources of water.

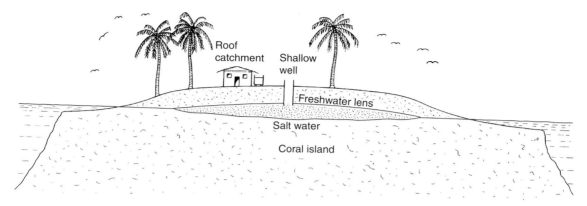

Fig. 3.6. Water catchment and the freshwater lens of coral islands.

Table 3.6. Sources of water, their advantages and disadvantages.

	Spring	Shallow well	Borehole	River	Lake	Catchment
Proximity	Distant	Near	Intermediate	Near	Near	Near
Reliability	Good	Variable	Good	Unreliable	Good	Unreliable
Quantity	Good	Moderate	Good	Variable	Good	Poor
Quality	Good	Moderate	Good	Poor	Poor	Good
Technology	Easy	Moderate	Difficult	Easy[a]	Easy[a]	Moderate
Cost	Low	Moderate	High	Low[a]	Low[a]	Moderate to high
Community preference	High	Moderate	Moderate	Low	Low	Moderate
Maintenance	Low	Moderate	High	Low	Low	Moderate

[a]These assessments are for taking water by hand from the river or lake. If a pump and supply system are used then the technology is difficult and the cost high.

Maintenance costs will therefore be low so greater capital expenditure can be allowed for protecting the spring and piping its water to the village.

Rainwater catchment is an underutilized source of pure water, either as a main method, or a subsidiary (for drinking water). So much good water runs to waste off large expanses of roof that have already been paid for in the construction of the building. For the additional cost of guttering and a tank, a family can have a good, safe source of water, inside or very close to their house. Storage tanks can either be close to the roof, or large concrete structures built underground. Their main danger is that if water is allowed to collect in poorly maintained gutters or uncovered tanks then mosquitoes can breed in them.

The ideal is to find a source that has both constant quantity and good quality, but where the latter is not achieved then quality can be improved by simple methods such as the three-pot system (Fig. 3.7). In this it is the action of allowing the water to settle and preferably exposing it to sunlight that purifies the water.

Filtering of water can be very effective and several commercial filters are available. They are particularly useful in emergency situations or for people moving from place to place. Several of the small filters used by travellers contain iodized salts, but an improved system uses silane-treated filters. When bacteria, including resistant organisms, touch the active surface the cell wall is destroyed by lysis.

Sunlight is very effective at disinfecting water and a simple method, appropriate for use in developing countries, and known as solar water disinfection (SODIS) utilizes plastic bottles filled with water. These are placed on the roof for 6 h to 2 days depending on the strength of the sun, after which the water is safe to drink. The sun's ultraviolet rays kill any pathogenic organisms while its heat has a pasteurizing effect.

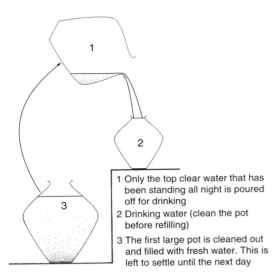

1 Only the top clear water that has been standing all night is poured off for drinking
2 Drinking water (clean the pot before refilling)
3 The first large pot is cleaned out and filled with fresh water. This is left to settle until the next day

Fig. 3.7. The three-pot system – a simple means of improving water quality.

3.3.4 Sanitation

With food and water supplies, the emphasis is on the prevention of contamination, but with sanitation it is on reducing the source of the contamination. Social habits concerned with excreta disposal are often strongly held and unless these are approached in a sensible manner then any system will fail. Sanitation is not just the provision of latrines, but a complex and interrelated subject involving the people, water supplies and all the other aspects of environmental health.

Health factors

As shown in Table 3.1, the main impact of sanitation is on disease groups 2, 3a, 4c and 5c. The installation of sanitation may produce a reduction in the infections shown in Table 3.7.

The provision of sanitation

When providing sanitation there is a sharp contrast with water supplies, everybody wants a water supply, but nobody wants to change their defecation practice. This is quite simple to explain in that substances taken into the body can be understood as a direct cause of illness, whereas excreting something from the body cannot. Defecation is a necessary but private business, not a matter for

discussion. There are also social practices that are set by religious, racial or cultural rules. These may dictate where and where not to defecate, will probably separate the sexes and define particular anal cleansing practices. With all these patterns and customs that have been taught since childhood, any change becomes a long and difficult process. If a family can see the benefits of a latrine then they will install and look after it, the health authority can then assist in technical specifications and subsidise costs. Any attempt to impose systems or even build them free of charge will cause resentment or non-use.

Like water, sanitation has to be paid for, but here costs are even less accepted by the population. People are only prepared to pay for the minimum possible in getting rid of their excreta. Only in urban areas will it be considered necessary to pay for the removal of excrement, in rural areas there is sufficient space. Cost is related to convenience, which is why people are prepared to pay for improved systems, their willingness to pay usually having nothing to do with health. A good pit latrine can be as effective in disease control as a conventional water-carried sewage system, the only difference being that the former is outside the house, while the latter carries excreta from within the house. The cost of this convenience is typically ten times that of a pit latrine.

In choosing the most appropriate excreta disposal system, the emphasis should be on simplicity. Only when a simpler method becomes outmoded because of rising standards and expectations will a more sophisticated system become appropriate. A simple incremental process, as illustrated in Fig. 3.8, can be planned. The first stage is to bury excreta, which will lead on to using a pit latrine. If pit latrines are already accepted by the community, then demonstrating the advantages of improved pit latrines will be the next step. The type of facility will also be determined by the availability of water. As mentioned in Section 3.3.3, the provision of water should precede any sanitation programme, as personal hygiene can only be taught if there is water at hand to wash with. The quantity and nearness of this water will then determine the type of sanitary system that can be used. In the second part of Fig. 3.8, the incremental progression of a water-utilizing sanitary system is shown. A pour–flush latrine can be installed where water is obtained from a village standpipe, but with a septic tank or sewerage, a water-flushing system requires in-house water connections.

Table 3.7. The expected improvements from the installation of sanitation.

Category	Infection	Through reduced contamination of	Possible reduction
1	Trachoma	The environment; flies (group 5c)	+
2	Enteric viruses (including hepatitis A)	Vegetables	+
2	*Hymenolepis*	Food and water	+
2	Amoebiasis	Vegetables	++
2	*Trichuris*	Food and water	+
2	*Giardia*	Food and water	+
2	*Shigella*	Food and water	++
2	Typhoid	Food and water	++
2	Other salmonellae	Food and water	++
2	*Campylobacter*	Food and water	++
2	Non-specific diarrhoeal diseases	Food and water	++
2	Cholera	Food and water	++
3a	*Ascaris*	Soil	+++
3a	Hookworms	Soil	+++
3a	*Strongyloides*	Soil	+++
3b	*Taenia*	Soil	+++
4b	Schistosomiasis	Water	+
4c	*Fasciolopsis*	Water	+
4c	*Opisthorchis*	Water	+
4c	*Paragonimus*	Water	+
4c	*Diphyllobothrium*	Water	+
5	Housefly-transmitted diseases	The environment, flies	±±[a]
5	Filariasis	Water and *Culex quinquefasciatus* breeding	+

[a]Sanitation, if not properly built or maintained, can be as responsible for increasing the fly nuisance as decreasing it.

Siting and contamination

The sanitation unit must be sited so that it does not contaminate the environment in such a way as to threaten the health of others. With a pit latrine, bacterial pollution can travel downwards for a distance of up to 2 m. If the contamination reaches the water table it will flow horizontally for up to 10 m. This means that any latrine should be sited at least this distance from a water supply, such as a well. The latrine should also be placed downhill to the well so that drainage is away from the well, although excessive pumping will draw water into the well from all directions, including possibly from a latrine. If a latrine is built less than 10 m from a river or stream, it can pollute it, as the water table will be flowing towards the stream. Latrines in this situation can be potent sources of pollution if the river is used for drinking water.

The effluent from a septic tank is highly charged with pathogens and must be disposed of properly. Running it into a storm drain, as often happens, is a bad practice and a considerable danger; instead, it should be led it into a soakaway, using the same precautions as with a latrine.

Pollution of the soil is a complex subject and the rough rule of 10 m distance between a latrine and source of drinking water is given as a guide. Contamination is dependent upon the following:

- the velocity of groundwater flow (should be less than 10 m in 10 days); and
- the composition of the soil (not fissured, e.g. as in limestone).

Expert advice should be obtained before embarking on a latrine programme.

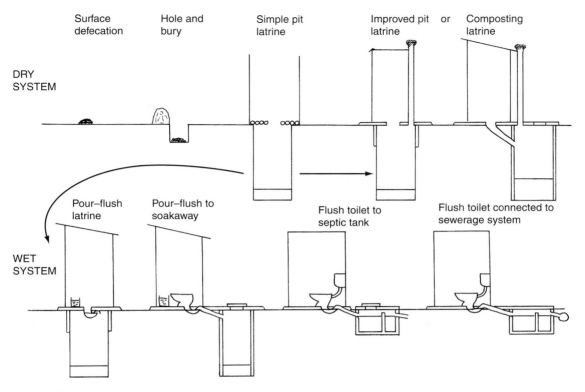

Fig. 3.8. Types of excreta disposal systems – incremental sanitation.

3.4 Vector Control

Parasites are transmitted from one host to another by vectors, often utilizing the stage in the vector to undergo multiplication or development. In some parasites, e.g. malaria, the vector is the definitive host, whereas in others, such as *Wuchereria bancrofti*, it is the intermediate host. Whichever part the vector plays it is a vital one for the parasite, which cannot continue if the vector is destroyed or reduced to sufficiently low numbers to prevent continuing transmission. The time of changing from one host to another is a precarious time for the parasite and considerable loss may occur. Malaria gametocyte development must coincide with a mosquito taking a blood meal and both male and female gametocytes are required for fertilization and maturation to take place in the insect's stomach. *W. bancrofti* suffers considerable parasite loss during the vector stage. The vector therefore does not have to be completely destroyed, but kept at levels too low for transmission to take place. So vector control means vector reduction not vector eradication.

3.4.1 Mosquito control

The various ways in which mosquitoes can be controlled are as follows:

- adulticides;
- repellents;
- personal protection;
- larvicides;
- biological control; and
- environmental modification.

These are all illustrated in Fig. 3.9.

Adulticides

Killing the adult mosquito can either be done while it is flying using a knock-down spray, or when it is resting with a residual insecticide. Knock-down insecticides will kill adult mosquitoes at the time of application only, whereas residual insecticides continue to have a lethal effect for a considerable period of time.

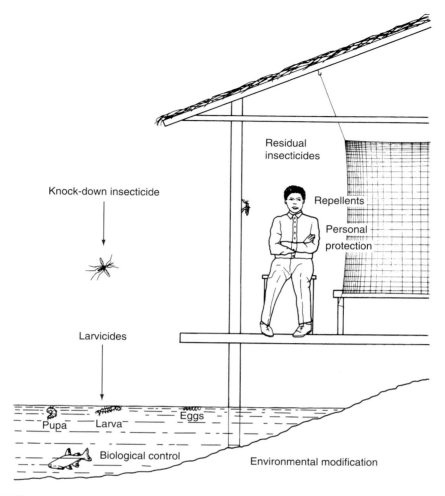

Knock-down insecticide

Larvicides

Residual
insecticides

Repellents

Personal
protection

Pupa — Larva — Eggs

Biological control

Environmental modification

Fig. 3.9. Mosquito control methods.

Knock-down insecticides

Knock-down insecticides are used to control epidemics of vector-transmitted disease where an explosive increase in the number of flying adults is responsible. They have been used in malaria epidemics, but have perhaps their greatest value in dengue and the control of arbovirus infections. They are used as space sprays (aerosols), in the house, for mosquito survey counts and for disinfecting aircraft. Knock-down sprays commonly contain pyrethrum, derived from a species of chrysanthemum grown in highland areas of East Africa. They can be dispersed in aerosols, smoke generators (fogging) or ultra-low volume (ULV) aerial sprays.

Residual insecticides

Residual spraying is the main method for control of mosquito-transmitted disease because the insecticide continues to remain active for 6 months or more. By careful organization, repeated applications, made at regular intervals can maintain a continuing killing effect. Ideally, the insecticide should be sprayed just before the start of the main transmission season, especially in areas where malaria is seasonal.

Residual insecticides act on the resting mosquito. Mosquitoes need to rest after they have taken a blood meal and generally choose the nearest place, which is the wall of the victim's house. If the wall is sprayed with residual insecticide then the mosquito will absorb a lethal dose through its legs while it is resting. The insecticide can either be sprayed as an emulsion or as a wettable powder, as few of the insecticides commonly used go into solution with a cheap and easily obtainable medium such as water. Emulsions are best on non-absorbent surfaces, while wettable powders are suitable for mud, leaf or other poor-quality walls. The wettable medium (generally water) soaks into the wall and leaves the powder on the surface. Some of the insecticide is taken into the porous surface, but this gradually comes out, maintaining a steady concentration. Once residual insecticide has been sprayed on a wall, then it must not be washed or painted.

Residual insecticide sprayed on to a surface depends upon a number of factors.

- the proportion of active insecticide in the preparation;
- the amount of insecticide mixed with the fluid medium;
- mixing, before and during application;
- the distance from the surface that is sprayed; and
- the speed of application.

These are all specified for a particular insecticide and spraymen must be trained to ensure that the right concentration is delivered. A measured area of plaster can be scraped and the insecticide content analysed.

Residual spraying is carried out by a team of spraymen with manually operated sprayers covering a village at a time. Houses are emptied and pets and domestic animals restrained in a suitable place some distance away (as they are sensitive to insecticides). Any insects, beetles and lizards that are killed should be swept up and disposed of before the domestic animals are allowed back into the houses. This takes a considerable amount of organization, with a strict schedule of notification, followed by spraying. The supervisor answers any questions, ensures that the work is done and arranges logistic support. If residual spraying is not adequately explained to people then organizational resistance will develop. The target is to spray every dwelling house, whether permanently or temporarily occupied.

Deterrents and repellents

Deterrents and repellents can be either smokes or applications to the body in the form of creams and solutions. They do not kill the insect but deter it from biting.

Mosquito coils or heated pads have a combined deterrent and repellent action. They are made with small quantities of pyrethroids in a slow burning base, but other insecticides can be added to enhance the activity. Used in a still atmosphere they can be most effective. If they do not prevent all the bites, they reduce the number, which is important in filariasis transmission. They reduce the probability of being bitten by an infective mosquito carrying any disease.

The most commonly used repellent is diethyltoluamide (DEET), which can be applied to the person, clothing, tents and mosquito nets. The solutions can either be dissolved in methylated spirit or emulsified with water and applied to the surface. DEET is not absorbed by synthetic fabrics and a cotton or wool base is essential if it is to remain for some time. Four weeks of activity are given if continuously exposed, but if the garments (such as a shawl or leg bands) are kept in a polythene bag, then repellent action can continue for 3–6 months. Precaution should be taken in applying DEET to the skin as some individuals are sensitive, while neurological toxicity can be produced in children. Natural repellents made from eucalyptus oil and other natural substances are preferable for application to the person.

Personal protection

Personal protection is a valuable precaution in reducing the number of mosquito bites. Clothing that covers the arms and legs, especially if combined with a repellent, can protect an individual most effectively. With the appearance of widespread insecticide resistance, greater reliance must now be placed on personal protection.

The use of mosquito nets is a well-tried method of personal protection. Mosquito nets are fitted to the bed and the edges tucked under the mattress. A knock-down spray applied prior to retiring will prevent any mosquitoes entering the net when the occupant goes to bed. Young children should be placed under nets before it gets dark. If the custom is to sleep on a mat on the floor rather than a bed, then mosquito nets can still be used. Insecticide-treated mosquito nets (ITNs) are now the main method of malaria control (see Box 3.1).

A less satisfactory alternative is to screen the whole house, which is expensive, and a torn area will destroy the whole effect. Air conditioning, by providing a sealed room, generally prevents mosquitoes from entering. Even so it is preferable to use a knock-down spray in the evening to prevent any mosquitoes that may have entered. The cost of these methods is considerably greater than using treated mosquito nets.

Box 3.1. **Insecticide-treated mosquito nets (ITNs).**

Although mosquito nets have been a method of protection against biting insects for some considerable period of time, their effectiveness has been improved considerably by treating them with insecticides. This has a double action of deterring the mosquito from the person, especially if the net is torn, and of killing mosquitoes that come in contact with the treated net.

Additional advantages of treated nets are that they provide some protection to other people in the same room and not sleeping under a net due to the repellent effect of the insecticide. They also kill fleas, lice, bedbugs and cockroaches and even if rolled up will still provide some protection. As well as in malaria they are also effective in other diseases: lymphatic filariasis, leishmaniasis, Japanese encephalitis, Chagas' disease and relapsing fever. A modification of this method is to treat curtains that are used to cover doors, windows or any opening. These methods are used in community malaria control programmes.

Nylon nets are better than cotton ones because they absorb less solution and are stronger, but this has to be offset by their greater cost. Nets are treated by soaking them in a solution of the insecticide when new or after they have been washed. The insecticide and dose required are given in Table 3.8.

The area of the net is measured and the amount of insecticide required calculated. This will depend on the absorbency of the net, which can be measured by weighing the net dry and then again after it has been soaked in water, the difference being the amount required for the calculated dose of insecticide. Some treated-net programmes use standard-sized nets all made of the same material, to avoid having to measure each one, but where this is not done a rough approximation can be made by weighing each net. Protective gloves should be worn and the excess fluid squeezed out before laying the net out to dry. Once nets have been treated they should not be washed again until just before retreatment as this decreases the effectiveness of the insecticide.

Some people suffer from nasal congestion when sleeping under a net that has recently been treated with deltamethrin or lambda-cyhalothrin and it is probably better to put it to one side for the first 2 days if either of these insecticides has been used. Otherwise they are perfectly safe and no long-term effects have been recorded.

One of the problems of treating mosquito nets is that they need to be retreated at annual or 6-monthly intervals, so advance has been made in the production of long-lasting insecticide nets (LLINs) where the insecticide is impregnated into the fibre of the net before it is woven. Because their action is maintained for at least 3 years these are now half the cost of ITNs and are the method of choice in malaria-control programmes. The annual cost is US$2.10 or, averaged out, US$1.05 per person per year.

There are three types of nets:

1. Permethrin-incorporated net (e.g. Olyset®) made of high-density polyethylene monofilament yarn blended with permethrin. A small proportion of the active ingredient is present on the surface so that when this is washed off it is replaced by a similar amount of insecticide giving it a protective efficacy of at least 5 years.
2. Deltamethrin-coated net (e.g. PermaNet 2.0®) made of multifilament polyester and the deltamethrin mixed with a resin that coats the netting, only releasing the insecticide progressively.
3. Alpha-cypermethrin-coated net made of multifilament polyester and a special coating that binds the insecticide within the fibres of the net.

Table 3.8. Dose of insecticide for treating mosquito nets.

Insecticide[a]	Dose mg/m^2
Alpha-cypermethrin	20–40
Cyfluthrin	50
Deltamethrin	15–25
Etofenprox	200
Lambda-cyhalothrin	10–15
Permethrin	200–500

[a]All the insecticides listed are synthetic pyrethroids.

Continued

Box 3.1. Continued.

While these manufactured nets are cost-effective there are a large number of conventional nets in existence that could be made to work in a similar way by treating them with special kits that incorporate a binder. This is mixed with the usual volume of water before the insecticide is added, so polymerizing the insecticide around the fibres.

There is some debate about the best way to provide mosquito nets to the population for malaria control. If given free of charge then not only will the cost be considerable, but people will take less care of them and perhaps not use them at all. If this method is adopted then pregnant women and those with young children should receive priority. Subsidized schemes, even in poor communities, have been shown to work well as it encourages people to be more responsible for their nets and to become more involved in their retreatment (Fig. 4.4). Local industry can be encouraged by supplying mosquito netting and paying local tailors to make the nets, generally in two or three standard sizes. It is preferable to not charge for the insecticide though and to organize retreatment on a regular basis, asking people to wash their nets beforehand.

The advent of LLINs, with their low recurrent cost and absence of retreatment, has changed the distribution requirements of mosquito nets, and recent research in Kenya has shown that giving them free of charge is the best strategy, with a 44% reduction in childhood deaths.

Larvicides

Substances that block the breathing apparatus of mosquito larvae, destroy the surface tension (so they sink to the bottom), or poison them, are known as larvicides. Kerosene spread on water covers the siphon of the larva so that it dies from asphyxiation. High-spreading oils have been developed which inactivate the force of surface tension that larvae use to float on the surface. Insecticides sprayed on collections of water will kill larvae as well as many other organisms (including fish), are expensive, and generally objected to by the public, so are rarely used as larvicides. Such preparations as temephos (Abate), with its very low toxicity, being a notable exception. Insect growth regulators such as diflubenzuron, methoprene or pyriproxyfen are non-insecticidal methods of larval control.

Larvicides are not efficient methods of mosquito control, their main use being in urban and peri-urban areas, especially against culicine vectors. Drains and gutters can be sprayed and temephos added to water containers and septic tanks. Surface sprays must be renewed at regular intervals.

To control *Culex quinquefasciatus*, the main vector of urban filariasis, which breeds in latrines or soakaways, expanded polystyrene beads can be placed in the pit. The beads float on the surface of the water so larvae are dislodged and prevented from breathing, while the function of the latrine or soakaway is not disrupted. The polystyrene is manufactured as fine granules and when placed in boiling water expands into beads.

Biological control

The term biological control is used to describe natural methods of reducing vectors. Various natural agents that have been tried include predators such as larvivorous fish, microbial organisms, e.g. *Bacillus thuringiensis* and *B. sphaericus*, or substances that interfere with growth (insect growth regulators). These are either juvenile hormone analogues (e.g. methoprene or pyriproxyfen) or chitin synthesis inhibitors (e.g. diflubenzuron, triflumeron or novauron) and are particularly useful for fly control (Box 7.1). Male insects can be sterilized by radiation or with chemosterilants and then released into the environment. If these sterile males compete successfully with the unsterilized males, then the females will not be fertilized. Unfortunately, this technique requires the preparation and release of a sufficient number of males to outnumber those in the natural habitat, which is generally impractical. An alternative technique is to breed mosquitoes that are refractory to the target disease. This can either be through genetic manipulation or by the introduction of a closely related natural species. Species replacement, as the method is called, offers some promise because similar, but competitive species can be obtained from different parts of the world.

The problem with any biological method is that nature continues in a balance. If a predator destroys all its food supply then it will die, so an equilibrium is reached whereby the number of predators and those they prey on remain in sufficient numbers for both to exist. Biological control is therefore more an aid rather than a definitive method.

Environmental modification

In some situations, it is possible to modify the environment to make it unsuitable for the vector. This can include simple methods such as burying tin cans or cutting holes in old tyres to drain water, to clearing vast tracks of forest for tsetse fly control. Any method of environmental modification on a large scale must carefully consider other systems that may be damaged. Clearing large areas of forest can affect the water retention of the soil and deforesting river banks can lead to severe erosion. Then again, filling in or draining a swamp can provide extra land. Eucalyptus trees, which absorb large amounts of water from the soil, can be planted and in time their wood can be used.

Specific methods of environmental modification, such as for trypanosomiasis, will be found under the section on the particular disease, while the emphasis here will be on mosquito control. One of the most successful methods for reducing surface water and preventing breeding places is the construction of subsurface drains. This should be within the ability of most health personnel. The system of drains should follow the contours and be at least 1.5 m below the surface. The gradient needs to be between 1 in 400 and 1 in 30. Various materials can be used for constructing the drains, such as stones, bamboo or poles laid lengthwise in the bottom of the drain. Another method of environmental mosquito control is to use a siphon, which flushes out mosquito larvae, or a simple dam, as shown in Fig. 3.10.

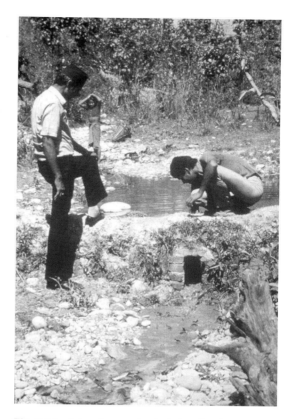

Fig. 3.10. A locally constructed dam for the control of *Anopheles fluviatilis* in Nepal. Every 3 days the bung is removed and the head of water rushing down the stream is sufficient to dislodge mosquito larvae.

3.4.2 Insecticides

Insecticides for vector control include the following:

- *Poisons*, e.g. Paris Green, which was used extensively as a larvicide. *Anopheles gambiae* was eradicated from Upper Egypt by this preparation. In view of the resistance to insecticides that has developed it could be reconsidered.
- *Fumigants*, e.g. hydrogen cyanide, methyl bromide and ethyl formate, can be used on grain or clothing to destroy infestations.
- *Knock-down* agents, e.g. pyrethrum, bioresmethrin and cyfluthrin.
- *Residual* agents, which are subdivided into organochlorines, organophosphates, carbamates and pyrethroids.

Organochlorines

The organochlorines were some of the first insecticides, but after the public outcry over the widespread use of DDT they were no longer used. However, DDT has been shown to be entirely safe for humans and so is being used again for medical purposes.

Organophosphates

The main organophosphates used for residual house spraying are malathion, fenitrothion and pirimiphos-methyl. They are volatile substances with an effective action of 2–6 months, and act by inhibiting cholinesterase at the nerve junctions, so can produce temporary paralysis (and respiratory failure) in man as well as in insects. They do not have a long residual action, or persist in the environment. Chlorpyrifos (Dursban) and temephos (Abate) are low-toxic compounds widely used as larvicides.

Carbamates

Carbamates act in a similar manner to the organosphosphates except that they compete with acetylcholinesterase rather than combining with it, making the action more easily reversed, so conferring an advantage to humans. The main carbamates are bendiocarb and propoxur.

Pyrethroids

Pyrethrum is a naturally occurring insecticide obtained from a species of chrysanthemum. It has been synthetically modified to produce a range of more active forms with good residual ability. These are stable substances, with low mammalian toxicity, and are widely used both for agricultural and medical control. All the synthetic pyrethroids mentioned in Table 3.8 can also be used as residual insecticides at the dosage recommended by the manufacturer.

3.4.3 Resistance

When an insecticide is being chosen for a control programme, the vector must be tested against various strengths of the insecticide to determine the discriminatory dose (this is when 99.9% mortality of the sample occurs). These tests need to be repeated from time to time during the course of the programme to determine whether the vector remains sensitive. If there are technical reasons why this cannot be done, then resistance will probably only be noticed by an increase in number of insects, or cases of the disease concerned. This result might, however, indicate deficiencies in the spraying programme and these should first be ruled out. Correct application of insecticide can be measured as mentioned above, while a simple field test for suspected resistance can be performed by placing a few of the insects in a glass jar held against the sprayed surface for a minute. If they are not all killed, then resistance should be suspected and entomological assistance obtained.

Resistance may be partial or complete. If partial, then increasing the concentration of insecticide may be sufficient to control the vector. Unfortunately, complete resistance is soon likely to develop. Resistance is a genetic character and resistant strains are selected out under pressure of insecticide use. Initially, resistance to single insecticides occurred, but subsequently cross resistance has developed, making several insecticides ineffective. Some species now have multiple resistance. Biological control or trying a completely different strategy may be effective in such cases.

3.4.4 Ectoparasite control

Ectoparasites, such as fleas, lice, bedbugs, mites and ticks, live on the outside of the body. They are responsible for transmitting a number of diseases and are covered in Chapter 16. There are various control methods:

- personal hygiene;
- reduction of interpersonal contact from overcrowding and clothes sharing;
- regular washing of clothes and bedding and the use of deep freezing;
- repellents;
- improved house construction; and
- insecticides.

Ectoparasites favour dirty dark places, whether they are searching for a suitable habitat on a person or a vantage place in the house from which to mount an attack. Fleas and lice are not removed by washing, but the continued use of warm water and soap considerably deters them. If this is combined with clothes washing, then fleas can rapidly be controlled. Where possible, clothes and bedding should be boiled or at least subjected to very hot water as fleas are not affected by cold water. A very effective alternative is to place clothes and bedding in plastic bags and leave in a deep-freeze overnight. Some communities practice head shaving to control lice, while short hair makes them easier to control.

Fleas and lice prefer overcrowded conditions such as occur during wars, famines or in refugee camps. Efforts should be instituted to reduce overcrowding, but where this is impossible then washing and laundry facilities should at least be provided. The wearing of other people's clothes or sharing combs are common methods of transferring ectoparasites in tropical areas.

Repellents have been used successfully in areas where infection is likely. Impregnated socks and trousers are effective when passing through microhabitats of scrub typhus or murine plague. Ticks, bedbugs and reduviids are repulsed by repellents.

Bedbugs, ticks and reduviid bugs live in cracks in the walls of poorly constructed houses, coming out at night to attack sleeping persons. Improving house construction or applying a layer of unbroken plaster to a wall discourages these arthropods permanently. Bed nets can protect the individual from being bitten.

Insecticides are especially useful in epidemic conditions. Dusting clothing, using a puffer to supply the insecticide up trouser legs and skirts and down collars and sleeves can quickly reduce the number of ectoparasites in concentrations of people. Insecticide solutions can be applied to the hair to kill head lice or to clothing if repellents are not available. Rat burrows and runs should be dusted with insecticides to kill plague-carrying fleas before rat catching. Benzyl benzoate or benzene hexachloride are effective against scabies mites. Unfortunately, many ectoparasites have developed resistance to insecticides so non-insecticide solutions containing silicone have been found useful with lice as they prevent the parasite from excreting water.

3.5 Treatment and Mass Drug Administration

Treatment of the sick is not only a humanitarian action but reduces the length of illness and therefore the period of communicability, so aiding control. However, where treatment is incomplete then it can actually prolong the period of communicability, encourage the development of carriers or, worst of all, resistant organisms. Case finding and treatment is the main method of control for leprosy (Section 12.6) and tuberculosis (Section 13.1), but careful follow-up is essential to ensure that treatment is taken for the whole period. Rapid diagnosis and treatment is particularly important in acute respiratory infections (ARIs, Section 13.2) and meningitis (Sections 13.6 and 13.7). The development of effective single-dose therapy for the treatment of the sexually transmitted infections (Chapter 14) has been one of the great challenges of chemotherapy, but the 'power of the needle' has also been the means of transmission of several communicable diseases. In many societies, having an injection (irrespective of what is given) is seen as the panacea of all ills but, unfortunately, improperly sterilized needles (including those for intravenous infusions) have been responsible for much of the transmission of HIV infection and hepatitis B.

Mass drug administration (MDA) is used as a method of control of filariasis (Sections 15.7 and 15.8). However an MDA needs to cover the entire population in the infected area and the full dose of treatment seen to be swallowed. This becomes an administrative exercise requiring a large number of assistants to ensure that the drug has been properly taken. One of the most successful campaigns, in the Pacific Island of Samoa, used women's groups, who are a very well-organized segment of society, with the result that the coverage was over 90%. Generally such organizations are not available, resulting in a lower coverage rate.

Mass treatment is also used in the control of trachoma (Section 7.8). Treatments and MDA regimes will be found under the relevant disease in Chapters 7–18.

3.6 Other Control Methods

The zoonoses often require specific control methods to reduce or eliminate the animal reservoir. Dogs are the major animal source of human disease (Table 17.1), so only those animals which are useful in the society should be kept, strays and unwanted dogs being destroyed. Laws to reduce dog fouling are reasonably effective in developed countries and could perhaps be applicable to urban areas of some developing countries.

Rats are a serious transmitter of disease, especially of plague (Section 16.1), leptospirosis (Section 17.8) and Lassa fever (Section 17.9). Methods of controlling rats are to be found in Box 16.1. Other methods of disease control and prevention will be found in the sections on specific diseases.

Summary

- Control methods can be against the agent, the means of transmission, by treating or protecting the host, or through modification of the environment.
- Vaccination stimulates the person to produce antibodies and is used against an increasing number of infections.
- Environmental control methods are personal hygiene, protection and preparation of food, protection of water supplies and proper methods of sanitation.
- Vector control is by personal protection, through the use of insecticides sprayed on surfaces, used as space sprays or larvicides or impregnated into netting, and by biological control or environmental modification.
- Mass drug administration can be used where none of the other methods are applicable and there is a safe and effective medicine.

Further Reading

Cairncross, S. and Feachem, R. (1993) *Environmental Health Engineering in the Tropics*. 2nd edn. John Wiley, Chichester, UK.

Feachem, R.G., McGarry, M.A. and Mara, D. (1978) *Water, Wastes and Health in Hot Climates*. John Wiley, Chichester, UK (out of print).

Feachem, R.G., Bradley, D.J., Garelick, H. and Mara, D.D. (1983) *Sanitation and Disease: Health Aspects of Excreta and Wastewater Management*. World Bank Studies in Water Supply and Sanitation 3. John Wiley, Chichester, UK (out of print).

World Health Organization (2006) *Pesticides and Their Application*, 6th edn. Document No. WHO/CDS/NTD/WHOPES/GCDPP/2006.1. WHO, Geneva.

World Health Organization (2007) *Long-lasting Insecticidal Nets for Malaria Prevention*, 3rd edn. WHO, Geneva.

Web resources

www.hpa.org.uk (UK vaccination recommendations from the Health Protection Agency; accessed 23 February 2012)

www.who.int/immunization/documents/positionpapers/ (Vaccine position papers from WHO; accessed 23 February 2012)

Control Strategy and Organization

The first two chapters covered the elements and theory of communicable diseases and the previous chapter how to interrupt transmission with the various methods of control available. This chapter puts all of this information into action when faced by an outbreak, or the instigation of control methods to an established endemic disease.

4.1 Investigation of an Outbreak

In any communicable disease outbreak the following sequence of events will need to be gone through:

- outbreak detection;
- investigation;
- confirmation;
- notification;
- analysis;
- treatment of cases;
- interruption of transmission;
- prevention of recurrence;
- analysis and writing of a report; and
- surveillance.

These are not mutually exclusive stages, and although they are in order of action, several can be carried out at the same time.

Excess cases, unusual deaths, exceeding the epidemic threshold or an unexpected clustering of cases will be indicators that an outbreak of a new or known epidemic disease is taking place. The cause will need to be identified and an estimate made of the magnitude and distribution of cases. Field investigations are organized and active surveillance set up to find any new cases. The disease can be confirmed by using an agreed case definition, specific laboratory test, or seroepidemiological technique. The disease must be notified as soon as possible, both nationally and possibly internationally (see Chapter 5). Judgement needs to be used in spending time on making an accurate diagnosis, or starting treatment with the information that is available. There will be great pressure to treat cases, which is a necessary humanitarian action, but until transmission is interrupted, more cases will occur. Once the disease is under control, methods must be implemented to prevent a recurrence. Finally the outbreak is analysed and written up. A surveillance system is on the lookout for the first indications of the communicable disease starting again. These stages will be considered in more detail.

4.1.1 Identification

The start of an epidemic can be dramatic, with a large number of cases being reported or many people dying. However, the cause may be anticipated as the agents of most communicable diseases are now known. The person reporting the outbreak will probably have made a provisional diagnosis, or it might be expected, having been reported in a neighbouring region. It will need to be confirmed by laboratory methods or by careful clinical judgement (e.g. measles). A case definition is a useful tool for ensuring that everybody understands what they are looking for.

Normally the confirmation of diagnosis is a relatively easy matter, but several laboratory specimens may be required and restraint exercised in rushing to a diagnosis (e.g. in typhoid). Alternatively, it may be a unique and rare disease for which the aetiology and transmission have not been worked out. If this is the case, expert assistance is sought, while general principles of control are carried out.

Enquiry and search are made to determine the extent of the outbreak, and whether there are many more cases, especially in areas where there are no medical facilities. Cases may be hidden or exaggerated, to avoid or attract medical attention. Is this the first case, or have there been several cases over a period of time? Have the cases come from another administrative area or country and is there a risk that they might infect other areas? Was notification received and should notification be given?

4.1.2   The epidemiological investigation

Collecting information on the cause and method of transmission utilizes the three pillars of epidemiology, *persons*, *place* and *time*. Information should be collected from as many angles and from as wide a field as possible. The more pointers there are to a method of transmission, the stronger will be the case.

It will generally not be possible to complete a detailed epidemiological investigation before starting some control methods, e.g. if the disease is diarrhoeal then emergency boiling of drinking water can be started. However, the full investigation must be made and completed, as quite often different factors come to light. A full investigation will help prevent a recurrence.

The method used in an epidemiological search is:

- Look for a common event that is shared by all the cases.
- Study exceptions to see if there are rational explanations.
- Base these findings on the population at risk.
- Elucidate changes that have occurred in the environment, which may have favoured the outbreak.
- Make a hypothesis of cause, route of transmission and method of control.

Ideally, information should be collected on every case, but this might be scant or absent on the first few cases. However, it is important to investigate these first cases thoroughly so that the start of the epidemic can be accurately fixed and an epidemic curve drawn (see Chapter 2). If the epidemic is a very large then it might be preferable to take a sample of cases and study these in detail, but some record of the total number of cases will always be required.

Information on *persons* should be available and sex and age classification can readily give an indication as to the cause of the epidemic. If it is just children that are involved then it is a common disease to which adults have obtained immunity, such as measles. If there are more cases in one sex than another this might indicate a division of duties, such as women (who are the main collectors of water) succumbing to a waterborne disease, such as cholera.

The address of each case should be plotted on a map and a note made of the most affected areas and whether there is any clustering. Look for associations, such as rivers, breeding places of vectors, forests which might harbour reservoir animals, or any other feature that the nature of the disease indicates is important. If maps are not available then constructing a simple sketch map might be necessary, especially if the epidemic is very well defined. Typhoid cases often occur in communities so the houses of individual victims will need to be identified on a sketch map of the village or town. Any clustering or association of cases might lead to the carrier from which the epidemic started. Exceptional cases can often provide definitive evidence of an association, such as the visit by a person resident in a different area that subsequently becomes infected. One of the crucial factors in John Snow's investigation of cholera in 19th century London was the woman from Highgate who sent her servant to the Broad Street pump to collect water because she liked the taste. Unfortunately, this practice led to her contracting cholera, but gave Snow the final piece of evidence to prove his case.

All calculations, such as the morbidity and mortality rates, must be calculated on the population at risk. Normally this is the population of the entire area, district, region or country, but in a very localized epidemic the population of the village, town or group of villages, might give a better estimate. Population figures are available from census data and malaria control programmes, and are often collected by the village authorities. Otherwise a sample needs to be taken of the number of occupants in a random number of houses, then all the houses counted in the area and multiplied by the average house occupancy in the sampled houses.

There is normally a reason why an epidemic has happened at a particular period in time. Diarrhoeal diseases often start at the beginning of the rainy season in tropical countries and influenza is more common in the winter months in the northern hemisphere. Religious gatherings or other large collections of people provide ideal conditions for transmission of disease. If there are strong indicators, then these can be used in future surveillance and the planning of preventive action.

A working hypothesis is established as soon as possible so that emergency control action can be commenced, but a detailed investigation must be completed. Search back within the maximum and minimum incubation period from the first case or cases, using other indicators gained from person and place data. Laboratory confirmation of cases might give a different pattern from clinical assessment, especially where several medical staff are involved. If available, samples might need to be taken from a suspect cause, such as a food item, or from the environment, such as a river used for drinking water, which will all take time to be analysed. However, a negative result will not necessarily alter the hypothesis, the specimen may have been collected too late or from the wrong place. It is the strength of association of all the different pieces of evidence that should be used to decide the cause.

4.1.3 Treatment of cases

The priority is to organize the treatment of cases rather than become involved in the clinical management, concentrating on investigating the outbreak and instigating control. This should be by:

- setting up emergency treatment centres or arranging transport of cases to hospital;
- mobilization of staff, medicines and equipment according to need;
- formulation of a standard treatment schedule; and
- making rules on period of quarantine, management of contacts, prevention of carriers and disposal of the dead.

As an epidemic is a large number of cases of a single disease, once the diagnosis has been made then the treatment of all the cases will be the same. There will be the complicated case that requires special attention, but the priority of the investigating doctor is to interrupt transmission and bring the epidemic to an end. A standard treatment schedule should be devised and all staff at every level made available to help with treating cases. Rather than trying to bring all the cases to a hospital it may be better to set up emergency treatment centres near to where the outbreak is taking place. Schools, community centres, religious buildings and warehouses can all be used. Not only does this avoid the problem of transporting cases, but frees the hospital from disruption and contamination.

4.1.4 Interruption of transmission

Once a hypothesis of causation is made from the epidemiological investigation, a method of control is commenced. This can be in three different phases:

- emergency;
- specific; and
- long-term prevention.

If the communicable disease is in epidemic form and threatening a large number of people, then emergency methods must be started as soon as possible. These are often non-specific and commenced before the detailed investigation has been finished. As an illustration of these three different strategies, an epidemic of dengue can be used. The emergency method would be a knock-down spray such as fogging, which kills all adult mosquitoes indiscriminately. This will control the immediate problem, but once the number of adult mosquitoes builds up again, the epidemic might recommence. The specific method will be a programme selectively against the *Aedes* mosquito vector by destroying all temporary breeding places and using larvicides in water containers. Long-term prevention will be by permanently altering breeding places, placing mosquito netting over water tanks, repairing broken guttering and all the techniques that are available for removing the mosquito permanently.

4.1.5 Analysis and report

A communicable disease outbreak should be analysed in detail and written down as a report. This will be based on the investigations made, the control methods used and the outcome. The numbers of cases and deaths are items of information that authorities are particularly interested in. The functions of a report are to:

- inform planning and organizing authorities what has happened;
- notify other workers who are or might soon be participating in a similar outbreak;
- make a record to be referred to in future outbreaks;
- evaluate actions taken and improvements that should be made;
- provide information for the general public;
- elicit funds for more permanent preventive measures;
- provide an illustration for teaching purposes; and
- if of an original nature, for the advancement of science.

4.1.6 Outbreak organization and community participation

Outbreaks occur suddenly and often with little warning, so there is no time to wait for help to arrive; the doctor, nurse or other health worker must take control. Generally the temptation is to become so involved in patient management and treatment that no investigation is done. But until the cause of the outbreak is investigated the cases will continue and generally increase in number.

Help in patient care can be obtained from many sources, such as other health workers, public health inspectors, hospital porters, even cleaning staff, but probably the main resource will be relatives. In most societies relatives will come with the patient and remain with them until they are cured. Care needs to be taken that they don't become patients themselves if the disease is highly infectious, so instructions on preventive methods will need to be given and enforced.

In many communities there is a local organization that should be involved at an early stage. This may be official – a village chief or headman; religious – the village priest; or just a respected member of the community, such as a schoolteacher. In some countries the local organization will have a person responsible for the health of the community or a village health committee. They will be of value in identifying cases, but even more useful in seeing that control measures, such as boiling drinking water, are enforced. They will also have a role in preventing the epidemic from starting up again in the future, such as ensuring that all children are vaccinated.

4.2 Surveillance

Surveillance is the continuous watching for any changes in known diseases and the monitoring of the environment for any new diseases to appear. The key to surveillance is reporting, developed in such a way that a continuous record is kept, not the desperate call of an established epidemic. Surveillance methods can be: routine or passive, active, sentinel, emergency, serological and virological, or in other forms.

4.2.1 Routine or passive

All health facilities collect data in their record keeping; at its simplest this is the name, age and sex of the individual and the symptoms or diagnosis of their illness. Considerable use can be made of well-kept records and it is worth doing an analysis of the type of information collected to determine the best system within the resources available. Hospital records will be more detailed than those of small clinics, but not representative of the population.

Additional categories can be added to the basic data collected, but care must be taken not to overload the health staff so that an unreasonable amount of their time is taken up with filling in forms. Every additional entry must be tested by a small pilot study to ensure it is collecting the information required and is within the means of the staff to collect it. If the task is too onerous there will be a tendency to either not bother to collect the information or, worse, to falsify the data. Even the routine data already collected should be looked at in detail. For example, staff may record many of their patients attending with headaches, which will not be a valuable criterion. Recording fever rather than headache (and taking a blood slide) is far more useful.

Accuracy of data collection can be improved by training, with regular refresher courses so that all staff are taught the same method at the same time. Regular feedback of an analysis of the data will encourage staff to be vigilant in their returns. Comparing one area with another will show up weaknesses, which can then be strengthened. Formulating case definitions encourages a more consistent diagnosis.

Where facilities are available laboratory confirmation is always desirable. Every fever case in a tropical area should routinely have a blood slide taken and sputum smears should always be made from persons with a chronic cough. In special circumstances, having a screening programme can enhance routine investigations. Examples are: antibiotic resistance patterns of sexually transmitted infections, an *Aedes aegypti* index in dengue susceptible areas, vaccine coverage in under-fives clinics and rainfall records to measure seasonality.

All data collected must be analysed or there is no point in collecting it in the first place. The well-established criteria of persons, place and time will be the basic model, but special techniques may also be required. Data from one level is sent to the next higher level where it is analysed and a copy of the analysis sent both to the level above and to those collecting the data in the first place. Special reporting may be required for notifiable diseases. Evaluations need to be made at regular intervals to modify and improve the system.

4.2.2 Active

Active surveillance is the deliberate search for target data. This has been used particularly in malaria control programmes, where contacts of malaria cases are visited and blood slides taken, as illustrated in Fig 4.1. Another example is a leprosy field worker who visits all the villages in his/her area and examines the population for any signs of early disease. Suspect cases are then sent to clinic or hospital for further tests.

4.2.3 Sentinel

Special health problems involving detailed or laboratory investigation are often best collected by using sentinel health services. These are selected by representative health centres that are given extra staff or facilities to enable them to identify the disease. Influenza information is often collected in this way as it is notoriously difficult to separate out influenza from the common cold and other causes of respiratory infection. Several sentinel health centres will then give a reasonable estimate of the problem in the entire area.

4.2.4 Emergency

Emergency surveillance is set up during an outbreak to monitor special risk areas, such as contacts, bacteria counts, etc. Suspect cases or contacts should be kept under observation. Monitoring of

treatment can detect the appearance of resistant organisms or an imbalance in the treatment regime. Utilization of staff and equipment can also be built into an emergency surveillance system.

4.2.5 Serological and virological

Where laboratory facilities permit, a record of certain diseases can be obtained from serological or virological studies. An example is the use of anonymous testing of blood samples collected at antenatal clinics for human immunodeficiency virus (HIV) and hepatitis B (HBV) infections. Care must be taken that the data is representative of the population and is measured continuously.

As the incidence of a parasitic disease declines it becomes increasingly difficult to detect the parasite and serological surveillance can be of more value. This method has been used in malaria programmes where the disease is nearing eradication.

4.2.6 Other forms of surveillance

Where all information reaches a single central authority then it is reasonable to assume that it is representative of the entire area from which it is collected.

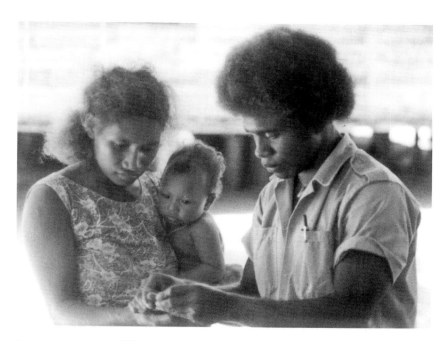

Fig. 4.1. An active case detection (ACD) technician taking a blood slide from a woman suffering from fever in a malaria eradication programme (Santa Isabel, Solomon Islands).

An example would be a public health laboratory, where more complex and standardized results are available.

Other allied disciplines may collect data that are relevant to health, such as veterinary and entomology services. Sleeping sickness is a more widespread and devastating disease in cattle than in humans so outbreaks in cattle are indicators to take precautions in associated human communities. Anthrax and bovine spongiform encephalopathy (BSE) are other examples.

Epidemics may first be reported by persons in authority, such as village leaders, schoolteachers, priests, etc. Indeed, they can often be relied upon to give continued and reasonably accurate information for the community they serve. It is often one of the functions of a village leader to collect data on births and deaths, which can be valuable in estimating the population.

More will be found on surveillance in Section 5.3 and under each disease in Chapters 7–17.

4.3   Control and Eradication

A communicable disease can be *controlled* or *eradicated*. By controlling a disease, it is kept at such a minimum level that it is no longer a health problem. Eradication, in contrast, sets out to eliminate the disease completely. The difference between control and eradication can be summarized as follows:

	Control	Eradication
Objective	Minimal incidence	Complete elimination
Duration	Indefinite	Time limited
Coverage	Areas of high incidence	Entire area
Method	Effective	Faultless
Reservoir	Animal or environment	Human only
Organization	Good	Perfect
Costs	Moderate for a long time	High for limited period
Complications	Acceptable	Extremely serious
Imported cases	Not important	Very important
Surveillance	Reasonable	Very good

The attraction of putting the entire health effort, funded by international support, into the eradication of a disease requires organization of the very highest order. There have been five global eradication efforts,

two successful, two almost successful and one not successful. The eradication of smallpox from the world has been one of public health's greatest triumphs against disease. This was only possible because the vaccine was extremely effective, there was no other reservoir but humans and the organization was very good. Recently, and with an entirely different kind of disease, guinea worm has been eradicated from all infected areas except for a small part of Africa by a programme of protected well construction. Poliomyelitis has been eliminated from all the World Health Organization (WHO) regions except Africa and Asia. The global yaws campaign eradicated yaws from large areas of the world, but it is still endemic in some places and on the increase in others. The tremendous progress of the malaria eradication campaign, followed by an equally impressive resurgence of the disease, has been a devastating setback to the doctrine of eradication. (There have been other localized eradication programmes such as that of *Anopheles gambiae* from South America.)

With eradication it is an all-or-none process; if it is not completed, then the disease can return to its former levels and all is wasted. In these circumstances, it is preferable to choose the alternative target of control, which will be the method used in the majority of infections.

A new terminology has been introduced by WHO: elimination. This uses a special programme and enhanced resources similar to an eradication programme, but accepts that eradication will not necessarily be achieved. Lymphatic filariasis, Chagas' disease, trachoma and neonatal tetanus have been designated as elimination programmes.

4.4   Campaigns and Integrated Health Care

(I am grateful to John Walley and Kirstie Graham for most of this section.)

Communicable diseases can be controlled by campaigns (called special programmes by WHO) or integrated into the general health services. A vertical programme (campaign or special programme) is generally organized and managed separately, with its own staff and funds. These programmes can be appropriate in outbreak, emergency and relief settings. Special campaigns have the attraction of putting all the effort into one particular disease, often with considerable initial success, but over the long term breaking down owing to an inability to sustain them. The advantages and disadvantages of the two approaches are as follows:

	Campaigns	General health services
Effectiveness	Initially very good	Only moderate
Continuation	Poor	Moderate
Duration	Short	Long
Staff	Special required	General health workers
Salary	Inflated	Average
Staff problems	No career structure	Addition to routine duties
Cost	High	Low
Integration	Low	High

If a campaign is then integrated into the general health services, difficulties over emphasis, staff absorption and resentment by the multi-purpose worker occur. Campaign workers are often specially recruited for the task, probably from non-medical backgrounds, and are paid an inflated salary to off-set the time-limited nature of the operation. The general health services are not used to dealing with the special disease and feel they are being given extra work, while still being paid the same.

4.4.1 Integration of health care

A fully integrated programme provides an effective and efficient alternative, if carefully planned. This type of health service provision has the potential to reach the whole population in a sustainable manner. Furthermore, general health services can participate in mass education, treatment or vaccination campaigns. Disease control programmes should work through, support and build the health system.

Where health care is provided by different organizations, it is still possible for such providers to work together when their services overlap. Integrated planning of these services will help prevent duplication of health care provision and allow resources to be directed to areas of need. This planning should cover both the area of work and the content of the service to be provided to ensure common policies and health education messages.

Integration is also needed for effective functioning of and referral between different levels of providers in a district health system. It is key that all health care providers use agreed case-management guidelines and referral criteria, and have a reliable system by which patient information is transferred. Figure 4.2 illustrates how a patient with chronic

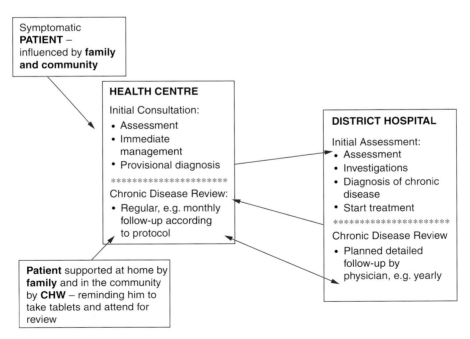

Fig. 4.2. The integrated care of patients with chronic disease within a district health service. CHW, community health worker. (Reproduced by permission of the World Health Organization, Geneva.)

disease could be managed across the different levels of facilities.

4.4.2 Integration of chronic care into primary care

With the increasing burden of chronic diseases, there have been efforts to integrate chronic care into routine health services, especially in countries affected by HIV and tuberculosis (TB). Integrated management of acute and chronic care requires that the immediate problem and an individual's ongoing illnesses are both taken into account. For example, if an adult presents with a chest infection, it is important for the health worker to check the case record for other associated problems. If the patient has recurrent diarrhoea, the health worker should consider the socio-economic situation and subsequently recommend an HIV test.

4.4.3 Integration across time

This refers to the continuity of care an individual patient will receive over a period of time. Ideally, the patient should be seen at the same health centre, preferably by the same health workers, for as long as a health-related intervention, or group of interventions are needed. For an infant, this would encompass all contacts with the health services from time of birth, to immunization, growth monitoring and treatment of childhood illnesses.

4.4.4 Integration of curative, preventive and promotive services as comprehensive care

Traditionally, curative services have been regarded as separate from preventive and promotive health care. Curative and preventive care may be the responsibilities of different health workers, or may be provided on different days. Integration of these services results in a more holistic package of care. Integrated curative and preventive maternal, neonatal and child health (MNCH) services are practised in health centres and hospital outpatient departments in many countries. All the essential interventions are available on the same visit. If a mother brings a sick child for care, she is counselled on the treatment to give her child and the signs of deterioration, and given a review appointment. However, preventive interventions are also provided, such as monitoring the child's weight and updating immunizations where needed. The mother is also offered antenatal care, family planning and nutritional education, if appropriate.

Within this wider integration of MNCH services, there are other integrated packages of care, such as WHO's 'Integrated management of childhood illnesses' (IMCI). The IMCI approach incorporates both preventive and curative services for children through improving the skills of health workers, strengthening health systems and addressing family and community practices. A similar WHO package exists for adolescent and adult illness, the 'Integrated management of adolescent and adult illness' (IMAI). The following case study exemplifies all aspects of integrated health care as discussed above.

Nthombi is a 28-year-old woman. She visits the health centre with a persistent cough and fever, which she has been suffering from for 5 weeks. She brings her 9-month-old child with her. The health worker at the clinic uses the specific page on cough within the IMAI case management guidelines and realizes that Nthombi may have TB. She tells Nthombi to go to the hospital for sputum tests the following day. However, before the family leaves, the health worker takes the chance to check the immunization and growth of the child. He is growing well, but has missed his measles vaccine. The health worker immediately gives this to him.

The next day, Nthombi goes to the hospital and is diagnosed with sputum-positive TB. She receives health education about TB and its association with HIV. She is counselled and accepts to have an HIV test, which is positive. She is given further counselling on using a condom and seeking advice early in the event of illness, and started on treatment. In order to treat her TB, Nthombi is enrolled in community-based TB treatment supervised by her community health worker. Every month, Nthombi visits the original health centre for a check-up and after 2 months is reviewed by the hospital doctor. After 6 months, the doctor says she is cured of TB but must continue on her HIV antiretroviral treatment. Nthombi is subsequently reviewed routinely by the health worker at the clinic every 3 months.

Nthombi is asked to bring her husband to the clinic where he is also found to be HIV positive, so is started on treatment. Over the coming months, Nthombi tells the rest of her family about her diagnosis and asks for their support. By this point, she is well and agrees to become a peer counsellor explaining to others the benefit of having an

HIV test, the use of condoms and the need to change behaviour.

4.5 Control Organization

During the malaria eradication campaigns a high level of organizational methodology was developed which is a useful model for any communicable disease control programme. The four stages are as follows:

- preparatory;
- attack;
- consolidation; and
- maintenance.

4.5.1 Preparatory

The preparatory stage is perhaps the most important, and time spent on collecting baseline data, trying to forecast problems and assessing the feasibility of the proposal, is always time well spent.

Surveys are made of the disease to measure its prevalence in as much of the area as possible. A good sample survey might be sufficient to measure the endemicity, but this will not reveal foci of infection, which normally cause the most problems. In addition, a surveillance system needs to be established, if there is not one already, to continually collect data on cases as the programme proceeds.

The population will need to be measured and it might be justified to spend money on carrying out a census if one has not been done recently. Maps are essential and if suitable ones are not available then they need to be drawn. They must contain up-to-date village locations, preferably with the population marked on them. Fig. 4.3 is an example of a map prepared in this way.

Every level of society must be committed, from the senior administrative head, through divisional chiefs and influential people, to the established health worker. This will require regular meetings with the establishment of key contacts. Without the complete and continued cooperation of the people, any special effort is doomed to failure.

Planning of the persons, money and materials (logistics) to be used in the programme is often the easiest part to initiate, but one of the most difficult to maintain. Utilizing existing staff that retain all their usual functions and continue in an established pattern of service is preferable to recruiting special staff, but this should not be at the expense of existing services. If special staff need to be recruited then conditions of service must be carefully worked out so that no conflict arises with existing staff.

Adequate funding is required, as no disease control programme has remained within estimates; they nearly always cost more than expected. Additions arise that were not foreseen, inflation increases faster than allowed for, and the programme takes longer than planned. If adequate finances cannot be secured and the programme has to be abandoned, then the net result is worse than doing nothing in the first place. More serious is the damage done to the existing health services by diverting funds from them.

Included in the preparatory stage is a *pilot programme* to try out the techniques and organization in a limited area. The pilot programme is a scaled-down version of the full programme, not a special effort to show what can be done. The area chosen should be fully representative of the larger area to be covered. If there are marked variations, then several different pilot studies may be required.

The pilot programme can be for a set period of time, or continued into the full programme after it has been assessed. If there are major difficulties, then the programme should proceed no further, and the whole strategy reworked. If there are minor problems then these are indicators of major problems in the future.

4.5.2 Attack

In the attack phase, the method that was found to be effective in the pilot programme is extended to the whole area. Alternatively, the area can be covered in sequence, but if this is done then measures may need to be instituted to prevent reinfection. Timetables and procedures are required to ensure that separate teams cover the area in a regular manner. Realistic targets are set and organization developed to make sure they are kept. The delay of one part of a programme will cause delay of everything else.

During the attack phase, the number of cases found by the passive surveillance services will rapidly diminish so progress is assessed by making serial surveys. Incidence is more useful than prevalence data so surveys are conducted at regular intervals in sample areas. However, this can pose a strain on relations with the population that is being sampled and areas of higher prevalence may be

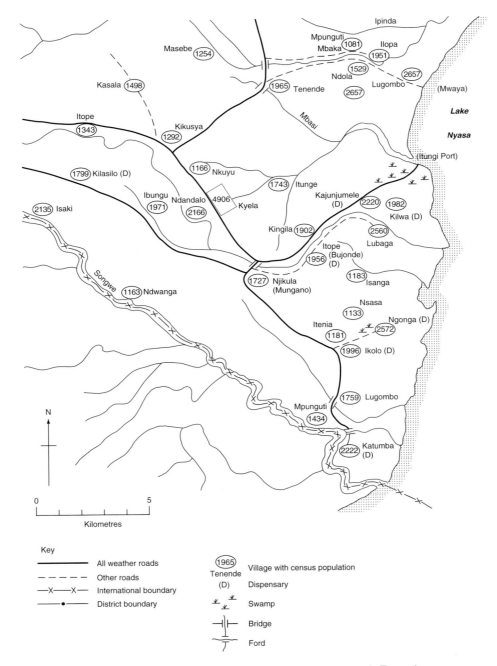

Fig. 4.3. Part of a village location map prepared for a disease control programme in Tanzania.

missed, so new sample areas may need to be used after a time.

To ensure that all the remaining cases are found an *active surveillance* system can be established. This involves special workers, each with an assigned area, which is visited on a regular basis. The active surveillance is not a substitute for passive surveillance, but the two should work closely together.

4.5.3 Consolidation

In the consolidation phase, the full apparatus of disease reduction is disbanded and reliance placed on small specialist teams that can rapidly respond to the active surveillance system. If a focus of malaria is found then focal spraying and radical treatment of cases is implemented. If a yaws or a polio case is suspected, then mass treatment or vaccination is given in the surrounding area. The essence of the consolidation phase is speed and efficiency. If rapid remedial action cannot be carried out, then the disease is liable to return.

4.5.4 Maintenance or a continuing level of control

If the target of the programme is to eradicate the disease then the maintenance phase will be an efficient monitoring system to ensure that any introduced cases are rapidly detected and treated. If it was to reduce the disease to an acceptable level, then this might need to be continued indefinitely. A limited control programme may be sufficient to reduce the burden of disease to allow a raising in the standard of living, which in the long term will have the most sustained effect of controlling the disease.

4.6 Social Factors in Control Programmes

4.6.1 The stigma of disease and traditional practice

Ever since ancient times, leprosy has been a feared disease, with the person doing all they could to hide any signs of their affliction. They generally risked being turned away from society and, even more tragically, from their own family. Trust had to be built up, not only with the affected person but also with society. Generations of committed health workers have overcome the stigma that surrounded this disease and fortunately it is now in decline.

Hopefully, lessons learnt from the long history of leprosy can be applied to the much more recent story of HIV infection. Except for the unfortunate cases obtained by blood transfusion, contracting HIV implies having had sexual contact with someone, probably not one's spouse or established partner, and then possibly passing it on to them. The infected mother who delivers an infected child carries considerable guilt even if she is not blamed by her family. As with leprosy, the person may be ostracized from family and society, with often the severest sanctions being applied to the unfortunate victim.

When HIV infection was first diagnosed it was in the homosexual community, a group of people often hidden from the rest of society by moral or religious constraints (with possible legal implications). First the awareness of such fringe groups, and then their sexual practices, were revealed to a shocked society, often with considerable resentment. Barriers have had to be overcome to allow for control and preventive strategies to be implemented. Similar, but to a lesser extent, was the revelation of the widespread network of commercial sex workers in the transmission of HIV in the heterosexual community. There were the more established prostitutes, who were an accepted, if unwelcome part of society, but others such as bar girls, divorced mothers and trafficked young and often underage women were also shown to be involved. It has been necessary to identify all these links and gain the confidence of those involved in developing the best strategies for control. (See further in Section 14.10.) At the same time, society has had to be educated that to turn a blind eye or, even worse, to ostracize these groups forces them to be more secretive and therefore more difficult for health authorities to provide preventive measures.

Certain diseases, with TB being a good example, have been hidden from medical help for other reasons. In many societies there is a practice of traditional medicine and this will often be tried in the first instance. With the prolonged course of TB such treatments might show some apparent success in the early stages of the disease with the result that considerable delay takes place before the person presents for conventional treatment. The delay means the disease has progressed, often with complications, making treatment difficult and making it impossible to restore the person to complete health. This only adds ammunition to the traditional healer in his practice.

Health promotion will be required alongside a search and treatment programme to make people aware of the serious nature of the illness and the need for early referral. However, not all alternative health practice is a problem; certain categories of traditional healers, especially traditional midwives, can be trained and incorporated into the existing health service as primary health care workers.

In many parts of the world, the regulation of medicines is poor with the result that potent medicines can be bought on the open market or prescribed by unqualified practitioners (quacks). Their only concern is making money, so the use of the wrong medicine or an incomplete course of treatment can lead to the development of resistant organisms, leaving the person in a worse condition than they were in before. The state control of medicines is the first priority, while the proper qualification and register of medical practitioners will instil security in the population not to use unqualified people.

Health promotion is of considerable importance, especially when a campaign or special programme is being planned. The groundwork may have been well laid before the main programme starts and initial response is good, but unfortunately as the programme proceeds complications begin to arise. In malaria control using residual insecticides, people are required to clear their houses and restrain domestic animals while the spraying is taking place. Initially people may see the advantage with the reduction in fever and illness, but as the programme continues the benefit is less apparent and people refuse to cooperate. While further discussion with the community may overcome some of the problems, in time the whole strategy may have to be changed.

4.6.2 Self-help and social marketing

To be able to do something for oneself is generally the best approach in all aspects of life, including health. To avoid illness by eating a healthy diet and taking regular exercise is something that can be done easily. Taking your children to be vaccinated, or an expectant mother attending antenatal clinic, require the active participation of the person, although the facilities are organized by the health services. Continuing with the malaria theme above, the promotion and use of insecticide treated mosquito nets (ITNs) changes the responsibility for the control of malaria from the health services to the individual. It is up to the person and the family to sleep under a mosquito net, but once this has become accepted and a regular practice, it is likely to be much longer lasting than an imposed programme.

Considerable success has been achieved in developing self-help programmes in the manufacture, treatment and distribution of ITNs. By using a rotating fund, nets can be purchased and sold to families at subsidized prices, with the aid donor providing the initial fund and the insecticide for the treatment of the nets. Women's groups are particularly good at running such schemes (Fig. 4.4). Where there is a local tailoring industry then netting can be bought in bulk and nets made in suitable sizes, depending on the traditional sleeping arrangements. However, it may be preferable to make them in two or three standard sizes to make the treatment of the nets easier. (See Box 3.1 for further information.)

The retail industry has developed a number of techniques, such as advertising and market research, to more effectively distribute its produce, so the same methods, called social marketing, can be used by health agencies. This has been widely used in the distribution of condoms for the

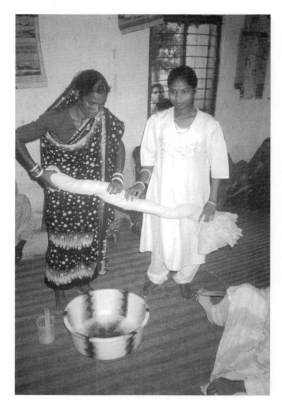

Fig. 4.4. Treatment of a mosquito net in a subsidized scheme in Orissa, India; aid worker on the right. Women's groups managed a revolving fund for the manufacture, sale and treatment of the nets.

control of HIV. All methods of advertising have been used, including television, and condoms distributed in markets, football grounds and any other gatherings of people. Small retailers, especially pharmacies, see this as a method of encouraging business, so are pleased to make condoms freely available in their shops. The Democratic Republic of the Congo (DRC) has successfully distributed condoms in this way under the brand name 'Prudence'.

Summary

- In the investigation of an epidemic the cause needs to identified, investigated, notified and the extent determined, while cases will need to be treated and transmission interrupted. The epidemic must be reported and a surveillance system developed to prevent the epidemic from starting again.
- Disease control should be integrated with the general health services but in special circumstances an eradication or elimination programme can be set up.
- Social factors such as the stigma of disease, alternative treatment by traditional healers and resistance to health interventions have to be sensitively approached with health promotion.
- Self-help schemes are good methods of involving the community in their own health care.
- Social marketing, using posters and advertising is an effective method of promoting disease control.

Further Reading

Abramson, J.H. and Abramson, Z.H. (2008) *Research Methods in Community Public Health: Surveys, Epidemiological Research, Programme Evaluation, Clinical Trials*, 6th edn. John Wiley and Sons, Chichester, UK.

Connolly, M.A. (2006) *Communicable Disease Control in Emergencies: A Field Manual*. World Health Organization, Geneva.

Green, A. (2007) *Introduction to Health Planning for Developing Health Systems*. Oxford University Press, Oxford, UK.

Heymann, D.L. (2008) *Control of Communicable Diseases Manual*, 19th edn. American Public Health Association, Washington, DC.

Lerberghe, W. and Lafort, Y. (1990) *The Role of the Hospital in the District: Delivering or Supporting Primary Health Care*. WHO/SIIS/CC/90.2. World Health Organization, Geneva.

Lucas, A.O. and Gilles, H.M. (2002) *Short Textbook of Public Health Medicine for the Tropics*. Hodder Arnold, London.

Noah, N.D. (2006) *Controlling Communicable Disease*. Open University Press, Milton Keynes, UK.

Vaughan, J.P. and Morrow, R.H. (2011) *Manual of Epidemiology for District Health Management*, 2nd edn. World Health Organization, Geneva.

Walley, J., Wright, J. and Hubley, J. (2009) *Public Health*, 2nd edn. Oxford University Press, Oxford, UK.

World Health Organization (2008) *A Systematic Review of The Effectiveness of Shortening Integrated Management of Childhood Illness Guidelines Training*: Final Report. WHO, Geneva.

World Health Organization/UNICEF (2008) *Integrated Management of Childhood Illness for High HIV Settings, Chart Booklet*. WHO, Geneva.

Wright, J. (1998) *Health Needs Assessment in Practice*. BMJ Books, London.

5 Notification and Health Regulations

Because of the serious nature of the disease or the ease by which it is transmitted some diseases are notified. Individual countries will have their own priorities as to which diseases these should be, whereas international agreement specifies certain diseases which must be notified to other countries, generally via the World Health Organization (WHO).

5.1 International Health Regulations

International health regulations require that certain diseases be notified. The purpose is to warn other countries and intended travellers to the country of the health risks involved. Assistance can also be requested, once the disease has been notified.

Diseases subject to the International Health Regulations (1969, 1974 and 1992) are:

- plague;
- cholera; and
- yellow fever.

Diseases under Surveillance by WHO are:

- louse-borne typhus;
- relapsing fever;
- paralytic poliomyelitis;
- malaria;
- influenza;
- human immune deficiency virus (HIV);
- meningoccocal meningitis;
- severe acute respiratory syndrome (SARS); and
- tuberculosis (TB).

The initial case is notified by e-mail to WHO's Global Alert and Response (GAR) Operations (www.who.int/csr/alertresponse), and subsequent summaries of the number of cases suspected and confirmed are sent at weekly intervals.

In 2005, the long-awaited International Health Regulations (IHR 2005) was approved, specifying that instead of the current list of three diseases, there is a requirement for all countries 'to notify WHO of all diseases or events of international public health importance'. This means that such events as the first cases of a new infection, such as SARS, must be reported.

The new regulations particularly emphasize the setting up of a national IHR focal point and the development of surveillance systems to detect, assess, notify and report any health event of international concern. Notification should be made within 24 h, including information on the number of human cases and any vectors or contaminated cargoes that may be involved. The regulations also give countries the facility to report this information from a public health risk identified outside their territorial limits. WHO will then request verification from the state mentioned and has the right to notify other countries of the risk when it becomes a public health emergency of international concern.

Regions such as the South Pacific Commission or Association of Caribbean States may initiate their own regulations, for example for the following:

- dengue;
- diphtheria;
- typhoid;
- whooping cough; and
- scrub typhus.

5.2 National Health Regulations

Countries have their own system of national notification of some diseases, including the following:

- tuberculosis;
- leprosy; and
- sleeping sickness.

5.2.1 Notifiable diseases for England and Wales

These are listed in the following table:

Very rare infections	Rare infections	Common infections
Anthrax	Leptospirosis	Food poisoning
Leprosy	Yellow fever	Viral hepatitis
Typhus	Cholera	Whooping cough
Relapsing fever	Diphtheria	Tuberculosis
Plague	Poliomyelitis	Malaria
Smallpox	Typhoid fever	Meningitis
Viral haemorrhagic fever	Paratyphoid fever	Meningococcal septicaemia
	Rabies	Ophthalmia neonatorum
	Tetanus	Measles
	Encephalitis	Dysentery (bacillary and amoebic)
		Rubella
		Scarlet fever

5.3 Special Surveillance

The principles of surveillance were mentioned in Section 4.2. A country at particular risk may be advised to set up a surveillance system of diseases of international or national importance. Some suggestions are:

- in plague areas, any case of fever, glandular enlargement and death;
- any person dying from diarrhoea (suspected cholera);
- any person dying of jaundice in the yellow fever zone (see Fig. 5.1);
- an *Aedes aegypti* index (the dengue and yellow fever vector);
- any case of acute flaccid paralysis following a feverish illness; and
- severe pneumonia with difficulty in breathing.

Any case coming within one of these categories is reported immediately to the responsible medical officer or doctor in charge who is required to investigate the report.

WHO has set up an international surveillance team to investigate any case of suspected smallpox reported. The suspected case must be isolated and WHO informed immediately. There is also concern about emergent diseases and the strengthening of surveillance systems, so the linking of one country's reporting with that of another will assist in detecting new diseases before they become a serious problem.

5.4 Vaccination Requirements

The only vaccination now required for international travel is for yellow fever in persons who come from or pass through a yellow fever zone. Although the risk of adverse reaction is small it is not necessary to insist on vaccinating all persons visiting an area where there is low potential for infection, so the yellow fever zone maps have recently been modified, as shown in Fig. 5.1. However, if within this area, the traveller is at increased risk of infection (such as from prolonged travel or extensive exposure from mosquitoes) then vaccination should be considered. Countries may insist that a person coming from or passing through a yellow fever area is vaccinated and, if not, the person can be retained for a period of 6 days.

A yellow fever vaccination must be recorded on the prescribed form with the signature of the doctor, the batch number and official stamp of the vaccination centre. The vaccination is valid for 10 years, 10 days after the date of vaccination or revaccination. Cholera vaccination is no longer required by international regulations.

Summary

- Any disease or event of international importance must be notified to WHO.
- Countries will have their own or regional list of notifiable diseases and may need to set up special surveillance systems to detect cases.
- Yellow fever is the only vaccination required for international travel.

Further Reading

World Health Organization (2005) *International Health Regulations*. WHO, Geneva.
World Health Organization (2011) *International Travel and Health, Vaccination Requirements and Health Advice*. WHO, Geneva.

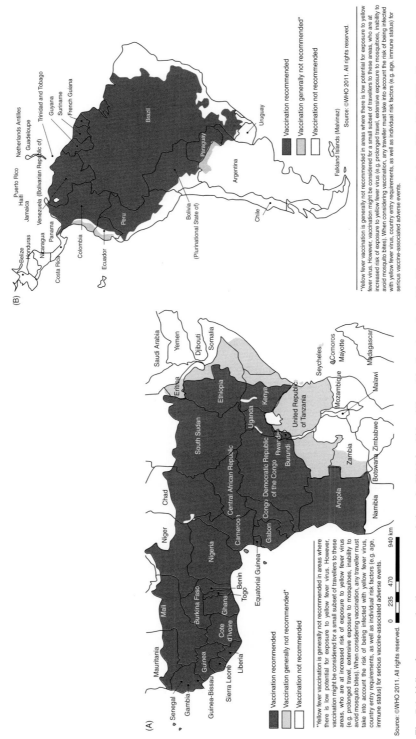

Fig. 5.1. Yellow fever vaccination recommendations in 2010 for Africa (A) and for the Americas (B). (Reproduced by permission of the World Health Organization, Geneva.)

6 Classification of Communicable Diseases

No biological system is perfect and communicable diseases in particular are not readily classified. However, any grouping makes it easier to understand and remember so the objective of this short chapter is to look at the different ways this can be done.

A disease is a morbid condition of the body, such as measles or plague, but as the causes of diseases were discovered then they became identified by the causative organism, and named accordingly – such as trypanosomiasis or pneumococcal meningitis. But straight away confusion arose because there are two forms of African trypanosomiasis and one of American, while the pneumococcus is an important cause of pneumonia as well as meningitis. This confusion continues, so rather than settle on one system or another I have tried to list communicable diseases by either the disease state or organism by which they are best identified. For example, gastroenteritis, one of the commonest causes of diarrhoea in developing countries, is a preferable definition rather than separately listing all the various organisms that can cause it. Conversely, the streptococcus is responsible for such an array of diseases that just to put down streptococcal infection would fail to reveal important diseases such as rheumatic fever or otitis media. William Farr (one of the founding fathers of epidemiology) first wrestled with this problem and out of his work has grown the International Classification of Diseases, now in its 10th edition. This is an unduly complex system and the World Health Organization (WHO) has now called for contributions to a new 11th edition. These can be from any interested party and, hopefully, a simplified system will develop, or at least a simplified version of the more complex classification. Rather than attempt to do this I have listed the majority of communicable diseases alphabetically in Chapter 20, at the end of the book, so quick reference can be made to them.

There are 353 diseases listed in Chapter 20, and of these the commonest causative organism is a virus, being responsible for 186 diseases, with arboviruses causing 118 infections. Bacteria and chlamydia account for 75 and the larger parasites 58, of which the nematodes cause 22 diseases, protozoa 18 and helminths 18.

The commonest method of transmission is the vector, with the mosquito incriminated in a staggering 77 infections, ticks in 31 and other or unknown biting insects in 40. Among methods of control, with disease vectors so frequent, vector control is the commonest, being useful in 147 of the disease conditions, but simple methods such as using repellents and sleeping under mosquito nets are all that is required much of the time.

Next comes personal hygiene, valuable in 102 infections, so just washing your hands and making an effort to be clean can be remarkably effective. Allied to personal cleanliness is food hygiene – ensuring that food is prepared properly, adequately cooked and stored under safe conditions; this accounts for 55 of the preventive methods. Animals, either in their farming or through our association with them as pets, account for 42 diseases that can be prevented by controlling those diseases in the animals concerned. The provision of good water supplies will reduce 40 conditions and sanitation 24, while the control of rats reduces 16.

Chemotherapy as a method of control is valuable in 40 diseases and vaccination in 34, but several of these are major disease problems such as tuberculosis (TB), measles and the sexually transmitted infections. The social and educational methods appropriate to controlling sexually transmitted diseases will be valuable in 21 conditions, while the screening of blood donors will avoid 15 diseases and the proper sterilization of needles, instruments and giving sets nine.

No attempt is made in the next few chapters to cover all 353 of the diseases listed in Chapter 20; the selection made covers only those that are of worldwide importance, are major problems in certain parts of the world, or illustrate a particular disease pattern. However, a brief synopsis is given for each of the 353 diseases in Chapter 20, and readers might find it useful to refer to this list before turning to the fuller descriptions in the following pages.

As already mentioned, diseases are normally classified by the causative organism, which has much to recommend it for the clinician and the pathologist, but different organisms can cause similar diseases, such as *Escherichia coli*, a bacterium, and *Giardia intestinalis*, a protozoan, both producing diarrhoea in the individual. Control methods are similar, so for the epidemiologist it is preferable to include them in the same group. In contrast, the closely linked group of viruses that cause hepatitis are very different in their means of transmission: hepatitis A is transmitted by the faecal–oral route and hepatitis B by blood and other body fluids, so it is preferable to separate these two diseases into different categories. In previous editions of this book, the endemic trepanematoses (yaws, pinta and endemic syphilis) were placed in the chapter on diseases transmitted by body fluids (Chapter 14) as this is the method of transmission, but mostly this is related to poor hygiene and improving hygiene, as covered in Chapter 7, is the main method of control, so they will now be found in this chapter.

Transmission is the key to the epidemiology of communicable diseases. Once the means of transmission is known it leads to the best method of control, so it is preferable to use this as the method of classification. Based on these criteria, all communicable diseases can be classified into 11 groups, as follows:

Disease group	Chapter
Diseases of poor hygiene	7
Faecal–oral diseases	8
Food-borne diseases	9
Diseases of soil contact	10
Diseases of water contact	11
Skin infections	12
Respiratory diseases and other airborne transmitted infections	13
Diseases transmitted via body fluids	14
Insect-borne diseases	15
Ectoparasite zoonoses	16
Domestic and synanthropic zoonoses	17

In earlier editions, Chapter 7 was called 'Water-washed Diseases', which is a very adequate description of the main method of control, while their cause and method of transmission results from poor hygiene, so this is the description that is now used. Diseases of poor hygiene could be called person-to-person diseases, but many diseases, including skin infections and respiratory diseases, are also transmitted from one person to another, so a preferable description is to include the main method of spread, which is due to poor hygiene. Faecal–oral is a very large group and could quite easily incorporate many of the diseases in the chapter on food-borne diseases, but it is easier to consider control methods if a separate chapter is made. There are important diseases that are acquired by contact with either soil or water, which means that methods of control are very specific. These divisions have already been mentioned in Chapter 3, originally developed by David Bradley, to whom I owe considerable thanks for the original idea of the classification system.

Skin infections are obvious in their presentation and most of them are transmitted directly by skin contact, but they also use other methods of transmission, so it is more convenient to classify them by their most common method of presentation. The respiratory infections are transmitted by the airborne route, which is also a method of transmission of several other infections that present in different ways. The chapter on diseases transmitted via body fluids is an attempt to bring together common themes in the transmission and control of diseases transmitted via blood, seminal fluid, cervical secretions, saliva and other less common methods of transmission. It includes the sexually transmitted diseases, which would warrant a chapter of their own, but other diseases that share many common features, such as hepatitis B (HBV) are better included with them. Insect-borne diseases not only include a large number of health problems, but also some of the most important diseases in the world, such as malaria. They already make up the largest chapter, which could be even bigger, but the combination of ectoparasite transmission (by fleas, lice, etc.) and zoonosis is a very specific one so a separate chapter has been included for this category. The rest of the zoonoses, where a vector is not included, form the last chapter in the classification.

No classification system is perfect and not every disease fits neatly into the 11 categories that have been used. For many diseases, there is more than one means of transmission and these can also be important in developing control methods. However, the categories are sufficiently broad to encompass minor differences. Bringing them together into such a system demonstrates similarities and associations, making it easier to understand the complexities of the many communicable diseases.

The fewer groups there are the easier it is to remember all of them, sparing the onerous task of learning each disease in detail. However, if each group is too broad much of the essential information is also lost, so defeating its purpose. For example, Vietnam had classified all its communicable diseases into just four groups, but this was found to lack the precision to work out the best control strategy for each group, so this was replaced by an abbreviated (longer) classification, as follows:

---

1. Person to person (skin and eye diseases)
2. Faecal–oral transmission
3. Soil contact
4. Airborne (respiratory infections)
5. Diseases transmitted via body fluids
   (includes sexually transmitted diseases)
6. Vector-borne diseases
7. Zoonoses

This simplification was due to the absence of such diseases as schistosomiasis and guinea worm, which are the only members of the 'Diseases of water contact' in the 11 category classification above, and also of several others, which allowed amalgamations. Any country might similarly like to draw up its own classification system based on the important diseases found there.

Summary

- Communicable diseases are grouped into their main methods of transmission enabling common control methods to be applied.
- The commonest causative organism is the virus, with arboviruses responsible for 118 diseases which, with other organisms transmitted by mosquitoes, make this numerically the commonest cause of infection.
- After vector control, hand washing and personal hygiene are the most important method in the prevention of communicable diseases.

Further Reading

World Health Organization (2010) ICD-10 Version:2010, International Statistical Classification of Diseases and Related Health Problems 10th Revision. WHO, Geneva. Available at: www.who.int/classifications/apps/icd/icd10online/ (accessed 27 February 2012).

Diseases of Poor Hygiene

The simplest disease transmission is by person-to-person contact (see Fig. 1.3). The diseases of poor hygiene arise from direct contact of the skin, conjunctiva or mucous membrane. Alternatively, organisms from the skin or in conjunctival secretions can be transported by an intermediate vehicle. The essential mechanism is contamination from lack of hygiene.

There are three groups of disease in this category: skin diseases, the tropical treponematoses (previously included in Chapter 14) and eye diseases. The skin diseases include infections of scabies, lice, the superficial fungal diseases and tropical ulcers. The tropical treponematoses are yaws, pinta and endemic syphilis, which affect both the skin and bones. The eye diseases of public health significance are trachoma, epidemic haemorrhagic conjunctivitis, epidemic keratoconjunctivitis and ophthalmia neonatorum.

The main method of control of the diseases of poor hygiene is to increase water *quantity*. These are the first category in Table 3.1, called the water-washed diseases. Providing an adequate volume of water for washing encourages personal hygiene.

7.1 Scabies

Organism. Infection of the skin is by a mite, *Sarcoptes scabiei.*

Clinical features. There is a skin rash and intense itching where the mite burrows into the superficial layers of the skin. It favours the wrists and hands, although in heavy infections it may be found in almost any area of the body, but not the head or face. Due to scratching, the affected skin can become thickened and discoloured, leading to a mistaken diagnosis of eczema. Secondary infection is common and this is often how the infection presents. Streptococcal glomerulonephritis can occur as a complication. Intractable scabies in adults, not responding to treatment, can indicate human immunodeficiency virus (HIV) infection. This may present in a crusted form (Norwegian scabies) or else as a hyper-infection.

Diagnosis is made from the clinical presentation, but skin scrapings can be made and the mite viewed microscopically.

Transmission of scabies is due to close personal contact permitting the mite to pass from one person to another. It can be transmitted by shared clothing and is commonly found in conditions of poor hygiene. Where possible, infected individuals should be prevented from infecting others, such as keeping children from school until they are clear. A careful search should be made for unreported or unrecognized cases in the community. Scabies can be spread among adults as a sexually transmitted infection.

Incubation period. 2–6 weeks.

Period of communicability. Infection can be passed on as long as there are viable mites on the individual, up until 1 week after the first course of treatment.

Occurrence and distribution. Scabies is found worldwide, but favours the hot moist tropics and flourishes in conditions of poverty. It mainly occurs in children, but anyone who comes in contact with infected individuals, e.g. mothers and schoolteachers, can catch scabies.

Control and prevention. Scabies is a community problem and treatment of an individual is insufficient unless the whole family, school or village is similarly treated. In communities with poor hygiene the provision of adequate water is the most effective method of controlling the disease. People should be encouraged to wash themselves with soap and water and to wash their clothes and bedding. Improving the water supply to provide an adequate quantity of water is the main method of prevention.

Treatment. Specific treatment is by benzyl benzoate, but this may need to be accompanied by an antibiotic if there is secondary infection. A 10% emulsion of benzyl benzoate is liberally applied to the whole body and left for 24 h before being washed off. Treatment is repeated after 7 days to kill off larvae that have hatched from eggs. The whole family is treated at the same time, while ensuring that only clean clothes and bedding are used. Alternatively, crotamiton 10% or sulfur 6% in petrolatum is applied to the entire body for 2–3 days before being washed off. The insecticide permethrin, used in the control of the mosquitoes that transmit malaria (Section 15.6), or the naturally occurring *Chrysanthemum* from which it is derived, are also effective. Reduction in scabies can be an additional benefit of insecticide-treated mosquito nets (ITNs). Otherwise, permethrin can be administered as a 5% cream or 1% lotion. Ivermectin, used in the treatment of filariasis and onchocerciasis (Sections 15.7 and 15.8), can be given systemically as a mass treatment on its own or can be a side benefit of these control programmes. If none of the special preparations is available, then repeated applications of oil to the skin can be effective. Any oil usually used by people to rub on the skin, such as coconut oil, can be effective. As the mite lives in a small burrow through which it respires, sealing off the opening with a film of oil asphyxiates it. This requires careful and repeated application to the whole body after washing.

Surveillance. Schoolteachers should be encouraged to regularly examine schoolchildren or do spot checks on any child found to be scratching.

7.2 Lice

Body lice are potential vectors of typhus (Section 16.2) and relapsing fever (Section 16.3) but the main worry of people is personal infestation.

Organism. *Pediculus humanus corporis*, the body louse, *P. humanus capitis*, the head louse, and *Pthirus pubis*, the crab louse. Lice glue their eggs to body hairs (nits) in which they are resistant to treatment until the nymphs hatch.

Clinical features and diagnosis. Intense localized itching at the site of bite will indicate lice, which can be found and identified with a hand lens. If *P. h. corporis* is not found on the skin it will be among body hair or in the clothes.

Transmission. Close contact between people, the sharing of clothes, hats and combs. Crab lice are generally transmitted during sexual contact.

Incubation period. Eggs hatch in 10–14 days.

Period of communicability is for as long as there are viable mites on the individual, up until 2 weeks after the first course of treatment. Body and head lice remain alive for up to 1 week and nits for 1 month on clothing not being worn.

Occurrence and distribution. Body lice are found worldwide in conditions of poverty or where people are forcibly driven together, such as in refugee camps. They are more common in colder regions of the world or in mountainous parts of the tropics, where people huddle together to keep warm. Head lice are found both in the tropics and colder regions, especially among schoolchildren. Girls appear to be more susceptible to head lice than boys.

Control and prevention. Washing with warm water and soap at frequent intervals is the main method of prevention. The clothes of an infected person should be boiled or insufflated with insecticide powder. The practice of pressing clothes with a hot iron might have originated as a method of controlling lice. Combs should be washed regularly and only used by one person.

Treatment is with 1% permethrin cream rinse and naturally occurring pyrethrins (from *Chrysanthemum*). The treatment should be repeated after 10–14 days to kill any young lice recently hatched from nits. If whole communities are infected then ivermectin can be given orally. This is also a side benefit of mass drug administrations such as for filariasis and onchocerciasis. Scabies will also be cleared (see Section 7.1). A non-medicated method uses a silicone-based solution which causes the lice to die because they are unable to excrete water. Shaving of heads is a rigorous but effective method of control of head lice, but not of body lice. In epidemic situations, whole communities should be treated irrespective of whether lice have been found or not (Section 16.2). Clothes and bedding can be treated with 1% malathion, 0.5% permethrin, 2% temefos (Abate) or 5% iodofenphos.

Surveillance. Parents or older siblings should carefully search through children's hair, looking for nits, if the child is found to be scratching its head. In situations such as refugee camps people should be encouraged to examine their clothes and those of their children at regular intervals.

7.3 Superficial Fungal Infections (Dermatophytosis)

Organism. Fungi of the genus *Trichophyton*, *Microsporum*, *Epidermophyton* and *Scytalidium*.

Clinical features. Also called tinea, the fungi attack specific sites on the body, the moist skin in the feet or groin, the nails, the scalp or the body. Tinea corporis (often called ringworm) produces well-defined circular lesions that spread out from the centre causing slight depigmentation as they proceed. Tinea capitis causes areas of baldness, hairs becoming brittle so that they break off. Pityriasis (tinea) versicolor (caused by *Malassezia furfur*) produces a blotchy hypopigmentation that can sometimes be misdiagnosed as leprosy. Tinea imbricata, found in South-east Asia, Western Pacific islands and Central America produces serpiginous scaly designs that can cover the whole body. Tinea nigra produces sharply marginated brown-to-black macules, commonly on the hands, that can be confused with melanomas.

Diagnosis is by clinical appearance. Infected hairs fluoresce in ultraviolet light or scrapings can be treated with potassium hydroxide, revealing hyphae on microscopic examination.

Transmission. Close bodily contact, the sharing of clothes, towels, etc. are the common means of transmission. Airborne spread can occur where there have been infected people. Dogs, cats, cattle and other animals also carry the fungus.

Incubation period. 4–14 days.

Period of communicability. Fungal material can persist on articles such as towels and clothing for considerable periods of time.

Occurrence and distribution. Superficial fungal infections are widely distributed throughout the world, being found in developed as well as developing countries. Children are most commonly affected.

Control and prevention. Prevention is by body washing with soap and water and not sharing clothes, towels, combs, etc. Towels should be boiled and antifungal agents, such as cresol, should be used to disinfect floors and common places, like changing rooms.

Treatment. Local applications of antifungals such as tolnaftate, miconazole, ketoconazole, clotrimazole, econazole, naftifine, terbinafine or ciclopirox can be used. Acetylsalicylic acid ointment or benzoic acid compound (Whitfield's ointment) are effective if applied regularly for some 3 weeks. In resistant cases, griseofulvin, itraconazole or oral terbinafine can be given by mouth for a sufficiently long period to clear all the fungal residue. Sodium thiosulfate 25% lotion or selenium sulfide can be used to treat pityriasis versicolor.

Surveillance. Schoolchildren should be examined regularly, especially the head, feet and groins.

7.4 Tropical Ulcers

Tropical ulcers are a common debilitating condition. They cause tissue loss and pain which temporarily invalids the person, making daily work an agonizing undertaking. The condition can last for several months and even when it heals, the victim is left with a scar that may lead to contracture. There are two types of tropical ulcers, one non-specific and one due to a mycobacterium, often called Buruli ulcer. These should both be differentiated from yaws (Section 7.5). Buruli ulcer will be covered in Section 11.3.

Organism. No specific organism is normally detected, but initial infection is often accompanied by cellulitis, probably caused by a streptococcus.

Transmission. Flies are responsible for contaminating small wounds and scratches or, occasionally, biting insects transmit infecting organisms directly. Scratching of the wound by the host can be a potent method of instilling organisms into the skin.

Clinical features. The initial wound becomes red and indurated, with cellulitis spreading to the regional lymph nodes, accompanied by systemic fever. An ulcer that refuses to heal then develops at the initial point of infection, producing increasing tissue loss. The diagnosis is made on clinical criteria.

Incubation period. Uncertain, but probably between 1 and 5 days.

Period of communicability. Unknown, but probably as long as there are moist lesions.

Occurrence and distribution. Tropical ulcers are found in the warm moist areas of the world where the temperature and humidity are fairly constant. All ages and both sexes are susceptible.

Control and prevention. Tropical ulcers can be prevented by taking scrupulous care over minor cuts and abrasions. As soon as any break in the skin surface occurs, it should be cleaned, have an antiseptic applied and be covered with a dressing. Flies should be controlled by the provision of sanitation (Section 3.3.4) and the disposal of garbage (see Box 7.1).

Treatment. During the invasive stage, antibiotics (penicillin is normally effective) should be given both systemically and locally, and the limb rested. Once the ulcer has formed, antibiotics have no effect and a cleaning solution, such as Eusol, should be applied. In coastal areas, soaking the affected limb in seawater is a cost-free method of cleaning out the ulcer. Skin grafting may be necessary.

7.5 Yaws

Organism. *Treponema pallidum* subspecies *pertenue*.

Clinical features. Yaws is a non-venereal treponemal disease affecting both the skin and bone. It commences as a primary papule which starts to heal, but after a period varying from a few weeks to several months it is followed by generalized lesions – multiple rounded papules – scattered all over the body. These lesions exude serum, which is highly infectious. There is also a mild periostitis in focal bony sites but these and the skin lesions normally heal with little residual damage. It is the tertiary stage that appears after an asymptomatic period, and some 5 years after the initial infection,

that results in gross damage to skin and bone, leading to hideous deformities. The opposite ends of the body are affected with destructive lesions of the nasal bones (gangoza) and scarring and deformity of the lower limbs (sabre tibia).

Diagnosis is by finding *T. p. pertenue* in the exudates of lesions. In the motile state, the spirochete can be seen by dark ground or fluorescence microscopy, or stained by Giemsa or silver salts. Serological tests for both endemic syphilis and venereal syphilis (Section 14.1) are positive.

Transmission. Yaws is a disease of poor hygiene, with close bodily contact being the manner in which infection commonly takes place. Flies may be involved in transmission from clothing and dressings that have become contaminated by fluid from sores. The spirochete cannot penetrate unbroken skin but requires a minor skin abrasion or cut by which to enter.

Incubation period is 2–8 weeks.

Period of communicability can be as long as moist lesions persist in the untreated case, which can be several years.

Occurrence and distribution. Yaws is predominantly an infection of children under 15 years of age with a peak in the 6–10 year age group. Mothers invariably become infected from their children if they did not acquire infection in childhood. The large overcrowded family with a poor standard of hygiene is the characteristic environment in which yaws so readily spreads. The need to stay indoors and keep close together for warmth in the rainy season might be the reason why the disease is more common at this time of year.

Yaws is restricted to the moist tropical areas of the world in a band that passes through Africa, South-east Asia and the Pacific Islands (Fig. 7.1). A resurgence of cases occurred in West Africa, South-east Asia and Pacific Islands after the World Health Organization (WHO) mass campaigns against the disease ended, but now some 5000 cases are reported annually, mainly from South-east Asia. The majority of these cases are from Indonesia and Timor-Leste (East Timor).

Control and prevention. Yaws, with its rapid response to a single injection of penicillin, has been the subject of successful mass treatment campaigns

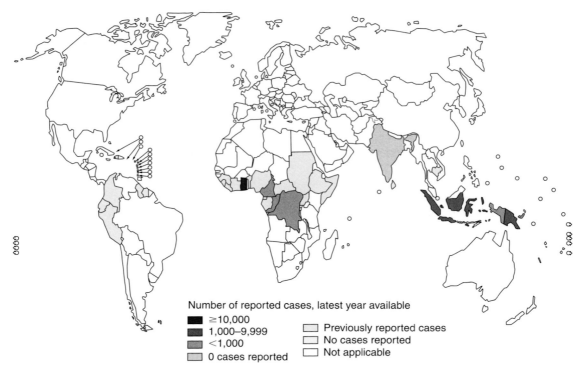

Fig. 7.1. Distribution of the endemic treponematoses worldwide, 2010. (Reproduced by permission of the World Health Organization, Geneva.)

Number of reported cases, latest year available
- ≥10,000
- 1,000–9,999
- <1,000
- 0 cases reported
- Previously reported cases
- No cases reported
- Not applicable

in the endemic parts of the world. Treatment in a mass campaign is to:

- all those with clinical signs of yaws;
- household, school and other close contacts; and
- any person suspected of incubating the disease.

The campaign is preceded by health education, encouraging all people to come forward with any suspicious lesions. Each village is visited in turn, everyone is examined and treatment given to cases, contacts or suspects. A follow-up surveillance service treats missed cases or new infections. This can readily be done by an effective rural health service.

The success of the WHO mass campaigns against yaws resulted in the virtual disappearance of the disease from many areas, followed by a resurgence. Newly trained health personnel are unaware of the disease and penicillin, once widely used (and successful in inadvertently treating of yaws), has been replaced by other antibiotics in the treatment of common infections owing to the development of penicillin resistance.

In the long term, improvements in the level of hygiene and socio-economic status will reduce the conditions in which yaws thrives.

Treatment is a single injection of benzathine penicillin G (1.2 million units for an adult, 0.6 million units for a child). Response is very satisfactory and lesions heal within 2–3 weeks.

Surveillance. Due to the possible appearance of new cases, a continuing awareness of the disease needs to be kept, with the taking of smears from any suspicious lesions. It is likely that searching will discover more cases, so cases and contacts should be treated along the same lines as in the eradication campaigns.

7.6 Pinta

Organism. *Treponema carateum.*

Clinical features. The disease has many similarities to yaws, commencing as a primary, painless papule. Secondary lesions, which develop in 3–12 months, are flat and erythematous but cover large areas of the body. Tertiary lesions result in pigmentary changes with often large patches of leucoderma. Unlike yaws, only the skin is involved in pinta, with lesions commonly on the face and extremities.

Diagnosis is made on clinical grounds with supporting evidence from positive serological tests for syphilis. *T. carateum* can be found in the serous exudates from lesions by dark ground or fluorescence microscopy.

Transmission. Direct contact or carriage by flies has been suggested as the means of transmission. Trauma, especially to the lower limbs, might facilitate entry of organisms.

Incubation period. 1–3 weeks.

Period of communicability is probably several years while secondary lesions are present.

Occurrence and distribution. Pinta is restricted to moist tropical areas of Central and South America occurring in communities with poor hygiene, such as in the Amazon and Orinoco basins (Fig. 7.1). Adults and adolescents are mostly involved. Recent surveys have found the disease to be naturally dying out.

Control, prevention and treatment. Mass treatment with penicillin in the same manner as for yaws (see above).

7.7 Endemic Syphilis

Organism. *Treponema pallidum* subspecies *endemicum*, which is indistinguishable from the *T. pallidum* that causes venereal syphilis.

Clinical features. The primary lesion is commonly found at the angle of the mouth, appearing as a raised mucous plaque. A more florid skin infection follows with moist papules under the arms and between the buttocks, and a maculo-papular rash on the trunk and limbs, resembling venereal syphilis. Destructive tertiary signs in the skin, nasopharynx and bones develop after months or years, but the nervous and cardiovascular systems are rarely involved.

Diagnosis is made on clinical grounds in endemic areas and by the finding of the organism with dark-ground microscopy. Serological tests for syphilis are positive and remain so for many years.

Transmission. Because of the site of the primary lesion on the mouth, transmission by shared drinking vessels and eating utensils is considered the most likely route. Direct contact with lesions is also a likely method of spread. The disease resembles venereal syphilis in many of its features except that it is not spread venereally.

Incubation period. 2 weeks to 3 months.

Period of communicability is for as long as moist lesions are present, generally several months.

Occurrence and distribution. The non-venereal form of syphilis is found in localized foci in Africa's Sahel region, and in Saudi Arabia and the Yemen where it is known locally as Bejel or Njovera (Fig. 7.1). Predominantly an infection of childhood, it thrives in conditions of poverty, overcrowding and where there is limited sanitation.

Control and prevention. This is a disease of low personal hygiene where crowding together and contact with lesions readily occurs. Cross immunity is shared with venereal syphilis, so to eradicate the disease by mass treatment generally means a replacement by the more serious and devastating venereal syphilis. Family planning, better housing, education and improving the general standard of hygiene might be a preferable control strategy in such situations.

Treatment is with penicillin in the same manner as yaws.

7.8 Trachoma

A common infectious disease, trachoma is the major cause of blindness in the world.

Organism. *Chlamydia trachomatis*, a microorganism that has features both of a bacterium and a virus.

Clinical features. Commencing as a keratoconjunctivitis, the first sign is *red eye*. There may be

---

Box 7.1. Fly control

Flies are important vectors of trachoma, bacillary dysentery (shigellosis) and other diarrhoeal diseases. The common housefly *Musca domestica*, the eye fly *M. sorbens*, the lesser house fly *Fannia canicularis* and the latrine fly *F. scalaris* are the main species involved. (Control of biting flies is discussed in Chapter 15.)

Flies are attracted to faecal material of humans and animals on which they feed and lay their eggs, as well as to any food, and it is this passive transfer of organisms on their feet and mouthparts that is responsible for the spread of infection. Any decaying matter, such as piles of rubbish, manure heaps, fish entrails and abattoir washings will attract flies, and every effort should be made to dispose of them. Rubbish should be stored in containers with well-fitting lids and emptied on a regular basis, to be incinerated or buried. Markets should be run on hygienic principles, with the removal of any unsold produce at the end of the day, all rubbish removed, and stalls and floors cleaned with an antiseptic solution. Proper latrine construction is covered in Section 3.3.4.

Young children should sleep under mosquito nets during the daytime as well as at night. Insecticide-treated mosquito nets (ITNs, Box 3.1) will effectively prevent flies from coming in contact with the person and even when folded will deter flies from the immediate neighbourhood. Whole houses can be screened, but this is costly, and flies entering through an open door get trapped inside. Particular care should be taken to protect the kitchen and areas where food is stored, covering food that is not wrapped or stored in a refrigerator.

Disasters can be dangerous times for health as well as physical damage because normal services are disrupted, houses are destroyed and decaying corpses (animal and human) are left to attract flies. Emergency methods may need to be implemented, such as the use of insecticides if uncontrolled fly breeding is taking place.

Where simple methods cannot be implemented to remove the fly problem then insecticides can be used, but this should not be regarded as a substitute as resistance will often develop. The first stage is to study the fly breeding, feeding and resting habits as well as sensitivity to insecticides. If possible, a targeted approach should be used, such as focal spraying or applying larvicides only at breeding sites.

All precautions should be observed, including the wearing of protective clothing and using gloves. Equipment must be properly maintained and care taken not to allow any insecticide to enter the aquatic environment.

Knock-down or space spraying using a portable or vehicle-mounted fogging apparatus is effective in killing adults but needs to be repeated on a daily basis for 1–2 weeks to kill off newly emergent flies. Most of the insecticides are the same as those used for mosquito control (Section 3.4.2) so should be used for the minimal amount of time so as to avoid resistance developing in any concurrent mosquito populations.

A preferable approach is to use insect growth regulators (IGRs) as larvicides. These are chemically unrelated to insecticides and generally cheaper to apply. Suitable IGRs are:

Insect growth regulator	Dosage in grams of active ingredient/m^2
Diflubenzuron	0.5–1.0
Cyromazine	0.5–1.0
Pyriproxifen	0.05–0.1
Triflumuron	0.25–0.5

---

irritation and discharge but this is passed off as a self-limiting infection. A follicular infiltration of the conjunctiva then takes place, particularly in the upper lid. Blood vessels grow into the periphery of the eye, forming pannus. However, it is at the late stages of the disease, when it is non-infectious, that scarring, particularly of the upper eyelid, turns the eyelashes inwards to rub on the eye, a condition called trichiasis. This constant rubbing of the eyeball, aided by the dryness of the conjunctiva, damages the cornea, leading to scarring and finally blindness. Trachoma is often further complicated by secondary infection.

Diagnosis is usually made on clinical grounds, but can be confirmed by finding the characteristic inclusion bodies in scrapings taken from the conjunctiva.

Transmission. Trachoma is a disease of poor sanitary conditions where a combination of close contact and dirty conditions encourages transmission.

Within the family unit, transmission is from child to child or by flies (mainly *Musca sorbens*) that are attracted to the discharges around the eyes. Cycles of reinfection and recrudescence continue to damage the eye and lead to blindness at school age. The usual method of wiping away secretions with hands, towels or clothing, which is then used by the adult on other children or themselves, is a typical pattern of transmission.

Incubation period is from 5 to 12 days.

Period of communicability continues as long as active lesions are still present. Once treatment commences infectivity ceases within 2–3 days, although the clinical disease persists.

Occurrence and distribution. Trachoma is found mainly in the dry regions of the world (Fig. 7.2), especially Africa, South America and the extensive semi-desert regions of Asia. A disease of antiquity, it was first described by the ancient Egyptians.

In endemic areas, 80 to 90% of children are infected by the age of 3 years. In conditions of improved sanitation there is a natural cycle lasting until age 11 years, with little residual damage. Females develop trachoma and blindness as adults more commonly than males, because they are directly concerned with looking after children. The chance of acquiring infection is increased by large families with short birth intervals, as there are more children of a young age living in close proximity.

Since the introduction of the WHO elimination programme there has been a reduction of trachoma cases from an estimated 360 million in 1985 to 41 million in 2009. Half the global burden of active trachoma is concentrated in Ethiopia, Guinea, India, Nigeria and South Sudan. It is hoped that active trachoma can be eliminated by 2020.

Control and prevention. The use of water to wash away secretions, the wearing of clean clothes and keeping the surroundings clean are the most effective methods. Face washing has been shown to reduce the risk of developing trachoma, so regular

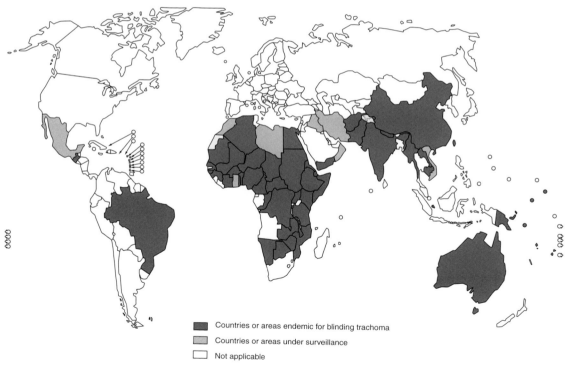

Fig. 7.2. Distribution of trachoma, worldwide, 2010. (Reproduced by permission of the World Health Organization, Geneva.)

Countries or areas endemic for blinding trachoma

Countries or areas under surveillance

Not applicable

Diseases of Poor Hygiene

daily face washing should be encouraged. Long-term preventive measures are to improve sanitation and provide water supplies.

Flies proliferate in rubbish and excrement, reaching their maximum numbers during the dry sunny period of the year. The damp, moist conditions in open pit latrines may be more important in encouraging fly breeding than non-use of latrines. Any flushing mechanism or improved latrine will discourage flies. (See also Box 7.1.)

A strategy for a control programme is as follows:

- Conduct a survey to find the worst affected areas.
- Give mass treatment.
- Conduct health education through schools, stressing regular face washing.
- Provide back-up services.

WHO has launched a programme for the global elimination of trachoma by 2020 and given it the acronym of SAFE. This stands for:

Surgery for trichiasis
Antibiotics
Facial cleanliness
Environmental improvement.

Treatment. Mass treatment is preferable, as the majority of the population in an infected area will have trachoma. This is given easily in schools, but is better done in the home, where the main transmission takes place. A single dose of azithromycin (20 mg/kg) is better than topical tetracycline and one dose a year may be sufficient to eliminate the blinding propensity of trachoma. Mothers can be taught to regularly treat all children in the household.

Preventing blindness once scarring and trichiasis have developed is very easily done by a simple operation that a medical assistant can be trained to do. This involves cutting through the scarred conjunctiva of the upper lid and everting it so that the eyelashes no longer rub on the cornea.

Surveillance. After the initial survey, follow-up surveys should be conducted at regular intervals. This is most easily done in primary schools.

7.9 Epidemic Haemorrhagic Conjunctivitis

First recognized in Ghana in 1969, epidemic acute haemorrhagic conjunctivitis has caused epidemics in a number of parts of the world, which have given their name to the disease, e.g. Nairobi eye.

Organism. Enterovirus 70 is the most important aetiological agent and has been responsible for tens of millions of cases. Coxsackievirus A24 has also been responsible for large outbreaks.

Clinical features. The infection starts suddenly with pain and subconjunctival haemorrhages. There is often much swelling and discomfort in the eye. However, this is a self-limiting condition, terminating within 1–2 weeks. In a few cases, there are systemic effects involving the upper respiratory tract or central nervous system (CNS). CNS effects are identical to those of poliomyelitis and residual paralysis can occur.

Diagnosis is clinical once the first few cases of an epidemic have been identified. Laboratory confirmation can be made by isolating the virus from a conjunctival swab.

Transmission is from one person to another from the discharges of infected eyes. Where there are systemic infections, transmission may be by the respiratory route. As with trachoma, intrafamilial transmission is common and in situations of poor hygiene and overcrowding large epidemics can occur.

Incubation period. 1–3 days.

Period of communicability. 4 days from start of symptoms.

Occurrence and distribution. The disease occurs in epidemic form infecting a large number of people in the immediate vicinity. Epidemics have been mainly in tropical cities of Africa, Asia, South America, the Caribbean and Pacific Islands.

Control and prevention. Careful hand washing, use of separate towels and sterilization of ophthalmological instruments are important in preventing transmission. Methods to improve hygiene and reduce overcrowding will prevent major epidemics.

Treatment. There is no treatment, so mass administration of eye ointment is not applicable.

Surveillance. The first cases of an epidemic should be notified centrally and neighbouring countries warned.

7.9.1 Epidemic keratoconjunctivitis

Organism. Adenovirus 5, 8 and 19.

Clinical features. Epidemic keratoconjunctivitis is similar to epidemic haemorrhagic conjunctivitis, but a keratitis also develops in some 50% of cases, 7 days after onset. This normally resolves in about 2 weeks, but a minority is left with conjunctival scarring. Upper respiratory symptoms and fever often accompany the eye disease.

Transmission. Similar to epidemic haemorrhagic conjunctivitis.

Incubation period. 5–12 days.

Period of communicability. 14 days from onset of disease.

Occurrence and distribution. Epidemics have occurred in Asia, North America and Europe.

Control and prevention are similar to methods used for epidemic haemorrhagic conjunctivitis.

Treatment and surveillance. As with haemorrhagic conjunctivitis.

7.10 Ophthalmia Neonatorum

Infection of the eye of the newborn infant can lead to blindness.

Organism. Neisseria gonorrhoea or *Chlamydia trachomatis.*

Clinical features and transmission. If the mother has gonorrhoea (Section 14.2) or non-gonococcal urethritis caused by *C. trachomatis* (Section 14.3), the infant's eyes can become contaminated with infectious discharges as it passes through the birth canal. This leads to conjunctivitis, and in gonococcal infection is an important cause of blindness, especially in developing countries.

Diagnosis is made by microscopic examination of maternal vaginal discharges.

Incubation period is 2–7 days in gonococcal infection and 7–14 days with *Chlamydia.*

Period of communicability. As long as genital or ocular infection persists.

Occurrence and distribution. Infection is found more commonly in sex trade workers and the sexually promiscuous. It is more common in developing countries where routine testing of expectant mothers is not performed.

Control and prevention. Detection and treatment of the initial infection in the mother (see Sections 14.2 and 14.3) is the best strategy. Any vaginal discharge occurring during pregnancy should be examined, cultured and treated.

Treatment. At delivery, all babies' eyes should be routinely wiped and a 1% aqueous solution of silver nitrate instilled. Wiping both eyes alone at delivery can reduce the incidence of infection if silver nitrate is not available and should always be practised. A 2.5% solution of povidone–iodine, tetracycline 1% or erythromycin 0.5% eye ointment can be used as alternatives to silver nitrate.

Surveillance. All vaginal discharges during the antenatal period should be examined and cultured. Where an infant is born with ophthalmia neonatorum (sticky eye), the parents and any sexual contacts should be fully investigated (Sections 14.2 and 14.3).

7.11 Other Infections

Many of the faecal–oral diseases covered in Chapter 8 and those due to soil contact covered in Chapter 10 are due to poor personal hygiene. Streptococcal and staphylococcal infections of the skin (Section 12.5) are also prevented by good personal hygiene. A full list of diseases prevented by good personal hygiene will be found in Section 3.3.1.

Summary

- Poor hygiene is responsible for a number of diseases which include skin infections, eye infections and tropical treponematoses.

- Conditions of poverty and large families, with the sharing of clothes, bedding and personal items are common factors.
- Flies, by their habits, are ready carriers of disease organisms and specific control measures may need to be undertaken to control them (Box 7.1).
- Adequate quantities of water, with frequent washing, especially of the face where trachoma is common, is the main control method.
- Long-term control is to provide water supplies with an adequate quantity of water. Good sanitation should also be practised.

Further Reading

Antal, G.M., Lukehart, S.A. and Matheus, A. (2002) Review: the endemic treponematoses. *Microbes and Infection* 4, 83–94.

Perine, P.L., Hopkins, D.R., Niemel, P.L.A., St John, R.K., Causse, G. and Antal, G.M. (1984) *Handbook of Endemic Treponematoses: Yaws, Endemic Syphilis and Pinta.* World Health Organization, Geneva (under revision).

World Health Organization/London School of Hygiene and Tropical Medicine/International Trachoma Initiative (2006) *Trachoma Control: A Guide for Programme Managers.* WHO, Geneva.

Chapter 7

Faecal–Oral Diseases

The faecal–oral group of diseases are transmitted by person-to-person contact, through water, food or directly to the mouth. The absence of a proper water supply, the presence of rubbish and dirty surroundings, with an abundance of flies, is the typical situation in which these diseases thrive. Breaking the faecal–oral cycle is the basis of control by personal hygiene, increase in water quantity, improvement in water quality, food hygiene and the provision of sanitation. The disposal of garbage and the control of flies are also important. (See Box 7.1.)

Many of the diseases in this group cause diarrhoea (Table 8.1).

8.1 Gastroenteritis

Gastroenteritis is a common form of diarrhoea that predominantly attacks children. It is endemic in developing countries, but seasonal epidemics occur. Attempts to find a specific organism are often unsuccessful and not essential as management and control are the same. Strains of enterotoxigenic, enteropathogenic and enteroaggregative *Escherichia coli*, as well as enteric viruses, are the main organisms. Rotavirus (Section 8.2) and *Campylobacter* (Section 9.2) are major causes.

Clinical features. Profuse, watery diarrhoea with occasional vomiting, but despite the fluid nature of the stools faecal material is always present. There is never the rice water stool characteristic of cholera. Water and electrolytes are lost which, in the young child, may be sufficient to cause dehydration and ionic imbalance, leading to death. Normally, a self-limiting condition but in unhygienic surroundings, or where babies' bottles are used, repeated infections occur leading to chronic loss of nutrients and subsequent malnutrition. A serious infection in neonates, mortality decreases with age until in adults it is just a passing inconvenience (travellers' diarrhoea).

Diagnosis is made on clinical criteria unless laboratory facilities sufficient to identify viral infections are available. Specific DNA probes are likely to be the most appropriate method of identifying causative organisms in developing countries if they can be made cheap enough.

Transmission. Epidemics occur in families or groups of children sharing similar surroundings. Infection is often seasonal, the beginning of the rains heralding an outbreak. This would suggest transmission by water, and simple control measures such as boiling of water can stop the epidemic. Improperly sterilized babies' bottles or their contents are a common method of infecting the neonate.

Incubation period. 12–72 h (generally 48 h).

Period of communicability. 8–10 days.

Occurrence and distribution. Gastroenteritis is found throughout the world, especially in developing countries and in conditions of poor hygiene. It is particularly common where bottle-feeding has been recently introduced, such as by unscrupulous infant-feed companies. A seasonal distribution suggests contamination of the water supply.

Control and prevention are by the following:

- promotion of breastfeeding;
- use of oral rehydration solution (ORS) in the community;
- improvement in water supply and sanitation;
- promoting personal and domestic hygiene;
- vaccination (rotavirus and other vaccines, e.g. measles); and
- fly control (Box 7.1).

Breastfeeding not only provides a sterile milk formula in the correct proportions (in contrast to

---

Table 8.1. Diarrhoeas.

Presentation	Disease	Organism	Characteristics
Acute watery diarrhoea	Salmonellosis	*Salmonella*	Sudden onset with vomiting in a group of people associated by food
	Food poisoning	*Staphylococci, Bacillus cereus, Clostridium perfringens, Vibrio parahaemolyticus*	
	Gastroenteritis (bacterial)	*Escherichia coli* or non-specific	Common, mainly in children, epidemic
	Gastroenteritis (viral)	Rotavirus and other enteroviruses, especially Noro virus	Occurs in children, often in institutions (hospitals, schools, etc.)
	Cryptosporidiosis	*Cryptosporidium*	Animal reservoir
	Cholera	*Vibrio cholerae*	Severe, dehydration, rice water stools, epidemic
	Yersiniosis	*Yersinia enterocolitica*	From eating meat
	Nosocomial	*Clostridium difficile*	Secondary to antibiotic use
Acute diarrhoea with *blood*	Bacillary dysentery	*Shigella* sp.	Severe, seasonal, all ages
	Enterohaemorrhagic and enteroinvasive	*E. coli* O157:H7	Severe, refugees, all ages
	Escherichia coli	*E. coli* serogroup O	Less severe, all ages
	Campylobacter	*Campylobacter jejuni*	Sporadic, from contaminated food, animal reservoir
Chronic diarrhoea	Giardiasis (Sprue or malabsorption syndromes)	*Giardia intestinalis*	Mainly children and travellers Adults mostly males nutritional deficiencies especially of folic acid
Chronic diarrhoea with *blood*	Amoebiasis	*Entamoeba histolytica*	Cooler climates, mainly adults
	Balantidiasis	*Balantidium coli*	Similar to amoebiasis, associated with pigs
	Schistosomiasis	*Schistosoma mansoni*	Endemic areas, characteristic eggs in stools

Diarrhoea is also a common condition in many other diseases, e.g. measles, malaria and tonsillitis.

the often-contaminated bottle) but also promotes lactobacilli and contains lactoferrins and lysozymes. Promoting breastfeeding and the administration of ORS solution in the community are the main control strategies. Improvement in water supplies and sanitation, with the promotion of personal hygiene, are long-term measures.

Rotavirus vaccination should now become part of the routine childhood vaccination programme (see Section 8.2). The oral cholera vaccine WC/rBS has been shown to be about 60% effective against enterotoxigenic *E. coli* so might have some place in control, although its protective effect in infants is considerably less than in adults. Preventing other childhood infections by vaccination, especially those associated with gastrointestinal disease, such as polio and measles, can reduce the severity of gastroenteritis.

Treatment is by the replacement of fluid and electrolytes using ORS in the moderately dehydrated and intravenous replacement in the severely dehydrated.

A suitable ORS is made by dissolving the following constituents in 1 l of water:

Sodium chloride (salt)	3.5 g (Na$^+$ 90 mmol)
Trisodium citrate dehydrate	2.9 g (citrate 10 mmol)
Potassium chloride	1.5 g (K$^+$ 20 mmol, Cl$^-$ 88 mmol)
Glucose anhydrous (dextrose)	20.0 g (glucose 111 mmol)

These ingredients can be obtained separately or in packets of ready prepared mixtures. In the absence of prepared packets, a simpler formulation can be made as shown in Fig. 8.1; this consists of mixing

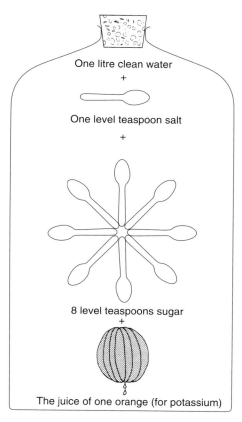

One litre clean water

+

One level teaspoon salt

+

8 level teaspoons sugar

+

The juice of one orange (for potassium)

Fig. 8.1. Preparing a simple oral rehydration solution.

salt and sugar in a litre of clean water. Potassium is not an essential constituent, but if the juice of one orange can be added, this is useful. Tea leaves also contain potassium, so the mixture can be prepared as tea, with salt and sugar added. Teaspoons vary in size and it is dangerous to give too much salt, so a useful check is for the mother to taste the solution before administering it to her child. If it tastes salty then more water is added.

A naturally available rehydration solution is the fluid from a green coconut. A 7-month-old coconut has been found to be the most suitable. Rice water made from a handful of rice boiled in a saucepan of water until it dissolves, plus the appropriate amount of salt for the volume of water, makes a simple rehydration solution. Carrot water can also be used.

If mothers are taught how to make up these solutions then they can treat their own children as soon as they start to get diarrhoea. The mother should use a cup and a spoon and sit with her child giving it small quantities of fluid at frequent intervals. Severe dehydration can usually be prevented by primary care from the mother.

There is no need to use an antibiotic or an antispasmodic, both of which are contraindicated. Lactobacilli, which inhibit *E. coli*, colonize the gut in the breastfed infant. Live yoghurt (curd) contains lactobacilli and can be quite effective, especially in adults, in reducing the severity and duration of diarrhoea.

Surveillance. In countries with a seasonal rainfall pattern gastroenteritis outbreaks often start with the beginning of the rains, so monitoring the weather can provide early warning of an impending outbreak.

8.2   Rotavirus Infection

Organism. The rotavirus has numerous serotypes distinguished by two surface proteins, glycoprotein G and protease-cleaved protein P. Specific serotypes vary widely from one area to another.

Clinical features. The main symptom is profuse watery diarrhoea, projectile vomiting and dehydration, with fever present in some 30% of cases. The disease is indistinguishable from other causes of gastroenteritis on clinical grounds.

Diagnosis. In the majority of cases, diagnosis is not required before treatment is started, but any of the immunological techniques, EM (electron microscopy), ELISA and LA (latex agglutination) can be used to identify the antigen in the faecal sample or from a rectal swab. These are available in commercial kits. In large outbreaks, confirmation of the diagnosis is necessary.

Transmission is by person-to-person contact by the faecal–oral route. Rotaviral disease is not waterborne. Following infection children acquire immunity with some 75% protection against reinfection. Infection occurs throughout the year in developing countries but is commoner in winter months in developed countries.

Rotavirus is also found in pigs, cattle, dogs and other animals but transmission to humans is uncommon.

Incubation period. 1–3 days.

Period of communicability. 2–8 days.

Occurrence and distribution. Rotavirus infection is the most common cause of severe diarrhoea among young children in the world. There are estimated to be 111 million cases and over half a million deaths every year. Asia and Africa have the majority of cases, with China, India, Pakistan, the Democratic Republic of the Congo (DRC), Ethiopia and Nigeria accounting for more than 50% of all rotavirus deaths.

The commonest age of infection is 2–3 years with peak incidence in children aged 6–18 months.

Control and prevention. Rotavirus vaccination (RV) is effective in young children and should be given at the same time as triple vaccine in the routine vaccination programme. The objective is to reduce severe illness and death rather than transmission as the animal reservoir remains as a potential source of reinfection and the development of new strains.

Treatment. ORS, in the same manner as gastroenteritis (see Section 8.1).

Surveillance. Where facilities permit, rotavirus should be identified from other forms of gastroenteritis and the pattern of spread determined. Collections of young children, such as in nursery schools, are places where infection rapidly spreads so preventive action can be taken.

8.3 Cryptosporidiosis

Organism. Cryptosporidium parvum is a coccidian protozoan parasite found in poultry, fish, reptiles and mammals, especially cattle, sheep, dogs and cats, from which the infection can be acquired.

Clinical features. Cryptosporidiosis presents as an acute watery diarrhoea associated with abdominal pain. Fever, anorexia, nausea and vomiting can also occur, especially in children. There may be repeat attacks, but these do not normally continue for more than a month. In the immunodeficient, especially those with human immunodeficiency virus (HIV) infection, the disease enters a chronic and progressive course and may spread to other parts of the body (gall bladder, pancreas and respiratory tract), with serious consequences. Pregnancy may predispose to infection.

Diagnosis is made by finding the oocyst in faecal samples. Alternatively, the intestinal stages can be looked for in intestinal biopsy specimens.

Transmission is from person to person via the faecal–oral route, from animals or from faecal-contaminated water. The disease is commonly transmitted from person to person where there are collections of people, such as in schools. Contact with farm animals, especially newborns, is a common means of transmission. Sexual practice involving oro–anal contact carries a high risk of infection. Explosive outbreaks occur where the water supply is contaminated with faecal material either from humans or animals. The oocyst is shed in the faeces of domestic animals and can survive in nature for a considerable period of time. The infecting dose is very low, with a single oocyst having a probability of 0.5% to cause infection, meaning that 200 oocysts will almost certainly do so; however, severity of symptoms is not dose related.

Incubation period. 1–12 days. Mean of 7 days.

Period of communicability. Up to 6 months in faecal material.

Occurrence and distribution. Cryptosporidiosis has a worldwide distribution, and is found particularly in conditions of poor hygiene. It is endemic in many developing countries, where infection is acquired at an early age. Massive epidemics have occurred in developed countries where the water purification system has failed (such as the 1993 Milwaukee (Wisconsin) epidemic where there were 500,000 cases). In other areas, cryptosporidiosis is a disease of animal handlers, homosexuals and institutions. There is a marked seasonality in the northern hemisphere with peaks of disease in spring and autumn.

Control and prevention are by personal hygiene, the provision of sanitation and safe water supplies. Domestic animals and pets can be important sources of infection so precautions should be taken when handling them.

Treatment is with oral rehydration to replace fluid loss (see Section 8.1).

Surveillance. Animals, particularly cattle, sheep and pigs, can be examined for *Cryptosporidium* infection.

8.4   Cholera

Organism. *Vibrio cholerae*. Classical cholera is caused by *V. cholerae* 01, while most of the recent epidemics have been due to the El Tor biotype. Two variant strains of the El Tor biotype have developed, 0139 Bengal, restricted to Asia, and an El Tor producing toxin of the classical strain (ETEC).

Clinical features. A profound diarrhoea of rapid onset that leads to dehydration and death should be considered as a case of cholera until proved otherwise. The diarrhoea contains no faecal particles but is watery and flecked with mucus (not cells), the so-called rice-water stools. The passage of large quantities of fluid and electrolytes leads to rapid and extreme dehydration, which can be fatal. Vomiting can also be present in the early stages. Blood group O is associated with more severe cholera.

Diagnosis. *V. cholerae* can be identified from the diarrhoeal discharge, vomitus or by rectal swab. Its characteristic mobility (it vibrates, hence being called a vibrio) can be seen by dark ground or phase contrast microscopy and is inhibited by specific antiserum. Confirmation of the diagnosis is made by culture on TCBS (thiosulfate-citrate-bile salts-sucrose) agar. A suitable transport medium is Carey Blair, or alternatively 1% alkaline (pH 8.5) peptone water, which can also be used for water samples. A dipstick rapid diagnostic test is under trial.

Transmission. Classical cholera is a disease of water transmission, whereas transmission of El Tor is by both water and food. Generally, epidemic cholera is transmitted by water, and endemic cholera by food. It may appear in a seasonal pattern, often in association with other causes of diarrhoea (Fig. 8.2). It is the endemic nature of El Tor and its persistence in the environment that has been responsible for its prodigious spread.

For every clinical case of El Tor cholera there can be as many as 100 asymptomatic cases, explaining how epidemics spread from one region to another, but not how infection remains in the environment.

One method may be the persistence of infection in the human population due to continuous person-to-person transmission in a subclinical asymptomatic cycle. When a susceptible person enters the cycle, or there is an environmental or climatic change, a fresh epidemic starts.

A natural cycle has now been established in an aquatic environment, with *V. cholerae* living in copepods, or in other zooplankton, as found in algal blooms. Vibrios are easily destroyed by sunlight, chemical action or competing bacteria; however, where these elements are not present they can survive in fresh water for some time and in saline for at least a week. The level of salinity needs to be between 0.01 and 0.1%, as is found in estuarine or lagoon water. *V. cholerae* in this saline environment can be taken up by shellfish or fish, which then form an alternative method of infection when eaten uncooked. Rising sea levels and increase in water temperature due to climate change makes cholera outbreaks developing from an estuarine environment more likely.

The isolation of *V. cholerae* from river water has been an enigma because epidemiological investigations show this source of infection to be important, but bacteriologists have not isolated organisms in sufficient numbers. One possible explanation is the presence of non-agglutinable vibrios (alternatively known as non-cholera vibrios), which are closely related to *V. cholerae*, except that they do not agglutinate antisera. These are known to be mutations, so that shifts between typical vibrios and non-agglutinable forms may occur. If this is a regular feature in nature, then it could help to explain where cholera goes to, (especially the classical form) during inter-epidemic periods. The appearance of non-01 cholera (vibrio 0139) supports this view.

V. cholerae has been found to remain viable in crude sewage for over a month and in sewage-contaminated soil for up to 10 days, thereby providing a possible source of infection to rivers or wells. It has been isolated from a number of foodstuffs, especially those with a pH of between 6 and 8, such as milk produce (e.g. ice cream), sugar solutions, meat extracts or articles of food preserved by salt. Uncooked fish and vegetables that have been washed or irrigated by sewage effluent have been responsible for outbreaks.

Direct person-to-person spread, or via fomites such as utensils or drinking straws (in home-brewed alcohol parties), do not appear to be as important as expected. Even in persons attending

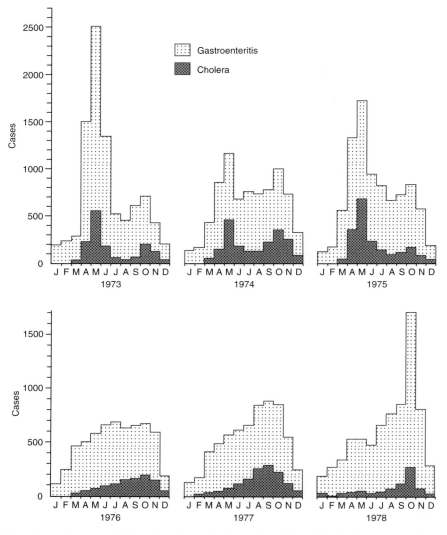

Fig. 8.2. Similar pattern of gastroenteritis and cholera in Calcutta (now Kolkata), India (1973–1978). (Reproduced by permission from the Indian Council of Medical Research (1978) *National Institute of Cholera and Enteric Diseases, Annual Report.* Indian Council of Medical Research, Calcutta.)

the death of a cholera case, it is more likely that infection will result from drinking water or consuming food that has been prepared for the mourning ceremony, rather than from the dead person or their shrouds.

A case of cholera can excrete between 10^7 and 10^9 *V. cholerae*/ml of diarrhoeal discharge and as the volume of this discharge may be in excess of 20 l/day, the potential for contamination of the environment is enormous. Clearly though, the severe case is unlikely to be anything but a transitory source; it is the asymptomatic case passing from 10^2 to 10^5 organisms/g of stool in a spasmodic manner that poses the greatest hazard.

A high dose of *V. cholerae* is required to infect the healthy subject. Some 10^6–10^8 organisms are needed, but if the person has a decreased gastric acidity then 10^3 organisms may be sufficient. Lowered gastric acidity is found more commonly than expected and may be related to malnutrition or diet. Cannabis smoking is also known to depress gastric acidity.

Carriers are of short duration. Seventy per cent of cholera cases are free of vibrios at the end of the first week and 98% by the end of the third. Long-term carriers are rare and of no epidemiological importance.

Incubation period. 1–5 days.

Period of communicability is until about 5 days after recovery, but prolonged excretion of organisms can continue in some individuals. Antibiotics reduce the period of communicability.

Occurrence and distribution. Humans are the only known reservoir, but the persistence of the organism in the environment, in possibly a changing form, as discussed above, may be another source. In endemic areas cholera is a disease of children (adults having developed immunity in childhood), whereas in its epidemic form adults are the more usual victims. The disease is associated with poverty and poor hygienic practices.

Classical cholera is restricted to South Asia and caused by *V. cholerae* 01. The El Tor biotype has infected Asia, Africa, Europe, Pacific Islands and South America, while the majority of cases are now found in Africa. First isolated from pilgrims to Mecca in the quarantine station of El Tor in West Sinai (now Egypt) in 1906, it differs from the classical variety by producing a soluble haemolysin. It is classified as either Ogawa, Inaba or Hikojima of the classical serotypes. The importance of the El Tor biotype is that it can survive longer in water, is more infectious, can cause mild infections and more frequently produces the carrier state. These characteristics have all assisted in the extensive spread of this organism. The more virulent El Tor *V. cholerae* 0139 has been responsible for epidemics in India, Bangladesh, Myanmar, Thailand and Malaysia, but is fortunately now on the decline. In 1992, a variant of the El Tor biotype but with toxigenic effects similar to those of classical cholera (ETEC) appeared in Asia and has now replaced the original El Tor strain in many parts of Asia and Africa. Antibiotic-resistant strains are appearing but proper management of cases should not require the use of antibiotics.

Control and prevention. Control is aimed at the cause. All too often a panic situation develops, foods are banned, vaccination given and quarantine instigated. If cholera is epidemic and preliminary investigations indicate that water is the vehicle of transmission, then the supply should be sterilized by super-chlorination (adding two to three times the calculated amount of chlorine required for the volume of water) or everybody told to boil their water. Boiling water is unpopular as it uses vital firewood and monopolizes scarce cooking pots, and the water has a flat taste. However, there is no reason why water cannot be boiled at the same time as the meal is cooked and simple clay pots used instead of metal ones. Boiled water can be re-aerated by shaking it up. A not so safe, but easier, method is to leave water to stand and then decant off the supernatant. A simple way of doing this is the three-pot system (Fig. 3.7). The solar water disinfection method (SODIS) using polythene bottles of water heated by the sun can also be used. Chlorine can be added to a well or communal water supply, but any vegetable matter in the water will inactivate chlorine, and several times the amount calculated may be required.

The banning or restriction of food should only be made on good epidemiological evidence. If fish are properly cooked before being eaten then they are unlikely to be a source. Disruption of a fish-eating practice may have dire consequences on other aspects of people's health. It is more often the fisherman rather than the fish, or the farmers rather than their produce, that are the purveyors of cholera.

Quarantine is rarely effective as bribery or evasion of the barricades by the few who might be carrying the infection negates the hardships borne by the many who are not. Giving tetracycline to immediate contacts of cases will reduce the number of asymptomatic carriers, but the widespread distribution of the drug will encourage tetracycline resistance.

The original inactivated *V. cholerae* vaccination gives about 50% protection and only lasts for 6 months. It does not prevent the asymptomatic disease state and can actively encourage the spread of infection, so is not recommended as a method of control.

Dukoral (WC/rBS) cholera vaccine consists of killed whole *V. cholerae* 01 in combination with a recombinant B subunit of cholera toxin. It confers protection of up to 90% for 6 months and has been found to be effective in preventing cholera in high-risk areas such as refugee camps and urban slums. Protection has been found to remain at about 60% for at least 2 years in adults and older children but declines rapidly in young children after 6 months. The vaccine is administered to adults and children over 6 years in two oral doses given 7 days apart. Children aged 2–5 years should have three doses each given 7 days apart. A booster dose to adults and children over 6 years can be given after 2 years. The vaccine has been found to be safe when given to pregnant women and those with HIV infection.

Dukoral can be used pre-emptively in high-risk areas, in epidemic situations and to protect travellers entering areas of high endemicity. Several mass vaccination campaigns have demonstrated its value in protecting populations at risk in an ongoing epidemic and in crisis situations where an outbreak of cholera has a high likelihood of occurring. It has also been found effective against ETEC.

Two other vaccines, Shanchol and mORCVAX, are based on serogroups 01 and 0139, but do not contain bacterial toxin B subunits so are not effective against ETEC. Shancol is produced in India for internal and international use, while mORCVAX will be used only in Vietnam. Shancol can be given to those over 1 year old and is administered in two oral doses given 14 days apart. These vaccines have been found to be as effective as Dukoral where ETEC cholera is not involved, providing longer term protection to children under 5 years of age, as well as being cheaper.

All these vaccines provide a herd immunity which is especially valuable in protecting young children. In high-risk areas, children as young as 1 year old should be targeted with Shancol or mORCVAX and 2 years olds with Dukoral, in periodic mass vaccination campaigns. Follow-up should be provided to give the second dose (and third with Dukoral) at 6 months. Booster doses should be given every 2 years. Pregnant women and HIV-positive persons should also be vaccinated.

In epidemic situations, oral cholera vaccines can be administered to populations in high-risk areas, but this is only a short-term option. Reliance should not be placed on vaccination to control an epidemic, but other methods of control such as sterilizing water supplies should mainly be used.

Persons dying from cholera should be buried promptly and the ceremony kept to a minimum. Disinfectants and hand-washing facilities should be provided at treatment centres and when bodies are prepared for burial. Flies should be controlled by disposing of or covering all faecal discharges, although they have not been shown to play a significant role in transmission.

Treatment. The vibrio binds to the cells and produces an enterotoxin, which activates adenyl cyclase, an intracellular enzyme that initiates a system of fluid and ion transport from the plasma to the intestinal lumen. There is no mucosal damage and increased permeability is unlikely, which explains why glucose and electrolytes can still be absorbed by the mucosa. This allows large quantities of low-protein fluid, bicarbonate and potassium to escape through an essentially undamaged intestine. Management is to correct dehydration in this otherwise self-limiting disease.

Fluid replacement must be rapid and adequate, the most easily available being the first choice. If rehydration can be started as soon as cholera symptoms begin, then oral rehydration will be all that is required. ORS can either be prepared from ready-mixed packets of salts (Section 8.1) or by making a sugar and salt solution (Fig. 8.1). Unfortunately, most cases have already lost a considerable quantity of body fluid on presentation, which means that they will require intravenous infusion. If available, Ringer-lactate solution (Hartmann's) contains the nearest approximation of electrolytes to that being passed in the diarrhoeal fluid. As a second best, a mixture of two units of normal saline and one of sodium bicarbonate can be used. The patient should be rehydrated intravenously as rapidly as possible, then oral rehydration solution substituted once the patient can swallow. This allows the body mechanisms to regulate electrolytes, as ionic imbalance can rapidly occur with intravenous infusion – from which many patients succumb. The body fluid deficit should be restored, followed by maintenance of one and a half times the equivalent amount of bowel loss. Fluid loss can be measured into a bucket under the bed. A bed or cholera cot is not essential though, and the patient can be nursed on a plastic sheet laid on the ground with the earth hollowed out under the pelvis to take a receptacle to collect the outpouring fluid.

Tetracycline is not essential in treatment, but shortens the duration of the illness and quantity of fluid replacement required. Tetracycline is given in a dose of 500 mg 6 hourly for 3 days, or doxycycline in a single dose of 300 mg. Sensitivity must be monitored as the development of tetracycline resistance will necessitate changing to another antibiotic.

The management of a cholera epidemic requires speed and good organization. Essentially, treatment is taken to the people by setting up treatment centres at strategic places in the vicinity of the epidemic. These can be dispensaries, schools, church halls or even tents that are supplied with staff and fluids. Cholera patients do not need to be treated in hospital.

Surveillance for cholera is both national and international. Under the International Health Regulations (2005) any outbreak is a health event of international concern so should be reported to the World Health Organization (WHO). This will provide an advance warning system to other countries, but neighbouring countries should be notified directly. Cases should be reported using the WHO case definition and not just laboratory-confirmed cases. Nationally, a warning system can be implemented for diarrhoeal diseases where an increase in numbers, or in persons dying from diarrhoea, may indicate an underlying outbreak of cholera (Fig. 8.2). There is considerable concern that *V. cholerae* 0139 has the potential to cause a pandemic so this serogroup should be tested for. Where cholera exhibits a seasonal pattern, then the population and health staff can be placed on the alert when the next season starts.

8.5 Bacillary Dysentery (Shigellosis)

Organism. Bacillary dysentery is due to *Shigella* invading the bowel. The species and strains of *Shigella* are numerous. There are four main species and serogroups:

S. dysenteriae with 15 serotypes	A
S. flexneri with 6 serotypes and 15 subtypes	B
S. boydi with 18 serotypes	C
S. sonnei with 1 serotype	D

Those causing the most severe disease are *S. dysenteriae* and the least *S. sonnei*, with *S. flexneri* the most common in endemic areas. A Shiga bacillus designated Sd1 (*S. dysenteriae* type 1) results in a more severe illness and is responsible for large outbreaks. Another form of bloody diarrhoea is due to enteroinvasive and enterohaemorrhagic *E. coli*, particularly serotype O157:H7.

Clinical features. Bacillary dysentery presents as an acute diarrhoeal illness with blood in the stools, resulting from invasion of the colonic epithelium.

This causes patchy destruction and the formation of micro-ulcers and inflammatory exudates. In mild infections, blood may be absent with a similar presentation to gastroenteritis. In severe cases, the stools are a mixture of pus and blood, and tenesmus is common. Fever accompanies the illness and nausea or vomiting can occur. Severity is determined by the strain of organism and age of the person, with a moderate mortality in the very young and very old. Serious complications are: metabolic abnormalities, sepsis, encephalopathy, toxic megacolon (in children with recent measles), rectal prolapse, intestinal perforation and haemolytic uraemic syndrome. Reiter's syndrome, a triad of arthritis, urethritis and iritis, can occur weeks to months after the acute infection. Case-fatality rate can be as high as 15% among people infected with Sd1.

Diagnosis. If bacteriological facilities permit, the organism should be cultured, identified, typed and sensitivity determined. A suitable transport medium is Carey Blair. Where this is not possible, then a specimen of fresh faeces should be examined by microscopy to detect polymorphonuclear leucocytes. A simple epidemiological investigation may provide sufficient information to indicate the mode of transmission. The case definition for reporting purposes is 'diarrhoea with visible blood in the stool'.

Transmission is by the faecal–oral route with either food or water as the main vehicle carrying the infection. Bacillary dysentery can occur in small outbreaks among families, suggesting food as the mode of transfer. Seasonal epidemics coinciding with the arrival of the rains indicate waterborne spread. Flies can be important in hot dry months when garbage accumulates and massive fly breeding takes place. Only 10–100 organisms are required to produce the disease, whereas the diarrhoea stool contains 10^6–10^8 *Shigella*/g.

Carriers can be important and sporadic epidemics in institutions might indicate a food handler with unsanitary habits.

Incubation period. 1–7 days.

Period of communicability. Infection is communicable for 4 weeks, but may persist for a longer time in the carrier.

Occurrence and distribution. Any outbreak of an acute diarrhoeal disease with blood should be considered to be bacillary dysentery until proved otherwise. Distribution is worldwide, with sporadic outbreaks occurring in both the developed and developing world. Infection is often carried from one area to another, or across international boundaries, by carriers. There are estimated to be at least 80 million cases of bloody diarrhoea, with 700,000 deaths per year, the majority of the deaths being in children under 5 years of age. Outbreaks of Sd1 have been particularly severe in refugees where conditions of overcrowding, poor sanitation and unsafe water supplies, with the resulting inadequate hygiene, provide ideal conditions. Major outbreaks have occurred in Africa and South Asia in the past two decades.

Control and prevention. Bacillary dysentery is likely to present as an outbreak so investigation and treatment will need to be implemented in the manner described in Section 4.1. Generally it is better to bring treatment to the site of the outbreak, setting up temporary treatment centres, unless the outbreak is a small one and the hospital has sufficient facilities to isolate cases. A seasonal outbreak will suggest that water supplies need to be improved. Searching for carriers is generally unsatisfactory and investigation should be restricted to food handlers.

Breastfeeding is protective for babies and infants and should be continued even by the sick mother. Hand washing with soap and water is the most effective method of interrupting transmission. The control of flies is covered in Box 7.1.

With widespread antibiotic resistance, *Shigella* infections could be controlled by vaccinating susceptible groups, especially if there is an outbreak in the vicinity. A live oral vaccine of *S. flexneri* (SC602) is currently under trial, while others are in the developmental stage. Children should be vaccinated against measles as this reduces complications.

Treatment. Management is the same as with other diarrhoeas, to replace fluid and electrolytes lost. ORS is adequate and effective in all but the severely dehydrated who will require intravenous rehydration. There is a place for antibiotics in bacillary dysentery, although sensitivity must be determined as resistance is common. Ciprofloxacin 500 mg (15 mg/kg in children) twice a day for 3 days

is the drug of choice. Second-line treatment can be with pivmecillinam, ceftriaxone or azithromycin. Reliance should not be made on antibiotic treatment though as resistance makes control more difficult and the disease can relentlessly spread though a country.

Surveillance is similar to that for cholera (Section 8.4), with notification of any outbreaks, and monitoring of the weather in seasonal occurrence.

There are many similarities between cholera and bacillary dysentery, especially in management and control, so further help can be found in Section 8.4.

8.6   Giardia

Organism. The small flagellate *Giardia intestinalis* (*lamblia*) is a common commensal of the human small intestine, but heavy infections can cause diarrhoea.

Clinical features. There are frequent and loose bowel movements which are greasy and have an unpleasant odour. Bloating and abdominal distension commonly occurs. Diarrhoea is uncommon, but the passing of loose stools can continue for 2–4 weeks unless treated, while 30–50% of cases will develop intermittent diarrhoea and chronic infection. These can produce partial villous atrophy, with a resulting malabsorption syndrome and loss of weight. Chronic infection in children can result in failure to thrive, impairing the uptake of fats and vitamins A and B_{12}. *Giardia* is one of the causes of travellers' diarrhoea.

Diagnosis. The characteristic 'face'-shaped flagellate is occasionally seen in the faeces, easily detected by its high motility, but the cysts are more commonly found (see Fig. 9.1). Jejunal biopsy or the duodenal string test may be performed in the differential diagnosis of the malabsorption syndrome.

Transmission is by person-to-person transfer of cysts from the faeces of an infected individual or by contamination of food or water. Infected food handlers are often responsible for infecting people in restaurants, while a poorly maintained water supply disseminates infection more widely. The cysts can survive for several weeks in fresh water and are not killed by normal levels of chlorine. An animal reservoir might also be responsible. There is a dose–response relationship, with asymptomatic infection resulting from the ingestion of only one cyst, but symptomatic disease requires many more. Other factors, such as age, other illnesses and previous infection will also determine the outcome. Asymptomatic carriers are common and are the main method of transmission.

Incubation period. 3–25 days; mean 6–15 days.

Period of communicability. It takes 12–19 days between infection and the appearance of cysts in the faeces. These can persist in the bowel for many months, and during all of this time the infection can be transmitted.

Occurrence and distribution. The infection is found worldwide, but is more common in the tropics and where conditions of hygiene are poor, ensnaring the unsuspecting traveller with chronic diarrhoea. Heavy infections occur in children, especially those in institutions or debilitated by other conditions.

Control and prevention. Individuals who are rigorous with their personal hygiene can largely avoid infection. Drinking water can be treated with 5–10 drops of iodine/l or boiled. Proper food handling and preparation, especially the washing of hands, is essential, while long-term prevention is through proper sewage disposal and the protection of water supplies.

Treatment is with tinidazole, either as a single dose of 2 g or with 300 mg a day for 7 days. Metronidazole 2 g a day for 3 days can also be used, as can praziquantal 40 mg/kg.

Surveillance. Giardia is a common infection in travellers and a routine stool examination after travelling to a less-developed area is advisable.

8.7 Amoebiasis

Organism. Amoebiasis is caused by the protozoan *Entamoeba histolytica*, which exists in an amoeboid form in the human large intestine and as a cyst in the environment. A non-invasive species identical to *E. histolytica* called *E. dispar* also occurs and should be differentiated from the pathogenic form by its characteristic of not ingesting red blood cells.

The pathogenic amoeba enters a mucosal fold and feeds on red blood cells. It frequently penetrates through the muscularis mucosae, forming an abscess with vascular necrosis at its base. This leads to tissue disintegration and the development of an ulcer (the so-called flask-shaped ulcer). Active amoebae can be found in the base of an ulcer.

Clinical features. Illness presents as acute diarrhoea with the passage of blood and chronic diarrhoea, or as an abscess with no apparent transitional period of diarrhoea. If the amoebic ulcer penetrates a blood vessel fresh blood is passed in the stool; this is a characteristic feature. Amoebae from the breached circulatory system are carried to various parts of the body, the liver being the commonest. In the liver, an abscess is formed, the right lobe being the predominant site. Liver damage is a predisposing cause, with liver abscess more common in males than females. The expanding abscess can track outwards through the peritoneum, through the abdominal wall and on to the skin, or upwards to form a subphrenic abscess. The most serious site of amoebic abscess development is in the brain. All these features are illustrated in Fig. 8.3.

Symptoms of an abscess are fever, weight loss and localized tenderness. Amoebic pus is characteristically a pale reddish brown colour (without odour) and can be discharged on to the skin from a penetrating ulcer, or coughed up from the lung. In a chronic infection, an amoeboma can be formed which may be confused with carcinoma.

Diagnosis is made by examining fresh stool specimens within half an hour of their production for motile amoebae with ingested red blood cells. Amoebae are occasionally found in amoebic pus which, similarly, must be examined as soon as possible as the active forms rapidly die off. Non-invasive motile amoebae without red blood cells are likely to be *E. dispar*. The finding of cysts indicates infection, but search must be made of fresh stools or pus for motile amoebae. Serological tests can be useful in indicating infection. Liver abscess is diagnosed by X-ray (raised diaphragm) or by ultrasound. The abscess is usually not tapped unless it is required to differentiate it from a bacterial abscess or it is about to burst.

Transmission. Cysts of *E. histolytica* are formed in the large intestines and passed into the environment

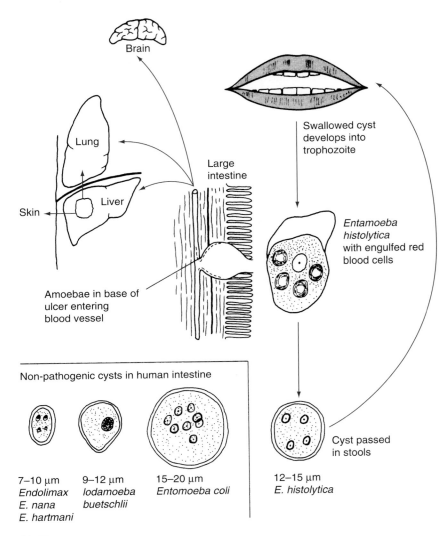

Brain

Lung

Large intestine

Swallowed cyst develops into trophozoite

Liver

Skin

Entamoeba histolytica with engulfed red blood cells

Amoebae in base of ulcer entering blood vessel

Non-pathogenic cysts in human intestine

7–10 µm
Endolimax
E. nana
E. hartmani

9–12 µm
Iodamoeba
buetschlii

15–20 µm
Entomoeba coli

12–15 µm
E. histolytica

Cyst passed in stools

Fig. 8.3. Amoebiasis.

in the faeces. They survive in faeces for only a few days but if they enter water they remain viable for considerably longer periods. Infection occurs through drinking contaminated water or eating salad vegetables irrigated with contaminated water. Flies can carry cysts for some 5 h. In circumstances of poor hygiene, direct faecal–oral transfer via food, or by utensils, can take place.

Cysts can survive in the cold for considerable periods, but they are killed by a temperature over 43°C, which must be obtained in any composting system where human faeces are used. Non-survival

of amoebic cysts is a useful indicator of effective decomposition (see Fig. 1.2).

Incubation period. 2–4 weeks.

Period of communicability. Cyst passing can continue for many years.

Occurrence and distribution. Amoebiasis is a disease of poor hygiene, more commonly found in cooler areas than hot areas. In the tropics, it predominantly occurs in highland areas or where there is a large temperature fluctuation. It is an infection of adult life and the longer the period of residence in an endemic area, the greater the chance of becoming infected. Some 100,000 deaths per annum are due to amoebiasis.

Control and prevention is by personal hygiene, food hygiene and the proper provision of water and sanitation. Sand filtration, especially if it is combined with alum flocculation, removes cysts from water supplies. A high concentration of chlorine is required to kill cysts (3.5 parts per million (ppm) residual), although they are more sensitive to iodine.

Treatment of all stages of the disease is by metronidazole 2.4g given as a single dose every day for 3 days or 2g daily for 5 days. Other derivatives of the 5-nitroimidazole group of compounds (tinidazole, ornidazole and nimorazole) can also be used. Cyst passers can be given diloxanide furoate (Furomate), 500mg 8-hourly for 10 days. Praziquantal in a single dose of 40mg/kg can be preferable to using metronidazole as only one dose is required, clinical signs rapidly disappear and it also clears cysts.

Surveillance. Routine stool specimens should be examined for amoebic cysts. Cysts of *E. histolytica* can be differentiated from other cysts by size and number of nuclei (Fig. 8.3).

8.8 Typhoid

Organism. *Salmonella enterica* serovar Typhi.

Clinical features. Although transmitted by the faecal–oral route, typhoid manifests mainly as a systemic infection, generally presenting as a fever. The fever starts gradually, increasing in a stepwise fashion over the first 1–2 weeks, producing a progressive malaise, disorientation and drowsiness. At the end of the first week, a rash of characteristic rose spots may appear (not seen in black skins).

The stools are normally constipated at first, but may later change to diarrhoea. If the organism localizes in the Peyers patches of the small intestine, ulceration, haemorrhage and perforation may occur. Other serious complications are cerebral dysfunction, delirium and shock.

Diagnosis is difficult and depends upon finding the organism in blood, stools or urine. A blood culture (3–5ml) taken in the first week is the most satisfactory method. Culture of the stools can be achieved if repeated examination is made from the start of the illness, with a greater likelihood of becoming positive as the illness progresses, provided antibiotics have not been used. Finding the organism from the urine, in which it is excreted spasmodically, is more difficult. Where the diagnosis has still not been made and further investigation is considered necessary, *S. enterica* can be cultured from the bone marrow or bile (by the duodenal string test). Bone marrow culture is more sensitive than blood culture and has the advantage of occasionally being positive even if the patient has received antibiotics. Sewage culture can be used in the investigation of epidemics.

The Widal test on the patient's serum can indicate infection, but a search for *S. enterica* must also be made to confirm the diagnosis. The Widal test has three components, the H (flagella), O (somatic) and Vi antigens, which are used to detect the corresponding antibodies in the patient's serum. The H antibody titre can be raised by any *Salmonella* infection and remain raised (giving an estimate of previous exposure), whereas the O antibody indicates recent infection. However both H and O levels will be raised by recent typhoid immunization, so a titre of 1/40 or higher is required. Added weight is given to the diagnosis by making a series of tests and demonstrating a rising titre. The Vi antibody is produced during the acute stage of the disease and persists while the organism is present, so has a value in detecting the carrier state.

Transmission. The main method of transmission is water, contaminated by faecal material from a carrier. These waterborne outbreaks may not always be explosive, and where low-grade infection of the water source is taking place groups of cases, spread over time, may occur.

S. enterica has been found to survive periods of 4 weeks in fresh water, but if the water is stored in bright sunlight (as in a reservoir) then the number of organisms rapidly dies off. It can survive in aerobic conditions with organic nutrient present, as found in contaminated streams. If the stream is polluted with raw sewage then the organism can survive over 5 weeks and within solid faecal material for considerable periods of time. Seawater is bactericidal, but where a sewage outfall is near a shellfish bed, then the organism is filtered and concentrated, providing a potent source of infection if the shellfish are eaten raw.

Milk and dairy produce provide ideal culture media and can become infected during handling by a carrier or rinsing of containers with polluted water. Contaminated ice cream has been responsible for several outbreaks. Pasteurization of milk at 60°C is effective in killing *S. enterica*. Infection of meat products and canned foods is less common, but can occur in the cooling process (if carried out in polluted water).

Flies can transmit the organism from faeces to food, whereas person-to-person infection is uncommon. Secondary cases form a very small proportion of an epidemic, so serial transmission in an unhygienic environment is not a feature.

Carriers. The carrier state is the most important epidemiological feature, with persistence of the organism in some individuals for periods in excess of 50 years. Three per cent of typhoid cases are found to still be excreting organisms after 1 year. People become more prone to act as carriers if they have a chronic irritational process such as cholecystitis, and especially the presence of gallstones (in which *S. enterica* is able to survive). *Clonorchis sinensis* has also been associated with the development of faecal carriers. Urinary carriers often suffer from an abnormality of the urinary tract, such as having a calculus, and *Schistosoma haematobium* is a predisposing cause.

Incubation period is 3–30 days, with a mean of 8–14 days. The length of the incubation period is inversely proportional to the infecting dose.

Period of communicability is from 1 week after the start of illness for a period of 3 months, except in the chronic carrier, where it continues for years.

Occurrence and distribution. In most tropical areas, the disease is endemic with seasonal outbreaks. Water is probably the main vehicle of transmission, but occurrences may be more related to collections of people gathering at scarce water sources (as occurs in the dry season), rather than manifesting as epidemics occurring with the early rains. Endemic typhoid is maintained by subclinical infections, especially in undiagnosed children, who obtain a degree of immunity. It has been suggested that these subclinical infections result from persons

swallowing lower bacterial doses than the critical threshold. In endemic areas the peak of infection is in children 5–15 years of age.

Typhoid is a worldwide disease and serious outbreaks, generally epidemic in nature, have occurred in developed countries from contamination of the water supply or of food produce. Repair work on water supplies or an accidental interruption of chlorination has led to epidemics. Typhoid organisms have persisted in canned meat cooled in infected water thousands of miles away from the outbreak. Many well-known outbreaks have been due to ice cream. The movement of carriers can be followed from the outbreaks they produce as they travel around. It is estimated that some 21 million persons suffer from typhoid each year and of these 1–4% die, the majority of these deaths being in Asia.

Control and prevention. Control relies on the protection of water supplies and the sanitary disposal of faeces. Placing latrines too close to wells, fractures in water mains and accidental contamination by sewage are ways in which outbreaks occur. Drinking water taken from polluted streams can be boiled, chlorinated or left to stand (the three-pot system shown in Fig. 3.7) and treated by solar disinfection (SODIS). Reservoirs and settling tanks can reduce the level of organisms below the infecting dose.

Where the outbreak can be traced to a food source then a search for carriers can be made. Stool specimens should be obtained from persons involved in the preparation of the food. If a carrier is discovered he/she should be prohibited from preparing food. This cannot always be applied to domestic catering, so careful instruction in personal hygiene should be tried. The organism can persist under the nails, so these should be kept short. Food must be protected from flies and stored only for limited periods (see also fly control in Box 7.1). All shellfish must be properly cooked.

An infecting dose of at least 10^3 organisms is required (except in persons suffering from achlorhydria), but this may need to be as high as 10^9. The main effect of vaccination appears to be to offer protection against lower dose infecting inocula (less than 10^5 organisms).

Typhoid vaccine has a variable effect, offering protection to persons who receive a low infecting dose, but none to those who ingest a high dose of organisms. It may, therefore, be useful for individual protection, but is limited on a mass vaccination basis, except to selected groups such as schoolchildren.

The live oral vaccine (Ty2la) gives protection for at least 3 years and may also give cross immunity against *S. enterica* Paratyphi B. It is available as a capsule taken orally every other day, with four doses in total. A vaccine containing the polysaccharide Vi antigen is administered parenterally by a single injection. These both produce fewer reactions than the whole-bacteria vaccine. A booster dose every 3 years is recommended in travellers or persons from non-endemic areas living in countries where typhoid is common. The Vi vaccine can be used to vaccinate children over 2 years of age and the Ty21a vaccine in those over 5 years in high incidence areas (such as slums) and in outbreak control. In some countries, vaccination is included in the childhood vaccination programme in areas of the country known to have a high prevalence of typhoid. It should be promoted along with health education and improvements of water supply and sanitation.

Treatment is with ampicillin or co-trimoxazole, but multiple resistant organisms have meant that more expensive antibiotics such as the quinalones (e.g. ciprofloxocin and ofloxacin) and third-generation cephalosporins are now required. Prolonged treatment of the carrier with ciprofloxacin 750 mg twice daily or norfloxacine 400 mg twice daily for 28 days has been successful. Relapse occurs in about 5% of treated acute cases.

Surveillance. Once carriers have been identified they should be warned of the danger they pose to others and told to report their condition to any medical people they come in contact with. Carriers are sometimes registered by health authorities.

8.8.1 Paratyphoid

Organism. *Salmonella enterica* Paratyphi A, B and C. Paratyphoid B is the commonest.

Clinical features. Paratyphoid is similar to typhoid, but with fewer systemic effects and diarrhoea a more important feature. A rash is less commonly seen, but when it does occur it is more extensive, involving the limbs and face as well as the body. Ulceration of the gut can occur, but less commonly than in typhoid.

Diagnosis. See typhoid.

Transmission. Infection originates from a carrier or a person with the illness, more commonly food borne than by other means (see under food poisoning, Section 9.1).

Incubation period. 1–10 days.

Period of communicability. 1–2 weeks.

Occurrence and distribution. Paratyphoid has a similar distribution to typhoid with an endemic pattern in developing countries and epidemic pattern in developed countries, but is less commonly detected.

Control and prevention. See typhoid.

Treatment. See typhoid.

Surveillance. See typhoid.

8.9 Hepatitis A (HAV)

Organism. Infectious hepatitis is a viral infection caused by hepatitis A virus (HAV).

Clinical features. The main pathology is inflammation, infiltration and necrosis of the liver, resulting in biliary stasis and jaundice. The infection generally starts insidiously; the person feels lethargic, anorexic and depressed. Fever, vomiting, diarrhoea and abdominal discomfort ensue, with the passing of pale-coloured stools, before the appearance of jaundice reveals the diagnosis. Once jaundice appears the person generally starts to feel better. Hepatitis A is a mild disease leading to spontaneous cure in the large majority, with only a few cases developing acute fulminant hepatitis and even more rarely severe chronic liver damage. There is an increase in symptomatic and severe cases with increasing age, while children may be virtually asymptomatic.

Diagnosis is made on clinical grounds and by the demonstration of IgM antibodies to HAV (IgM anti-HAV) in serum. For differential diagnosis of jaundice see Table 8.2.

Transmission. The early case is highly infectious, contaminating food and water. Infection can also be transmitted directly from poor personal hygiene, such as by handshaking. Intrafamilial transmission

Table 8.2. The causes of jaundice.

Disease	Clinical indicators	Occurrence
Hepatitis A (HAV)	Fever, lethargy, abdominal discomfort	Worldwide, epidemic in institutions
Hepatitis B (HBV)	More severe than HAV	Worldwide, endemic
Hepatitis C (HCV)	Prolonged course of chronic active disease	Worldwide, blood contact
Hepatitis delta (HDV)		Associated with HCV
Hepatitis E (HEV)	Epidemics	South and South-east Asia
Yellow fever	Fever, haemorrhages	Africa and South America
Rift Valley fever	Fever, haemorrhages	Africa
Infectious mononucleosis	Glandular fever	Young adults
Leptospirosis	Fever, haemorrhages	Rat-infested watercourses
Malaria	Periodic fever	Tropics, worldwide
Babesiosis	Fever and anaemia	Worldwide, with cattle
Amoebiasis	Diarrhoea and abscess	Africa, Asia, South America
Hydatid disease	Abdominal discomfort	Close contact with dogs
Clonorchiasis (Opisthorciasis)	Dull pain over liver	East and South-east Asia
Hookworm	Anaemia	Worldwide, children
Toxoplasmosis, congenital	Lymphadenopathy, including central nervous system	Associated with cats
Cytomegalovirus, congenital	Hepatosplenomegaly and purpura	Worldwide
Physiological jaundice of the newborn	Jaundice soon after birth or in premature infants	Worldwide
Glucose-6-phosphate dehydrogenase deficiency	Birth or drug reaction	Africa, Mediterranean
Hepatocellular carcinoma	Mass, weight loss	Africa, East Asia
Cholecystitis	Pain in right hypochondrium	Obese females
Gallstones	Pain in right hypochondrium	Obese females
Pancreatitis	Abdominal pain, vomiting	Underlying neoplasia
Pancreatic carcinoma	Weight loss, pain	Mainly Polynesians
Cirrhosis	Ascites	Following hepatitis or alcoholism
Drug reactions	Following the taking of drugs	Numerous drugs

is the commonest pattern, generally due to contamination of food and utensils by a food handler, but large epidemics can occur where a person in the early stages of the illness prepares communal food. Because of its insidious nature, the disease is not generally recognized until jaundice appears, by which time infection may have been widely transmitted.

Hepatitis is mainly a disease of poor sanitation, with water and food as the principle vehicles of transmission, but it can also occur when sanitation is good. Salads, cold meats and raw sea food are common vehicles of transmission.

The carrier state is not important but a large number of asymptomatic cases are produced. Epidemics occur when sewage contaminates water supplies producing infection in people who have previously acquired some immunity, suggesting that the disease may be dose dependent. Where there is a large infecting inoculum then infection can occur despite previous experience of the disease. Chimpanzees and other animals have been found infected, but probably have no epidemiological significance.

Incubation period is from 15–50 days, generally about 28 days.

Period of communicability is the latter half of the incubation period until about 1 week after jaundice appears, so that most cases have already transmitted the virus to family and contacts before they report to medical attention.

Occurrence and distribution. Hepatitis is endemic in most tropical countries, children coming into contact with it early in life and developing a degree of immunity. Non-immune persons, such as those from an area of good sanitation, coming into this environment are likely to develop the disease.

Epidemics occur in developed countries, especially in institutions such as schools and prisons, owing to poor food hygiene.

Control and prevention. During an outbreak of hepatitis A extra effort should be made to encourage scrupulous personal hygiene with hand washing. Anybody who starts to feel unwell should be temporarily relieved of preparing food. In an epidemic situation, a search should be made for the origin of the outbreak and preventive measures taken. In the long term, water supplies and sanitation should be upgraded.

Hepatitis A vaccine protects the individual at risk, and should be mandatory for those going from an area of good sanitation to one of poor sanitation, such as tourists and expatriates. Two doses are required given 6–18 months apart although one dose still gives high levels of immunity. Immunity from a two-dose regime may be lifelong, but a booster at 10 years is currently recommended. As most of the population in an endemic area will have met the infection as children and either had no symptoms or just a mild infection there is no case for mass vaccination, except for high-risk groups. Some countries in the Americas now include hepatitis A in the routine childhood vaccination programme.

Treatment. There is no specific treatment and supportive measures should be undertaken. Fatty foods should be avoided and a good fluid intake maintained.

Surveillance. Once hepatitis has been detected, health authorities should notify central authorities and surrounding areas.

8.10   Hepatitis E (HEV)

Organism. Hepatitis E virus (HEV).

Clinical features. Hepatitis E is very similar to hepatitis A except that it nearly always occurs in large epidemics. Symptomatic infection, with jaundice, anorexia, nausea, vomiting and fever, with a large tender liver, is most common in young adults. Infection is particularly severe in the pregnant woman and can result in a high mortality (up to 20%). In children it is mostly asymptomatic or causes a mild illness without jaundice.

Diagnosis is by the detection of IgM and IgG anti-HEV in serum or by the reverse transcriptase polymerase chain reaction (RT-PCR).

Transmission. This is similar to hepatitis A although the main means of transmission is via water. Contaminated water or food supplies, especially raw or inadequately cooked shellfish, have given rise to epidemics. A reservoir has been found in wild and domestic pigs, cattle, sheep and goats as well as rodents, suggesting a zoonotic pattern of transmission.

Incubation period. 3–9 weeks (mean 40 days).

Period of communicability. From 14 days after the appearance of jaundice and for a further 2 weeks.

Occurrence and distribution. Hepatitis E has been responsible for large epidemics in South and South-east Asia, especially Myanmar and Vietnam, where it appears to be endemic. Epidemics have also occurred in North and West Africa, Ethiopia, China and Mexico.

Control, prevention and treatment. The same as HAV, but extra precautions should be taken to protect pregnant women. There is no specific vaccine.

Surveillance. Epidemic hepatitis should be reported to WHO as an event of public health importance, and neighbouring countries warned.

8.11   Poliomyelitis (Polio)

Organism. Poliovirus (*Enterovirus*) types 1, 2 and 3.

Clinical features. Infection commences with fever, general malaise and headache, the majority of cases resolving after these mild symptoms, but approximately 1% proceed to paralytic disease. The virus has a predilection for nerve cells, especially those with a motor function (the anterior horn cells of the spinal cord and the motor nuclei of the cranial nerves). These cells are destroyed and a flaccid paralysis results.

In general, the paralysis is more common in the lower part of the body, becoming less common the higher up it affects. Unilateral lameness is commoner than bilateral lameness. The severe form of bulbar poliomyelitis is generally fatal in poor countries where respirators and intensive nursing care are not available. Site of paralysis is associated with injections or operations and such procedures should be avoided if there is any suggestion of poliomyelitis.

Diagnosis of the disabled case is made on clinical grounds, differentiating from the spastic paralysis of birth injury with which it is commonly confused. In polio, there will be a history of normal birth with commencement of walking, followed by a feverish illness and the development of flaccid paralysis. The paralysis is limited to well-demarcated muscle groups and there is no sensory loss. A similar history may be given for meningitis, but the damage will be central with accompanying mental deficiency. Virus may be recovered from throat swabs in the early stages of the illness or from rectal swabs or faeces later on. A rise in the antibody level of serological tests is not diagnostic due to the widespread use of polio vaccine.

Transmission is generally via the faecal–oral route, although the virus initially multiplies in the oropharynx so airborne transmission can also occur. The virus then invades the gastrointestinal tract, where it is excreted for several weeks.

A disease of low hygiene, young children (4–5 months) meet the virus with only a small proportion showing overt disease; 80–90% have an inapparent subclinical disease, 5–10% suffer from fever, headache and minor clinical signs, with 1% only going on to paralysis. Paralysis is more common with older age, so a non-immune person going into an endemic environment is at far greater danger of developing paralytic poliomyelitis. Raising standards of hygiene will also have the same effect because it spares people from meeting the virus as young children and allows a pool of susceptibles to develop. In time, the number of non-immunes will be sufficient for an epidemic to take place. There will also be a higher proportion of paralysed cases (peak age 5–9 years), and many deaths. So, sadly, the raising of living standards will change polio from an endemic disease with a few paralysed cases to an epidemic disease of increased severity. In epidemic poliomyelitis, where sanitation is good, pharyngeal spread becomes a more important method of transmission.

Poliovirus strains vary in their neurovirulence, with the more virulent strains having a greater tendency to spread. This could be due to a lower infective dose of the virulent virus being required to produce disease.

Incubation period is from 5–30 days with a mean of 10 days.

Period of communicability. This is from 2 days after exposure up until 6 weeks.

Occurrence and distribution. Poliomyelitis formerly occurred throughout the world, and was endemic in the poorer regions and epidemic in those with good sanitation, but this has changed considerably with the WHO programme of eradicating polio from the world. The Americas, Europe and Western Pacific are now free of infection, but cases still persist in Africa (Angola, Chad, Central African Republic (CAR), DRC, Ethiopia, Niger, Nigeria and Sudan) and Asia (Afghanistan, India and Pakistan), and previous targets have had to be revised.

Control and prevention. The main method of prevention and control is with polio vaccine. Two types of vaccine are available: the inactivated polio vaccine (IPV) (Salk) and the attenuated live vaccine (Sabin). The Salk vaccine is given by intramuscular injection, inducing a high level of immunity that is not antagonized by inhibitory factors in the gut, but is expensive to produce because it contains many organisms. The Sabin vaccine is administered orally (oral polio vaccine, OPV) making it easier and cheaper, as well as producing intestinal immunity which can block infection with wild strains of poliovirus. Multiplication of the OPV virus in the intestine makes it very useful in preventing epidemics and allows it to spread to non-vaccinated persons in conditions of poor hygiene, so protecting them as well. Unfortunately, the inhibiting action of antibodies in breast milk and colonization of the gut by other enteroviruses can reduce its effectiveness. Increasing the dosage and telling mothers not to breast feed for at least an hour after administration can help.

Because there are three strains of the poliovirus the vaccine should be given on three separate occasions, separated by periods of at least 1 month to ensure that immunity develops to each of the strains. Polio vaccine is conveniently administered at the same time as diphtheria, tetanus and pertussis (DTP). Where there is a high risk of poliovirus and importation or the transmission potential is high then a first dose should be given soon after birth.

In countries nearing eradication, a monovalent polio vaccine has been found to be more effective than the trivalent one, with type 3 virus predominating in the Indian subcontinent and type 1 in the remaining endemic parts of the world. A bivalent oral polio vaccine (bOPV) containing just type 1 and 3 viruses gives a higher rate of protection and is easier to administer. Unfortunately, the use of monovalent and bivalent vaccines has led to the development of vaccine-derived poliovirus (VDPV) outbreaks, mainly in Africa and the Indian subcontinent. This has been a particular problem in the immunodeficient, leading to the risk that they will develop paralytic disease, while also being reservoirs for the spread of poliovirus. Where incomplete vaccination programmes are occurring then the full triple vaccine should be used.

There is a slight risk of a live attenuated virus becoming more virulent, and as an alternative strategy to the development of VDPVs, many countries where polio has been eradicated now use IPV in their routine vaccination programmes. A high level of vaccination must be maintained to produce 'herd immunity' as there is still a risk of introduced cases from parts of the world where wild virus is still circulating.

Schoolchildren and adults who have received a full course of childhood vaccinations should have booster doses every 10 years. Maintenance of vaccination coverage should continue even in countries now free of infection and is essential for travellers going to parts of the world where polio has not yet been eradicated.

The long-term aim of prevention should be to raise standards of hygiene with the provision of water supplies and sanitation, but as mentioned above this must proceed at the same time as an adequate vaccination programme.

Treatment. There is no specific treatment for the acute stage, but rest and the avoidance of physical activity are beneficial. Specific supportive measures can be given to those with disabilities.

Surveillance developed for poliomyelitis eradication looks for cases of acute flaccid paralysis (AFP) in children under 15 years of age. These are investigated by stool examination, inquiry and search for other cases in the area. Remedial measures are carried out around the case, vaccinating all contacts.

8.12   *Enterobius* (Pinworm)

Organism. A nematode worm, *Enterobius vermicularis.*

Clinical features. The main symptom is intense pruritis ani. Heavy infections can rarely cause appendicitis, or salpingitis in the female.

Transmission. The gravid female migrates out of the anus at night to lay her eggs on the perianal skin before dying. This activity of the female causes the patient to scratch so that eggs are transferred to the fingers from which they are swallowed or passed on to someone else. Eggs are thrown into the air, such as in bed making or sweeping, so are often inhaled. Masses of eggs are liberated at each occasion so that infection of family groups, dormitories of schoolchildren, etc. occur at the same time.

Diagnosis. Eggs can be collected from the perianal skin by using an adhesive tape slide. This is examined directly by microscope, the characteristic oval egg with flattened side measuring 50–60 μm by 20–30 μm (Fig 9.1) being seen.

Incubation period. 2–6 weeks.

Period of communicability. As long as adult female worms discharge eggs until 2 weeks after treatment.

Occurrence and distribution. This very common infection is more prevalent in the temperate than tropical regions of the world, favouring conditions where poor hygiene prevails.

Control and prevention. Good personal hygiene, particularly the cutting of fingernails and hand washing are the means of control. Bedding and underclothes need to be washed frequently at the same time as treatment is given.

Treatment is with piperazine 65 mg/kg for 7 days, pyrantel pamoate in a single dose of 10 mg/kg (maximum 1g), repeated after 2 weeks, or albendazole or mebendazole 100 mg single dose repeated after 2 weeks. It is preferable to treat everyone in the group at the same time to break the transmission cycle.

Surveillance. Regular checks in an institutional situation, especially on individuals with repeat infections, will prevent spread throughout the establishment.

Summary

- A large number of infections are transferred by faecally contaminated fingers, food or water.
- Many of these infections produce diarrhoea, often adequately treated by oral rehydration solution.
- In cholera and bacillary dysentery outbreaks, emergency treatment centres should be set up, standardized treatment and rehydration regimes instigated and the outbreak fully investigated.
- Vaccinations are available for the prevention of rotavirus, cholera, typhoid, hepatitis A and poliomyelitis.
- The prevention of faecal-oral transmitted infections is by the improvement of water supplies, provision of safe sanitation and hand washing, especially before preparing or eating food.

Further Reading

Olsen, B.E., Olsen, M.E. and Wallis, P.M. (2002) *Giardia: the Cosmopolitan Parasite*. CAB International, Wallingford, UK.

Ravdin, J.I. (2000) *Amebiasis* (Tropical Medicine: Science and Practice Vol. 2). World Scientific Publishing, Singapore/Hackensack, New Jersey/London.

World Health Organization (2004) *Cholera Outbreak, Assessing the Outbreak Response and Improving Preparedness*. WHO, Geneva.

World Health Organization (2005) *Guidelines for the Control of Shigellosis, Including Epidemics Due to Shigella dysenteriae type 1*. WHO, Geneva.

Web resource

www.who.int/cholera/en (Global Task Force on Cholera Control: accessed 28 February 2012.)

Chapter 8

9 Food-borne Diseases

The faecal–oral mechanism for transfer of infection often includes food as a mechanism of infection, but in addition there are other diseases that are only transmitted by food. These can infect foods in general, such as with food poisoning, or be very specific in the particular food, such as with certain helminth infections. As the method of infection is so specific so is its method of control, which is through food hygiene, the proper cooking of foods and sanitary methods to prevent the food from being contaminated.

9.1 Food Poisoning

9.1.1 Food poisoning due to bacteria

Organism. Food poisoning can be due to bacteria, viruses and organic or inorganic poisons (Table 9.1). The most common form is that produced by bacteria. The main types of bacterial food poisoning are due to *Salmonella*, *Staphylococcus* or *Clostridium*.

Clinical features. Due to the similarity of presentation it is more convenient to consider all the causes initially as a group. Onset is sudden, with fever, vomiting and/or diarrhoea in a family or group of persons who have shared the same meal. Sometimes a subnormal temperature or lowered blood pressure is the presenting symptom. The incubation period is very short and sufficiently precise for the type of food poisoning to be suspected by the length of time since the food item was eaten.

Incubation period. The length of time from eating the suspect food to the onset of symptoms can give a good indication of the organism responsible. If it is 1–6 h, the food poisoning is likely to be staphylococcal, while over 6 h, usually 12–36 h, it is more likely to be *Salmonella*. *Clostridium* has a similar range of 12–24 h but this can reach several days. Less commonly, food poisoning may be due to *Bacillus cereus* (1–12 h) and *Vibrio parahaemolyticus* (12–48 h).

Transmission is through the consumption of food contaminated with the bacteria or its toxins. Infection can sometimes result from a contaminated water supply and via milk that has not been pasteurized. *Salmonella* generally infects the food in the living state, such as cattle, poultry or eggs, but unhygienic practice in the slaughtering of animals or preparation of foodstuffs can also be responsible. The bacteria are killed by proper cooking and no toxins are produced, so examination of the meal should reveal an improperly cooked source.

Staphylococcal food poisoning results from toxin produced by the bacteria so the food may be adequately cooked and no bacteria isolated from the suspected food source. It is commonly transmitted by food handlers with an infected lesion or unhygienic habits, such as transferring bacteria from the nose. *V. parahaemolyticus* is particularly associated with seafood or food that has been washed with contaminated seawater.

Clostridial food poisoning can be caused by several types of organisms. *C. botulinum* infection results in a severe disease, botulism, which is characteristic of home-preserved foods (see further in Section 19.6). *C. perfringens* generally produces a mild disease of short duration, but in New Guinea and Western Pacific Islands it is responsible for enteritis necroticans or pigbel, in which there is an acute necrosis of the small and large intestines with a high fatality rate. This is associated with feasting, generally on pig meat, but also on meat from other animals such as cattle. Children, particularly males, are mainly affected. The disease is probably accentuated by a protease inhibitor contained in sweet potato preventing breakdown of the toxin.

Table 9.1. Food poisoning.

Agent	Period of onset (h[a])	Symptoms	Types of food
Bacterial food poisoning			
Staphylococcal	1–6	Sudden, vomiting more than	Stored food
Bacillus cereus	1–12	diarrhoea	
Salmonella	12–36	Vomiting, diarrhoea and fever	Improperly cooked meat, eggs and milk produce
Clostridium perfringens	9–24	Abdominal cramps, diarrhoea, shock	Cooked meat, especially pig
Clostridium botulinum	9–24	Ptosis, dry mouth, paralysis	Preserved foods
Vibrio parahaemolyti-cus	12–48	Abdominal pain, diarrhoea and fever	Undercooked or raw fish
Fish poisoning			
Ciguatera	1–30	Paraesthesia, malaise, sweating, diarrhoea and vomiting	Barracudas, snappers, sea bass, groupers
Scombroid	1–12	Burning sensation, nausea, vomiting	Tuna, mackerel, salmon or in cheeses
Tetraodontoxins	0.5–3	Hypersalivation, vomiting, paraesthesia, vertigo, pains	Puffer fish
Shellfish, paralytic	0.5–3	Paraesthesia and paralysis	Clams and mussels
Shellfish, diarrhoeic	0.5–3	Diarrhoea and vomiting	Clams, scallops, etc.
Plant foods			
Akee (*Blighia sapida*)	2–3	Vomiting, convulsions, death	Unripe fruit
Cassava (cyanide)	Hours	Vomiting, diarrhoea, abdominal pain, headache, coma	Improperly processed root
Contaminants			
Triorthocresyl phosphate	Days	Neuropathy	Cooking oil

[a]Unless otherwise indicated.

Clostridia have resistant spores, which can remain in the soil for long periods, and their contamination of partly cooked and reheated food allows multiplication and production of the toxin.

There is often a seasonality of food poisoning, *Salmonella* in the summer months and *C. jejuni* in spring and autumn. *C. perfringens* occurs throughout the year.

Diagnosis and investigation of the outbreak. The epidemiologist is concerned with diagnosing the cause of the outbreak, so a search is made to discover a common food that has been eaten by all the persons that have succumbed to the illness. The foodstuff is likely to be one particular ingredient of the meal, rather than the whole meal, and samples should be taken for culture. If nothing is grown, this does not rule out a staphylococcal or clostridial cause of food poisoning, and finer questioning on foodstuffs consumed might be the only way to discover the offending item. (See Section 2.2.5 on how to analyse the relative importance of different foods eaten.)

Period of communicability. In *Salmonella* infection organisms can be excreted for up to 1 year although it is generally just for a period of weeks.

Occurrence and distribution. Food poisoning is found worldwide with large outbreaks associated with gatherings of people, such as celebrations and weddings. Many small outbreaks and those occurring in the home go unreported unless individuals are sufficiently ill to be hospitalized. Sometimes a batch of food is infected and distributed to several outlets.

Control and prevention. All suspect food must be destroyed and if it is part of a common foodstuff, then all of it must be traced and disposed of. The source of contamination, such as an abattoir, must be looked for and control measures implemented.

Prevention is by proper cooking of food and personal hygiene. Where repeated attacks occur, a search for a carrier should be made among food handlers. Anyone with a septic or discharging sore should be banned from handling and preparing food.

Food must be stored, prepared and cooked properly (Section 3.3.2). Establishments that prepare food, such as restaurants and hotels, should be regularly inspected and certified. Gloves should be worn by those preparing food in these establishments, and the bad practice of licking fingers and tasting food – as shown by celebrity chefs – should not occur.

Treatment. The treatment of cases of food poisoning is supportive, with fluids and electrolytes (either given orally or intravenously). Antimicrobials may be required in a severe case, but their use should be limited to those with complications as the development of drug resistance is a serious problem.

Surveillance. Food handlers should be checked by supervisors and food establishments visited on a regular basis by health inspectors. Outbreaks of food poisoning should be fully investigated (including identification and phage typing of the organism) and reported.

9.1.2 Salmonellosis

Although it is probably easier to understand all the main causes of food poisoning when they are grouped together, salmonellosis has become the most important cause of foodborne disease in the world. The problem is made more complicated by the number of serotypes (2.501 having been identified up to 2004) and the presence of drug resistance.

Case definition. Clinical: an illness with diarrhoea, abdominal cramps, fever, vomiting and malaise. Details of the person's address, time and day of onset plus recent meal information should also be recorded. Laboratory confirmation: isolation of *Salmonella* spp. from the stool or blood. This should be identified by species and phage type to assist in the investigation of the outbreak.

Clinical complications. The majority of cases are not life threatening, but in the very young or the elderly there can be dehydration and spread in the bloodstream. There has also been an increase in cases, often with complications, due to the widespread use of antibiotics in other infections such as those of the respiratory tract. These alter the intestinal flora and make the person more susceptible to a *Salmonella* infection (see further in Section 19.5). Drug resistance has also been a severe problem, leading to prolonged duration of illness, increased severity and the infection more likely to terminate in bloodstream spread.

Transmission. Infection is generally acquired from eating contaminated food of animal origin, mainly meat, and especially poultry in which 50–60% of chickens may be infected. Eggs are also a potent source of infection as well as contaminated cow's milk. Salmonellosis has also been acquired with increasing frequency directly from pets, such as dogs and cats which have become infected in the same way as humans. *S. enteriditis* and *S. typhimurium* are the most important serotypes, evolving in importance as a result of the intensive farming of domestic animals for consumption. A peak due to *S. enteriditis* occurred in 1992 in Europe, while *S. typhimurium* is now becoming more common.

Control and prevention. While the proper cooking and protection of foods is the main preventive action, the development of multi-drug-resistant organisms has developed owing to the excess use of antibiotics, especially in animals. These are often given in a routine process to encourage meat production, but pose considerable risk to humans, such as the use of fluoroquinolones in animals; this led to the development of resistant organisms that subsequently spread to humans, seen particularly in *S. typhimurium* phage type DT104 which is now a global multi-drug-resistant organism. Such practices need to be strictly controlled or outlawed.

While the control of antibiotic use in animals might reduce the risk of resistant organisms developing, good abattoir practice and food hygiene will prevent meat from becoming contaminated should they develop. Farmers and those working in the meat and poultry production industry need to be taught that human health rather than profit is the more important objective.

Much of the spread of food-borne diseases has been due to the globalization of the food supply, resulting in the widespread dissemination of suspect food items and the failure of national mechanisms to check their quality and safety. If it is not the food item that is doing the travelling the widespread movement of people through tourism, immigration or the deployment of work forces exposes these people to unfamiliar foods and to foods whose safety is in doubt. The danger is increased where the young, the elderly or those with conditions that compromise their resistance are either the recipients of the globally distributed food or are doing the travelling. International and national food controls therefore need to be of the highest level, and where food-related outbreaks occur they need to be fully investigated and control measures modified to prevent their recurrence. Health advice to travellers should be mandatory, not only for vaccination requirements but for every aspect of preventive health, including food consumption.

Treatment. In the majority of cases, the treatment is with oral rehydration, but in the severe case antimicrobials will be required. In adults, the optimal treatment is with one of the fluoroquinolones, while in children a cephalosporin is preferred. Chloramphenicol, ampicillin, amoxicillin and trimethoprim-sulfamethoxazole can be used where there is no resistance to these.

Surveillance is a laboratory-based exercise with identification and phage typing of the *Salmonella* spp. Samples should be collected from all cases, suspect foods or other sources and, if necessary, referred to a specialist laboratory for phage typing. A network of laboratories might have been set up to test food samples on a regular basis.

Outbreaks should be reported nationally, to neighbouring countries and internationally to the World Health Organization (WHO) Global Database on Foodborne Diseases Incidence.

9.1.3 Fish poisoning

Organism. Fish poisoning is a specific form of food poisoning caused by toxins either present in the fish or shellfish when they are caught, or developing owing to partial decomposition taking place if they are not refrigerated or eaten straightaway. Ciguatera toxin is produced by the dinoflagellate *Gambierdiscus toxicus*, which is present in algal blooms, often called red tides, while shellfish poisoning can de due to the dinoflagellates *Gonyaulux*, *Gymnodinium*, *Dinophysis* or *Alexandrium*.

Clinical features. Symptoms are normally mild with paraesthesia (tingling and burning sensations or pain and weakness), malaise, sweating, diarrhoea and vomiting, but in the young or those who have consumed a large quantity of poison the condition is more serious. Respiratory and motor paralysis can occur, often resulting in fatalities. Neurological symptoms can persist for some time after the original illness.

Transmission is through eating fish that has not been refrigerated or already contains the toxin. At certain times of the year and when hurricanes, seismic shocks or similar disturbances of the coral reef occur, an algal growth containing the dinoflagellate develops. Fish feed on the algal bloom, or it is inadvertently filtered by shellfish, and their flesh becomes poisoned. Fish that are normally quite edible, such as barracudas, snappers, sea bass and groupers become poisonous at these periods. The commonest poison is ciguatoxin, which is not destroyed by cooking.

Incubation period. 0.5–3 h after eating fish or shellfish.

Period of communicability. Not transmitted from person to person.

Occurrence and distribution. Fish poisoning is commonly found among island communities or coastal people for whom fish is a major item of diet. It is an important problem in Pacific Islands, the Caribbean, South-east Asia and Australia.

Control and prevention. All freshly caught fish should be gutted and refrigerated as soon as caught, unless cooked and eaten straight away. Red tides (algal blooms) occur as a result of some disturbance of coral reefs such as hurricanes, earthquakes and El Niño climatic disturbances. Algal blooms, and hence fish poisoning, are related to the surface temperature, so where this is abnormally increased during an El Niño event there is an increase in fish poisoning, with the converse when the temperature is less than expected.

Some poisons are water soluble so water in which fish is cooked should be thrown away. Shellfish should not be eaten when there are red tides.

Treatment. There is no specific treatment; supportive therapy being given.

Surveillance. When red tides are reported, eating reef fish or shellfish should be avoided. Outbreaks of fish poisoning should be reported.

9.1.4 Food poisoning due to organic or inorganic toxins

More generalized outbreaks involving large numbers of people not necessarily associated with each other and presenting with bizarre symptoms, such as paralysis, may be caused by an organic or inorganic poison contaminating the food. Examples are cyanide poisoning from poorly processed bitter cassava, eating unripe akees (a fruit popular in the Caribbean) or contaminants in cooking oil.

Although very localized, such outbreaks can be serious with considerable morbidity and sometimes mortality, so the source needs to be identified as a matter of urgency and banned from human consumption.

9.2. *Campylobacter* Enteritis

Organism. *Campylobacter jejuni* is the main species but *C. coli*, *C. laridis* and *C. upsalensis* may also cause infections. There are 16 species and six subspecies.

Clinical features. *Campylobacter* infection produces an acute diarrhoeal disease with abdominal pain, malaise, fever and vomiting. It is often self-limiting within 4–7 days, but in severe cases pus and blood are found in the stools, with a presentation similar to bacillary dysentery. Because of its association with a food source the disease is often thought to be a case of food poisoning until the organism is identified. *Campylobacter* enteritis is an important cause of gastroenteritis (Section 8.1) and travellers' diarrhoea. In a small proportion of cases, post-infection arthritis can develop or, more seriously, Guillain–Barré syndrome. This is a polio-like paralysis with respiratory and neurological dysfunction.

Diagnosis. The organism can be isolated from the stools using selective media. A preliminary diagnosis can be made by examining a specimen of stool with phase contrast (dark ground) microscopy, where a spiral or curved rod-shaped bacteria will be seen. The presence of faecal material and absence of cholera-like symptoms will differentiate the disease from cholera.

Transmission. Domestic animals including poultry, pigs, cattle, sheep, cats and dogs are reservoirs of the organism and their consumption or man's close association with them is responsible for much of the transmission. Most infections are due to faecal contamination by animals or birds, especially of unpasteurized milk and unchlorinated water. Water can be contaminated by bird droppings in which the organism is able to survive for several months at a temperature below 15°C. Many infections are transmitted by pets, especially puppies, and person-to-person transmission can occur in a similar way.

Incubation period. 1–10 days. The larger the dose of organisms ingested the shorter the incubation period.

Period of communicability. This is 2–7 weeks, but human-to-human transmission is uncommon.

Occurrence and distribution. Children under 2 years of age are most commonly infected in developing countries, immunity developing to further infection in those over this age. There is a worldwide distribution, with many of the cases in developing countries not being identified. There has been a progressive increase in *Campylobacter* enteritis due to the increased consumption of infected chickens and the globalization of food, as has been responsible for the increase in salmonellosis (Section 9.1.2). *Campylobacter* is one of the commonest causes of gastroenteritis (Section 8.1).

Control and prevention. Proper cooking of foodstuffs and control of pets are the main preventive methods. Wherever possible, water should be chlorinated and milk pasteurized. Good personal hygiene should be practised in the preparation and consumption of food. See also under salmonellosis (Section 9.1.2) on the globalization of food distribution and the importance of travel. Vaccines are being developed but there is a concern that Guillain–Barré syndrome could be a problem. An oral live multivariate vaccine containing *Campylobacter*, shigellas and enterotoxigenic *Escherichia coli* is being developed to protect the traveller from the most common causes of diarrhoea.

Treatment is with oral rehydration, an antimicrobial not being required in the majority of cases, but erythromycin, tetracycline or one of the quinalones can be used where there are complications.

Surveillance and investigation. An outbreak of *Campylobacter* should be investigated in the same way as a food-poisoning outbreak and remedial measures taken around the source.

9.3 The Intestinal Fluke (*Fasciolopsis*)

Organism. The large human fluke *Fasciolopsis buski*.

Clinical features. The adult worm lives in the small intestines and produces damage by inflammatory reaction at the site of attachment. This sometimes leads to abscess and haemorrhage, but as well as these local effects the parasite produces toxins. These can lead to oedema, weakness and prostration, ending fatally in the debilitated child.

Diagnosis is made by finding the egg in faeces. The egg is a giant among parasites (Fig. 9.1), although it is indistinguishable from that of *Fasciola hepatica* (see Section 9.4).

Transmission. The eggs are passed in faeces either directly into water or are washed there following rains. They hatch in water and each liberates a miracidium, which must find a snail of the genus *Segmentina*. Developing first into a sporocyst, then a redia, numerous cercaria are produced. On leaving the snail the cercaria encyst on water plants that are subsequently eaten raw by humans (Fig. 9.2). These plants include the water calthrop (*Trapa* sp.), the water chestnut (*Eliocharis tuberosa*) and the water bamboo (*Zizania aquatica*). Beds of these water plants are often grown in ponds fertilized by human sewage so there is considerable opportunity for transmission. Even if the foods are subsequently cooked they are often first peeled with the teeth so that cercariae are still swallowed.

A reservoir of infection is maintained in pigs, sheep, cattle and other domestic herbivores. Infection is particularly high in pig-rearing areas. Humans also act as reservoirs.

Incubation period. 2–3 months.

Period of communicability is 12 months but animals act as a permanent reservoir.

Occurrence and distribution. East Asia, especially China, Taiwan, Thailand, Borneo and Malaysia, in some 15 million people.

Control and prevention is by the proper preparation and cooking of water plants. Much can be done to reduce transmission by regulating the use of human faeces as a fertilizer. Domestic animals should be kept away from water plant cultivation ponds.

Treatment is with praziquantel 25 mg/kg three times a day for 2 days or 40 mg/kg as a single dose.

Surveillance. When a case is diagnosed other members of the family should be investigated and a common food source looked for.

9.4. The Sheep Liver Fluke (*Fasciola hepatica*)

Organism. The sheep liver fluke *Fasciola hepatica*. Less commonly *Fasciola gigantica*.

Clinical features. The parasite has a predilection for the liver, piercing the gut wall and migrating through the liver substance to lie in the biliary passages. This migration and residence in the liver causes extensive damage, leading to fibrosis and cirrhosis.

Initially there is prolonged fever and pain in the right hypochondrium, leading in time to hepatomegaly. There is also a marked eosinophilia.

Diagnosis is made by finding the very large egg in the stool; this is almost identical to that of *Fasciolopsis* (Fig. 9.1).

Transmission. The life cycle is similar to that of *Fasciolopsis* in that eggs passed in the faeces each liberate a miracidium on contact with water. The miracidium searches for and invades snails of the genus *Lymnaea*. After passing through sporocyst and redia stages, the cercaria encyst on grass or water plants (e.g. water cress). The normal life cycle is in sheep, with man becoming incidentally infected when he eats contaminated water plants (Fig. 9.2). Cattle and goats also act as reservoirs.

Incubation period. Probably 2–3 months.

Period of communicability. Not transmitted from person to person.

Occurrence and distribution. Worldwide distribution in sheep-rearing areas, especially the Andean highlands of Bolivia, Ecuador and Peru, the Nile

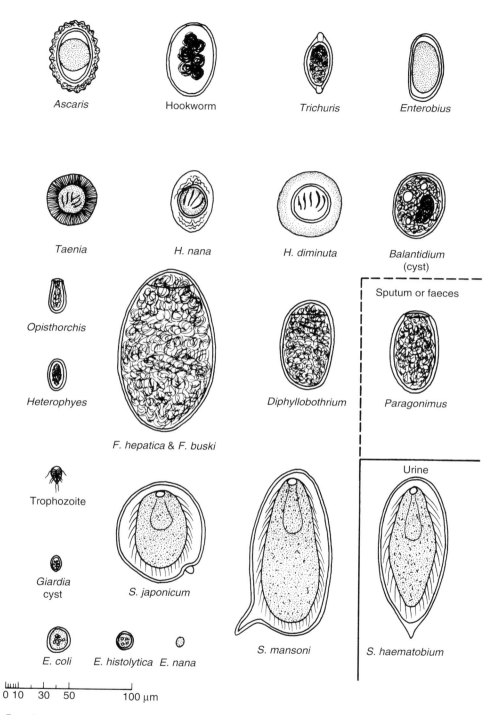

Fig. 9.1. Parasite eggs found in faeces, urine and sputum: *E.* (*nana*), *Endolimax*; *E.* (*coli*), *E.* (*histolytica*), *Entamoeba*; *F.* (*hepatica*), *Fasciola*; *F.* (*buski*), *Fasciolopsis*; *H.* (*diminuta*), *H.* (*nana*), *Hymenolepis*; *S.* (*haematobium*), *S.* (*japonicum*), *S.* (*mansoni*), *Schistosoma.*

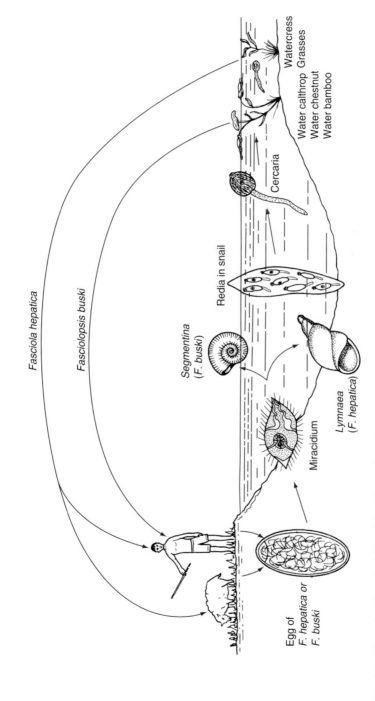

Fig. 9.2. Life cycle of intestinal (*Fasciolopsis*) and sheep liver (*Fasciola*) flukes.

delta region of Egypt and northern Iran. *F. gigantica* is found in Africa and the Western Pacific. Some 2.5 million are probably infected in the world, with up to 60% of the population infected in highly endemic areas.

Control and prevention. In known endemic areas careful control is required in the growing and consumption of water plants such as cress. Animal faeces should not be used to fertilize water plants. The close association of man and sheep or other domestic animals, greatly increases the opportunity for infection.

Treatment. Praziquantal 25 mg/kg three times a day for 2 days or 40 mg/kg as a single dose. Alternatively, triclabendazole at 10 mg/kg single dose, which can be repeated after 12 h.

Surveillance. Sheep should be examined at regular intervals and treated.

9.5 The Fish-transmitted Liver Flukes

Organism. The trematode fluke *Clonorchis sinensis*.

Clinical features. The adult fluke lives in the branches of the bile duct, resulting in trauma and inflammation. Dilation of the biliary system causes a distortion of the liver architecture, which can lead to biliary stasis, hepatic engorgement, fatty infiltration and finally cirrhosis. *C. sinensis* is a risk factor for cholangiocarcinoma. Migration of the flukes up the pancreatic duct can damage the pancreas, leading to recurrent pancreatitis.

The main feature is pain in the right hypochondrium, intermittent at first but then continuous. There is often a hot sensation felt over the skin of the abdomen. An enlarged liver is felt and gall stones or an enlarged gall bladder are seen on X-ray.

Diagnosis. The small operculated egg is found on faecal examination and is identical to that of *Opisthorchis* (Fig. 9.1.).

Transmission. Man is infected by eating raw fish, which includes pickled, smoked or undercooked fish. Eggs passed in the faeces develop into miracidia, which are swallowed by snails of the genera *Bulimus*, *Bithynia* or *Parafossarulus*. These pass through the sporocyst and redia stages in the snail and produce free-swimming cercaria. Having sought out a suitable fish, they penetrate between the scales and encyst in the flesh. The parasite also attacks dogs, cats, rats and pigs, which form reservoirs of infection (Fig. 9.3).

Incubation period. Approximately 4 weeks.

Period of communicability. Eggs may be passed for as long as 30 years, but reservoir animals are also an important source of human infection.

Occurrence and distribution. Distribution is very similar to that of *Fasciolopsis*, with *C. sinensis* being found in China, Japan, Korea, Taiwan, Thailand, Laos, Cambodia and Vietnam (lower Mekong valley). Some 30 million suffer from the disease.

Control and prevention. Control is by the proper cooking of fish. Members of the carp family (Cyprinidae), the so called 'milk fish', are eaten raw as a delicacy. They are grown in fish farms as part of a system of aquaculture, which is fertilized by human faeces. Regulation of this practice is required to reduce this unpleasant infection. Other foods such as fish paste, often added to food after it has been cooked to improve the taste, are made from raw fish and are a potent source of infection.

Treatment. Treatment is with praziquantel 25 mg/kg three times a day for 2 days or 40 mg/kg as a single dose.

Surveillance. When a case is identified search should be made for the culprit food source.

There are a number of less common trematodes that have the same life cycle as *C. sinensis* (Fig. 9.3). *Opisthorchis viverrini* is found in Thailand and Laos where raw fish paste is a favourite food additive. *O. felineus* occurs in Central and Eastern Europe, similarly causing disease of the liver; as suggested by its name, this is mainly a disease of cats, but humans can become infected. *Heterophyes heterophyes* and *Metagonimus yokogawai*, found in Asia and the Far East, do not attack the liver, but remain in the intestines. The eggs of all of these flukes are very similar (Fig. 9.1).

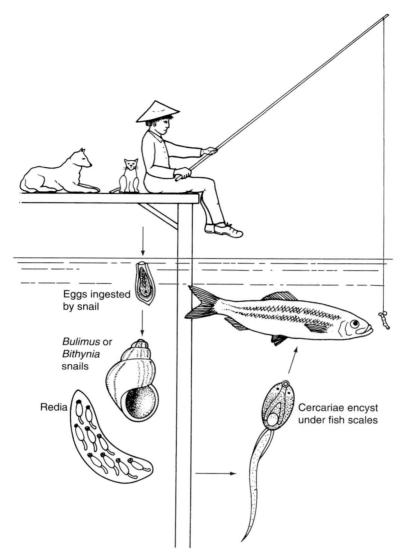

Fig. 9.3. The life cycle of the fish-transmitted liver flukes, *Clonorchis sinensis, Opisthorchis felineus, O. viverrini, Heterophyes heterophyes* and *Metagonimus yokogawai*.

9.6 The Lung Fluke

Organism. Unique among all the helminths, the trematode *Paragonimus westermani* selectively inhabits the lung.

Clinical features. Foreign body reaction to the parasite in the lung results in fibrosis, compensatory dilation and abscess formation. Haemoptysis is often an important feature, mimicking tuberculosis.

Symptoms include cough and chest pain. If the parasite migrates to a site other than the lung it can cause central nervous system (CNS), liver, intestinal, genitourinary or subcutaneous disease.

The first symptoms are diarrhoea and abdominal pain, followed by fever, chest pain, dyspnoea and a chronic cough. Blood-stained sputum results from coughing bouts, but there is no weight loss and the patient can live with the symptoms for many years.

Within the figure:
Eggs ingested by snail

Bulimus or *Bithynia* snails

Redia

Cercariae encyst under fish scales

Diagnosis is by finding eggs in the sputum or, if swallowed, in the faeces (Fig. 9.1). Any case of haemoptysis without other signs of tuberculosis should have a sputum examination on which an acid-fast bacteria (AFB) stain has not been used as this destroys the eggs.

Transmission. The egg, on reaching water, softens and a miracidium frees itself from the egg capsule and searches for a snail of the genus *Semisulcospira*. Passing through the sporocyst and redia stages, the cercaria encyst in the gills and muscles of freshwater crabs and crayfish. Humans are infected by eating uncooked, salted or pickled freshwater crab (*Eriocheir* and *Potamon*) or crayfish (*Cambaroides*), while an animal reservoir (mainly cats and dogs) helps to maintain the disease. The liberated metacercaria pass through the intestinal wall and penetrate the diaphragm to enter the lung. Adults develop in the lungs to produce eggs, which are liberated into the sputum. Occasionally they find their way to unusual sites, the brain being particularly serious (Fig. 9.4).

Incubation period. 6–10 weeks.

Period of communicability. Up to 20 years.

Occurrence and distribution. P. *westermani* disease is found mainly in China, other parts of Asia, Africa and the Americas. Closely related species are *P. africanus* and *P. uterobilateralis* in West Africa, *P. pulmonalis* in Japan, Korea and Taiwan,

P. philippinensis in the Philippines, *P. heterotremus* in Thailand and Laos, and *P. kellicotti, P. caliensis* and *P. mexicanus* in Central and South America. In all, it has been calculated that some 30 million people suffer from the lung fluke.

Control and prevention. Control is most effectively achieved by ensuring that all crab and crayfish meat is properly cooked. Much can be achieved by teaching people about the life cycle of this and other trematode infections, stressing that all food must be cooked and faeces disposed of properly. Spitting should be outlawed.

Treatment is with praziquantel 25 mg/kg three times a day for 2 consecutive days or 40 mg/kg as a single dose. Alternatively, triclabendazole 10 mg/kg, repeated in 12 h, can be used.

Surveillance. It is a focal disease so identifying a case will often lead to a focus of infection and preventive action can then be instituted.

9.7   The Fish Tapeworm

Organism. The large tapeworm *Diphyllobothrium latum*.

Clinical features. Such a large worm (10 m or more), when present in the intestines, can consume a considerable quantity of nutrients, but its main pathology is due to its selective absorption of vitamin B_{12}, resulting in a megaloblastic anaemia in the host.

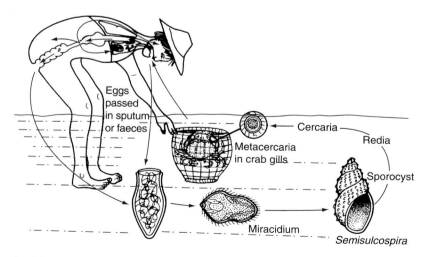

Fig. 9.4. Life cycle of the lung fluke, *Paragonimus westermani*.

This is a long-lasting complaint and symptoms of pernicious anaemia appear 3–4 years after infection, commonly in 40 year olds. These symptoms are paraesthesia and disturbances of motility and coordination, often accompanied by fever, glossitis, oedema and jaundice, but gastric secretions contain the intrinsic factor necessary for vitamin B$_{12}$ absorption, thus differentiating it from true pernicious anaemia.

Diagnosis is made by finding the egg in the faeces (Fig. 9.1). Sometimes worm segments (proglottids) are also passed.

Transmission. The adult worm is found in the intestines of humans, dogs, cats, foxes and bears, and in a number of other mammalian hosts. Eggs are passed in the faeces, which on contact with water liberate a coracidium, which is ingested by a copepod (*Cyclops* and *Diaptomus*). The coracidium develops in the copepod to a larval form, a procercoid, which when eaten by a freshwater fish finds its way into the muscles and develops into a plerocercoid. When the raw or improperly cooked fish is eaten the liberated plerocercoid attaches itself to the intestinal wall and develops into an adult tapeworm (Fig 9.5).

Incubation period. 3–6 weeks.

Period of communicability. Humans can continue to liberate eggs into the environment for many years but most of the infective source is from the animal reservoir.

Occurrence and distribution. The parasite is found in the cooler parts of the world, around the lakes of Europe, America, China and Japan. It is also found in indigenous tribes living in the Arctic and subarctic. It is a disease of some 13 million people.

Control and prevention. Control is by ensuring that fish are properly cooked. Deep-freezing fish will also kill the parasite. Sanitation will decrease the human cycle and animal faeces should be prevented from entering water sources.

Treatment. Praziquantel as a single dose of 5–10 mg/kg or niclosamide as a single dose of 2 g. The pernicious anaemia is treated with folic acid and vitamin B$_{12}$ and can produce remission of the anaemia even without expulsion of the parasite.

Surveillance can be conducted in areas where the parasite commonly occurs. Any case of anaemia should be examined for the presence of the parasite.

9.8   The Beef and Pork Tapeworms

Organism. *Taenia saginata*, the beef tapeworm, and *T. solium*, the pork tapeworm.

Clinical features. The adult worm of both species can live in the intestines producing little pathology, being diagnosed often by accident. It does however share the food supply of its host so that debility can occur. The serious problems are due to the *Cysticercus cellulosae* (from *T. solium*). The cysticerci die and calcify, those in the brain being a common cause of epilepsy or mental disorder.

Gastric disturbances can occur, often with mild pain, or the patient may notice the proglottids being discharged. If people are unfortunate enough to be infected with cysticercosis they may suffer from convulsions, intracranial hypertension (vomiting, violent headaches and visual disturbances) or psychiatric disorders (confusion, apathy or dementia), there being a 50% mortality in untreated cases.

Diagnosis is made by finding the proglottids in the faeces, with patients often making their own diagnosis. It is very important to distinguish between *T. saginata* and *T. solium* in view of the danger of inducing cysticercosis: *T. saginata* has 18–30 compound branches of the uterus on each side whereas *T. solium* has only 8–12 (Fig. 9.6).

Transmission The adult worm lives in the small intestine of man and as it matures gravid segments break off and are passed in the faeces. Cattle or pigs inadvertently eat the proglottids (the mature segments), or the discharged eggs contaminate the pasture. Alternatively, the animal can become infected by drinking water polluted by sewage. It has also been found that birds feeding on sewage can carry eggs long distances and then deposit them on pasture land. Flies might have a place in transmission as well. The eggs develop into cysticerci in the muscles, favouring the jaw, heart, diaphragm, shoulder and oesophagus. Humans acquire the disease by eating improperly cooked beef or pork containing the cysticercus.

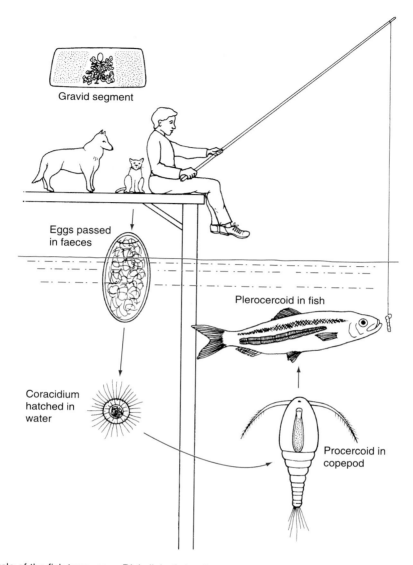

Gravid segment

Eggs passed in faeces

Plerocercoid in fish

Coracidium hatched in water

Procercoid in copepod

Fig. 9.5. Life cycle of the fish tapeworm, *Diphyllobothrium latum.*

The beef tapeworm (*T. saginata*) and the pork tapeworm (*T. solium*) have the same life cycle except that the intermediate stage, the cysticercus of *T. solium*, can also occur in humans. This happens by swallowing eggs directly, either by autoinfection from eggs in food or water, or through sewage contamination. Also, any gastric disturbance that might cause the regurgitation of proglottids into the stomach (including improper treatment) can lead to the liberation of vast quantities of eggs, with the result that cysticerci are produced anywhere in the body, including the brain, orbit and muscle.

Incubation period. 8–12 weeks.

Period of communicability. Adult worms can live for as long as 30 years, their eggs contaminating the environment for this period of time.

Occurrence and distribution. These are the commonest and most cosmopolitan of all the tapeworms,

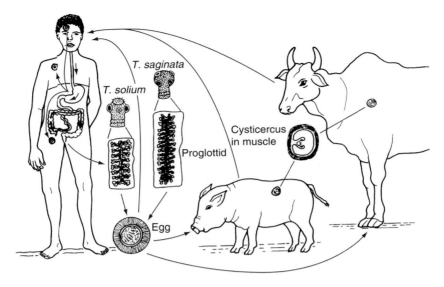

Fig. 9.6. Life cycle of the tapeworms *Taenia solium* and *T. saginata*.

with a worldwide distribution in beef- and pork-eating areas, especially in the tropical belt and Eastern Europe. Over 60 million people are thought to be infected.

In such areas of beef and pork eating, there is a ready transmission cycle in operation. Finding the worm in humans means that transmission is probably reasonably common in that area, whereas in other places where beef and pork eating are just as much part of the usual diet, but food hygiene is adequate, they are not found. *T. saginata* is increasing in Europe, probably because of human sewage contamination of animal drinking water. *T. solium* is common in Mexico, Chile, Africa, India, Indonesia and Russia.

Control and prevention. The main means of control is the proper cooking of meat. The underdone steak or joint of meat where internal temperatures are not high enough to kill the cysticercus are common ways in which transmission can still take place, despite cooking. Proper control of slaughtering in official abattoirs, with meat inspection, can prevent the dissemination of infected meat. Condemned carcasses must be burnt.

Treatment for both worms is with niclosamide 2 g as a single dose. Alternatively, praziquantel as a single dose of 5–10 mg/kg can be given. Praziquantel at a dose of 50 mg/kg for 15 days can be used for

cerebral cysticercosis in conjunction with corticosteroids, as an inpatient.

Surveillance. Where a localized cycle of infection is occurring, investigation may reveal a sewage leak or other source of contamination that could easily be rectified.

9.9 Trichinosis

Organism. *Trichinella spiralis, T. nelsoni, T. nativa, T. britovi* and *T. pseudospiralis,* nematode worms.

Clinical features. The severity of the disease depends upon the dose of larvae that have encysted in the tissues. During the second week of infection there is headache, weakness, muscle pain (particularly in the masseter and extraocular muscles), pyrexia, subconjunctival haemorrhage with oedema of the orbit and eosinophilia. If the symptoms are sufficiently severe death can occur (generally due to invasion of the CNS or heart); otherwise once the attack is over the cysts cause no further trouble, gradually die and calcify.

Diagnosis is made by muscle biopsy of the deltoid or thigh muscles where the encysted larvae are found.

Transmission The life cycle is a simple one (Fig. 9.7). Encysted larvae in the muscles are eaten by another animal and the liberated larva develops into an adult to produce numerous new larvae, which are then carried to all parts of the body in the circulation. Only the larvae that reach striated muscle survive, the diaphragm, tongue, throat, eye and thorax being favoured sites.

In the different climatic zones of the world, where different groups of animals live off each other, several transmission cycles have evolved. In Africa, the warthog and the bush pig form the vital link in the cycle. Being the favoured prey of lions and leopards, these carnivores, with the hyenas and jackals that finish off the remains, all become infected. The general scavenging nature of the warthog and pig, which inadvertently eat the remains of dead animals, allows the cycle to be completed. Humans come in as intruders, a dead end to the cycle when they feast on a recently killed bush pig.

In Europe and Asia, the rat is the reservoir of infection, but in its scavenging nature the pig acquires infection and when cooked on a spit or otherwise eaten in an improperly cooked way humans become infected. Sausages made from food scraps or hamburgers contaminated with bits of pork can be potent sources. In the Arctic, the seal and polar bear are involved in the transmission cycle, and the latter acquires very high levels of infection. The demise of some Arctic explorers has been blamed on killing and eating polar bears infected with trichinosis. This has been speculated as the reason that Franklin and his party died.

Incubation period. 8–15 days.

Period of communicability. Not transmitted from person to person, but animals are probably infectious for the rest of their lives, sometimes acquiring very heavy infections from eating other infected animals on a regular basis.

Occurrence and distribution. Approximately 40 million of the world's population are affected, although trichinosis commonly occurs as localized outbreaks with a group of people all contracting the disease at the same time. A classic example is for a wild pig to be killed and cooked over a fire by turning it on a spit. By this means, only the outside meat is well cooked; inside, the temperature has not been sufficient to kill the larvae. Outbreaks in industrialized countries and in the urban areas of developing countries are commonly caused by eating sausages, especially of the salami type.

Control and prevention. All meat for human consumption should be inspected by cutting into the muscle in several places, where the calcified cysts can be detected with the naked eye. Where

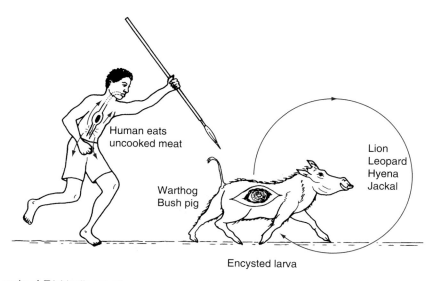

Human eats
uncooked meat

Warthog
Bush pig

Lion
Leopard
Hyena
Jackal

Encysted larva

Fig. 9.7. Life cycle of *Trichinella spiralis*.

an outbreak occurs, such as with eating sausages, the source should be investigated and food hygiene practices enforced.

All meat must be properly cooked until there is no redness in any part of the joint. Cooking slowly for a long time is preferable to cooking quickly or on an open fire where the outside gets overcooked while the inside remains almost raw. Deep-freezing of meat for 20 days, or irradiation, can kill the cysts.

Treatment is symptomatic, with steroids. Mebendazole or albendazole should also be given for 4 days.

Surveillance. Where an outbreak occurs, the participants at the feast will all start having symptoms at much the same time. By counting back 2 weeks from these cases, the source of infection can be localized.

9.10 Other Infections Transmitted by Food

A number of other infections are also transmitted by food although their principal method of transmission is by other means. Any of the faecal–oral diseases covered in Chapter 8 can be transmitted this way, bacillary dysentery, typhoid, hepatitis A, *Giardia* and El Tor type cholera being spread by eating salad vegetables, raw fish or other food. The parasitic worms transmitted by soil contact, *Trichuris*, *Ascaris*, *Strongyloides* and the hookworms (Chapter 10) can also be transmitted by food, especially that grown in soil, such as root crops and vegetables. Hydatid disease (Section 17.2) and toxoplasmosis (Section 17.5) can be acquired through food. Brucellosis (Section 17.6) is often transmitted in goat's milk or cheese made from it, while anthrax (Section 17.7) can (rarely) be caught by eating the meat of a cow that has died from the disease.

Summary

- Infections such as food poisoning can cause disease in any kind of food, whereas helminth diseases and trichinosis result from specific foods in which the organism has a developmental cycle.
- Where food poisoning is suspected, questioning of those involved and a relative risk assessment will determine the likely cause.
- There has been an increase in foodborne diseases due to the globalization and international transportation of foods, particularly meat and poultry.
- Helminth diseases can nearly always be diagnosed by finding the specific egg in the faeces.
- Preventing the contamination of food by good hygiene and its proper cooking are the main methods of control.

Further Reading

Cheesbrough, M. (2005) *District Laboratory Practice in Tropical Countries, Part 1*, 2nd edn. Cambridge University Press, Cambridge, UK.

Cheesbrough, M. (2006) *District Laboratory Practice in Tropical Countries, Part 2*, 2nd edn. Cambridge University Press, Cambridge, UK.

Chiodini, P.L., Moody, D.H. and Manser, D.W. (2001) *Atlas of Medical Helminthology and Protozoology*, 4th edn. Churchill Livingstone, Edinburgh, UK.

Muller, M. (2001) *Worms and Human Disease*, 2nd edn. CAB International, Wallingford, UK.

Pasvol, G. and Peters, W. (2006) *Atlas of Tropical Medicine and Parasitology*. Mosby-Wolfe, London.

10 Diseases of Soil Contact

The soil can be a source of infection for several diseases, particularly those caused by nematodes and the bacterial infection of tetanus. Transmission can either be direct from contamination with the soil as with tetanus bacilli, by swallowing nematode eggs, or from larval penetration of the skin when it comes into contact with the soil. Developmental stages often take place in the soil and this is a necessary environment for the life cycle. The promotion of personal hygiene and preventing contamination of soil through sanitation are the main methods of control for the nematode infections, while vaccination is the main method for tetanus.

Because there is a common mode of transmission for the three main nematode infections (*Trichuris*, *Ascaris* and the hookworms) they nearly always go together, so if the person is infected with one they are likely to have all three (Fig. 10.3). It is this combined effect that causes considerable morbidity in children in developing countries, and if one looks again at Table I.1 it will be noticed that having all three infections brings their importance in terms of DALYs (disability-adjusted life years) to 11th position.

10.1 *Trichuris* (Whipworm)

Organism. The nematode *Trichuris trichiura*, which has a characteristic egg (elongated and with a knob at each end) when seen in faecal specimens (see Fig. 9.1).

Clinical features. A large number of people carry this infection quite asymptomatically, but it has been realised that its debilitating effect, especially in children in developing countries, can be quite considerable. This is especially the case when trichuriasis is associated with other common infections, with the combined effect leading to much ill health. When there are over 16,000 eggs/g of faeces, a chronic bloody diarrhoea, anaemia, rectal prolapse and occasionally appendicitis can result. These infections tend to occur where the child eats earth (pica), which can be a result of iron deficiency. Heavy infections are more likely when there are nutritional deficiencies, especially of zinc.

Diagnosis. The characteristic egg is easily seen in a fresh faecal specimen (Fig. 9.1).

Transmission. The egg develops in the soil and, when swallowed directly or as a contaminant of food, changes into an adult in the caecum. Eggs are most commonly carried on the fingers, or swallowed when the fingers are licked. The soil is readily contaminated from indiscriminate defecation, especially where the faeces are not buried or a latrine is not used. Villages often have traditional places for defecation so the potential for infection is greater when such customary practices are the rule.

Incubation period. It takes 2–3 months for eggs to be found in the faeces after eggs are first swallowed, with symptoms occurring about a month after ingestion.

Period of communicability. Persons can remain infected for several years if not treated, continually contaminating the environment if they have poor defecating practices.

Occurrence and distribution. *Trichuris* is a very common parasite (an estimated 795 million people are infected) and causes far more disability than was formerly thought to be the case (see Table I.1). Most of the infection with debilitating consequences occurs in developing countries, but the parasite is found worldwide (Fig. 10.3).

Control and prevention. Hand washing before meals and the careful preparation of food are the main methods of control. Vegetables and root crops, in particular, must be washed carefully to remove all earth. Parents should discourage their children from eating earth and have anaemia treated with iron supplementation. Proper sanitation should be installed to prevent soil contamination.

Treatment is with mebendazole or albendazole. (See under Hookworms, Section 10.3, for dosage.)

Surveillance. Routine stool investigation of children admitted to hospital will discover a number of nematode infections.

10.2   *Ascaris*

Organism. The nematode worm *Ascaris lumbricoides*.

Clinical features. The fertile egg, when swallowed, hatches in the stomach and the larva penetrates the intestinal mucosa to enter the bloodstream, passing through the venous and pulmonary circulations to the lungs where it breaks through the alveolar wall to emerge in the bronchiole. Migrating to a main bronchus, it ascends the trachea and is swallowed back into the gastrointestinal tract. By the time it reaches the intestines, it has developed into an adult, with the fertilized female laying eggs in the excrement (Fig. 10.1). This common intestinal parasite can occur in considerable numbers without causing any symptoms and is often found when a routine stool examination is performed. When the larvae pass through the lungs, pneumonitis and possible haemoptysis can occur; otherwise, the sheer number of worms can cause intestinal obstruction or blocking of vital structures, such as the common bile duct. Where nutrition is marginal, the loss of nutrient can be sufficient to tip a child into malnutrition. It has been calculated that 25 worms can produce a loss of 4 g protein daily from a diet containing 40–50 g protein. Deficiency of vitamins A and C can also occur. Performance in school is reduced with heavy ascaris infections.

Diagnosis. Direct smear examination of the stool is sufficient for diagnosis (Fig. 9.1). The egg has a strong outer coat, which is stained brown from bile pigments, differentiating it from hookworm eggs, which are of a similar size.

Transmission. The eggs are not infective until they have undergone development in the soil for 1–2 weeks. They require warmth and moisture to develop and will remain viable in the soil for a considerable period of time, awaiting the right conditions. The infective larva goes through stages of development within the egg casing and, if swallowed, infection occurs. Eggs are normally swallowed in polluted water, on vegetables that have been washed with polluted water or by swallowing earth directly. Eggs are passed during indiscriminate defecation.

Incubation period. 10–20 days.

Period of communicability is from 2 months after infection up until about 1 year.

Occurrence and distribution. Ascaris is a very common nematode infection found in all parts of the world and in all strata of society (1.221 billion people are estimated to be infected). Children aged 3–7 years have the highest prevalence.

Control and prevention is with personal hygiene, food hygiene and proper sanitary facilities. The egg is extremely resistant, being unaffected by cold, drying and disinfectants. A temperature of 43°C or over is required to kill the eggs so any composting process using human excreta must maintain this temperature for at least a month (Fig.1.2).

Treatment is with pyrantel pamoate or mebendazole. (See under hookworm, Section 10.3 for dosage.)

Surveillance. As with *Trichuris* infection, it is worth doing routine stool examination on children admitted to hospital as any lessening of the worm burden will improve health.

10.3   Hookworms

Organism. Ancylostoma duodenale and *Necator americanus* cause the two common hookworm infections of humans.

Clinical features. The infective (filariform) larvae directly penetrate the skin and migrate to a blood or lymphatic vessel where they are carried in the circulation to the lungs. Here they break out of the alveoli, find their way up the trachea and enter

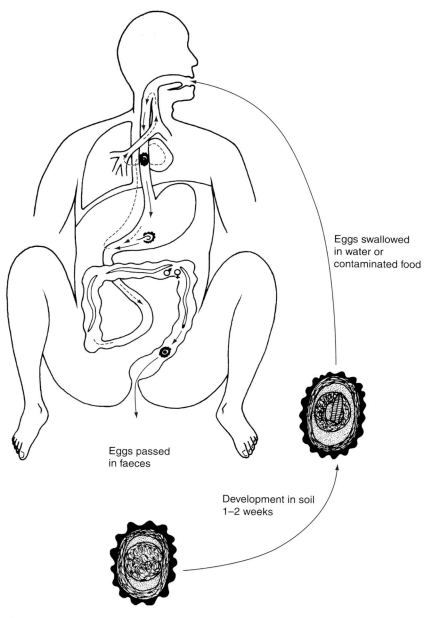

Eggs swallowed
in water or
contaminated food

Eggs passed
in faeces

Development in soil
1–2 weeks

Fig. 10.1. *Ascaris lumbricoides* life cycle.

the gastrointestinal tract. The adult stage is finally reached in the duodenum or jejunum, where the male and female worms mate and produce eggs (Fig. 10.2).

Despite its extensive journey through the human body, like *Ascaris*, the hookworms are very well adapted to their host and only produce symptoms when heavy infections occur. The passage through the skin can result in a transient urticaria (ground itch), while that through the lungs can cause pneumonitis and haemoptysis. Occasionally the haemoptysis can be sufficient to suggest a diagnosis of

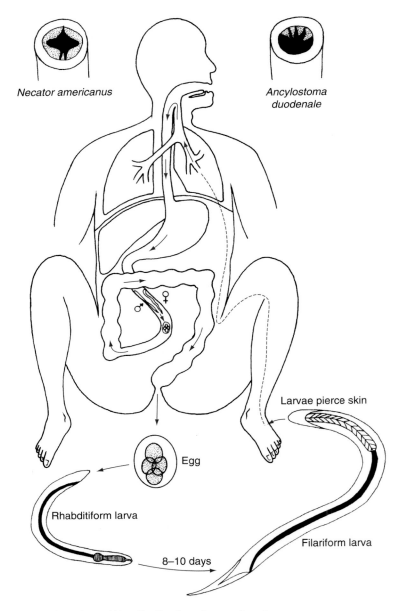

Necator americanus

Ancylostoma duodenale

Larvae pierce skin

Egg

Rhabditiform larva

Filariform larva

8–10 days

Fig. 10.2. The hookworm life cycle and identification from the mouthparts.

tuberculosis. The main effect results from the adult worms attaching to the intestinal wall where they invaginate a piece of mucosa and extract blood and nutrients. Anaemia results from continued blood loss and depletion of iron reserves. The degree of anaemia produced depends upon the worm load, and one estimate calculates that 60–120 worms (measured by 30 worms excreting 1000 eggs/g faeces) will result in slight anaemia, whereas over 300 worms (10,000 eggs/g faeces) will cause severe anaemia. The newly established worm may produce several bleeding points and if the sexes are unbalanced the search for a mate can result in increased activity. These effects will naturally be most profound in the growing child and the pregnant woman. It is the combination of malaria, malnutrition and other intercurrent infections with hookworms that accentuates the seriousness of this infection.

On the plus side, recent research suggests that low-level infections may have a protective effect from the child developing asthma, inflammatory bowel disorders and even diabetes type 1. So long has the parasite been in association with humans that the anti-inflammatory substances secreted by the worms are used to desensitize the body. So a few worms may be an advantage.

Diagnosis. Eggs are found in faecal examination. They are oval and have colourless thin walls that differentiate them from *Ascaris*, which has a thick brown exterior (Fig. 9.1). The eggs of the two hookworm species are identical and only the adults can be differentiated, mainly from their characteristic mouthparts (Fig. 10.2).

Transmission. The eggs are passed in the faeces and hatch within 24 to 48 h to liberate an intermediate (rhabditiform) larva. After some days, it moults to produce the infective filariform larva. In suitable conditions of moist, warm but shaded soil (30°C for *N. americanus* and 25°C for *A. duodenale*) this stage of the larva can live for several months awaiting the opportunity to penetrate through the skin of a new host. (The ingested third-stage larvae of *Ancylostoma* can also produce infection.) The larva commonly penetrates the foot of the unshod person and intense infection can occur where areas of beach or bush are demarcated for defecation purposes. Non-human hookworms can also penetrate the skin and produce cutaneous larva migrans (Section 17.4).

Incubation period is 8–10 weeks.

Period of communicability is from about 2 months after infection to up to 5 years; generally 1 year.

Occurrence and distribution. N. *americanus*, despite its name, is the more widely distributed, being found extensively throughout the tropical belt and well north of the tropic of Cancer in America and the Far East. *A. duodenale* is found in the Far East, the Mediterranean and the Andean part of South America (Fig. 10.3). It has been

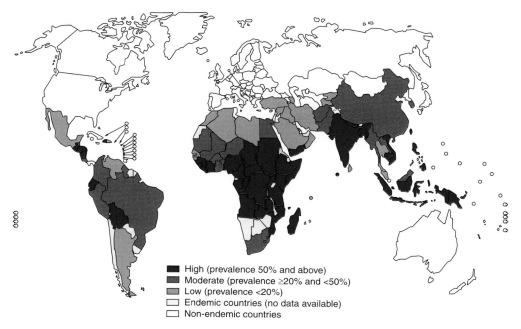

■ High (prevalence 50% and above)
■ Moderate (prevalence ≥20% and <50%)
■ Low (prevalence <20%)
☐ Endemic countries (no data available)
☐ Non-endemic countries

Fig. 10.3. Global distribution of soil-transmitted helminthiasis, 2008. (Reproduced by permission of the World Health Organization, Geneva.)

suggested that *N. americanus* was carried from Africa to the Americas as a result of the slave trade. Altogether some 740 million of the world population have hookworms.

Control and prevention is by use of pit latrines or other methods of sanitation. The wearing of footwear effectively prevents penetration by the larvae. The open sandal type of footwear often worn (thongs, flip-flops) are not effective and infection can readily occur. Mass treatment can be given to reduce the parasite load, but without health education and the proper use of latrines this will only produce a temporary improvement.

Treatment. A number of drugs are effective in treatment: albendazole 400 mg single dose, mebendazole 500 mg single dose or 100 mg twice a day for 3 days; levamisole 2.5 mg/kg daily for 3 days; oxantel 10 mg/kg daily for 3 days; or pyrantel pamoate 10 mg/kg daily for 3 days. The treatment should be repeated 12 weeks after the original course of treatment. There is concern that resistance could develop, as has happened in veterinary practice, so combinations such as mebendazole + levamisole or pyrantel + oxantel have been advocated. In the debilitated child, supportive therapy will need to accompany deworming. Iron supplementation, or in the severe case blood transfusion, will be required to treat the anaemia.

In the treatment of filariasis and onchocerciasis a combination of albendazole plus ivermectin or albendazole plus diethylcarbamazine are used (see Sections 15.7 and 15.8), so treatment of helminths often occurs as an extra benefit. The albendazole plus ivermectin combination is more effective for *Ascaris* and *Trichuris*.

Surveillance. When mass treatment is planned an initial survey will delineate the size of the problem. Follow-up spot checks of individual stool specimens can be made to assess progress.

10.4 *Strongyloides*

Organism. The nematode *Strongyloides stercoralis*, which is morphologically similar to the hookworms. Far less common is *S. fülleborni*.

Clinical features. There are several alternative cycles of development and it is the type of cycle which determines the nature and degree of pathological change, and hence the clinical features.

An infective filariform larva develops in warm moist soil, penetrates the skin and follows the same internal route as the hookworms to the final resting site in the small intestine. However, no eggs are passed to the outside, only rhabditiform larvae are found in the faeces. If environmental conditions are favourable, a free-living cycle takes place, with the rhabditiform larvae developing into adults in the soil. This cycle can be repeated, and the number of potential parasites increases with each completed cycle. If conditions change, filariform larvae are produced, or if unsuitable for the free-living cycle, then the rhabditiform larvae passed in the faeces change directly into filariform larvae. Direct auto-infection can also occur, with the rhabditiform larvae penetrating the intestinal mucosa to enter the bloodstream, without ever leaving the body. In addition, swallowed larvae can complete their development by entering the body through the intestinal mucosa (Fig. 10.4). Achlorhydria, as occurs in malnutrition, makes infection easier by the oral route.

The chronic disease commonly presents as abdominal pain, diarrhoea and urticaria. It is the abnormal cycle of auto-infection that can lead to wandering larvae producing linear urticaria (larva currens) or 'eosinophilic lung'. Larva currens can persist for periods in excess of 40 years. Immunocompromised persons, such as those with human immunodeficiency virus (HIV) infection or malignant disease can develop widespread dissemination of worms, resulting in fever, abdominal distension, shock, jaundice, cough, wheezing and dyspnoea. Pneumonia or meningitis are serious outcomes.

Diagnosis is made by finding the rhabditiform larvae in the faeces or in the aspirate of the duodenal string test. Serological tests can be of value but, where positive, repeat stool examinations should be made to confirm the diagnosis.

Transmission is from direct penetration of the skin by infective stage (filariform) larvae or being swallowed from contaminated food, water or fingers. Soil is contaminated from faeces deposited directly on the ground or inadequately buried.

Incubation period is 2–4 weeks.

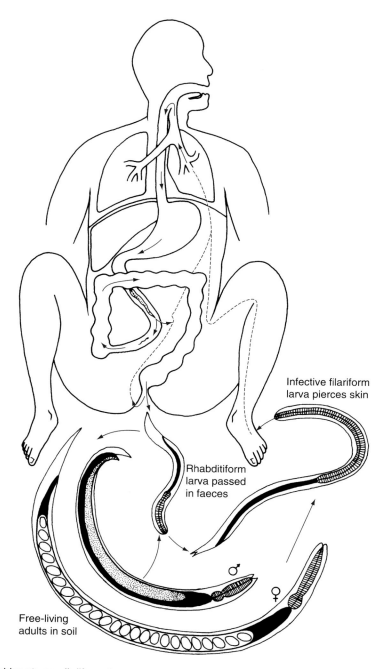

Fig. 10.4. *Strongyloides stercoralis* life cycles.

Infective filariform
larva pierces skin

Rhabditiform
larva passed
in faeces

Free-living
adults in soil

Period of communicability. Due to auto-infection and long-living adult worms, once infected, a person can continue to produce larvae for 30–40 years.

Occurrence and distribution. Mostly found in the warm wet tropics, the parasite also occurs in temperate areas. *S. fülleborni* has only been reported from Africa and Papua New Guinea. Adults rather than children manifest the clinical symptoms, having either acquired the parasite when they were children or in adult life.

Control and prevention. All the methods applicable to the other soil-based nematode infections are applicable, such as personal hygiene, careful washing and preparation of vegetables, and the wearing of adequate footwear. Soil contamination can be prevented by good sanitation.

Treatment is the same as for hookworm.

10.5 Tetanus

Organism. The bacillus *Clostridium tetani* is the causative organism of tetanus. It is a Gram-positive rod with spherical, terminal spores that give it a characteristic drumstick appearance. It produces spores which can remain in the soil for considerable periods of time.

Clinical features. Infection results from the organism entering an abraded surface, such as a cut or scratch. It favours anaerobic conditions, liberating toxin, which produces severe muscle spasms. It is a serious condition in the neonate due to infection of the umbilical cord stump.

The adult presents with muscle spasm and rigidity. There may be trismus, in which the muscle of the jaw and later the back become rigid, leading to lockjaw and opisthotonos. Muscle spasms can produce the characteristic half smile, half snarl of 'risus sardonicus' or the arched back of opisthotonos. These spasms are initiated by external stimuli such as touch or attempts at intubation and every care must be taken to protect the patient from such stimuli. Neonatal tetanus generally presents as a difficulty in sucking, then the rigidity of muscles and generalized convulsions develop. It usually commences within 5–10 days of birth.

Diagnosis is on the clinical presentation.

Transmission. The organism is introduced into a wound from soil, dust or animal faeces. Cutting the umbilical cord with an unsterile instrument, such as a bamboo knife, or traditional practices of treating the umbilical stump are potent methods of causing neonatal tetanus. These can involve the use of unsterile dressings or customary practices using cow-dung or earth poultices.

The bacillus is found naturally in the soil where it survives in anaerobic conditions. Many types of soils have been found to harbour *C. tetani*, but it is more common in cultivated soils, especially those manured with animal faeces. The organism is found in horse and cattle dung, and, less commonly, in pig, sheep and dog faeces. It is occasionally found in human excreta, particularly in people associated with animals.

The vegetative form of the organism is sensitive to antibiotics, disinfectants and heat, but as a spore it is resistant to all but the superheated steam of an autoclave. Indeed, the spores of *C. tetani* are used to test the effectiveness of the sterilizing process because if it cannot survive, then no other organism can (apart from anthrax).

Spores can survive for considerable periods of time, but when they enter a wound or umbilical stump in which there is a low oxygen-reduction potential they release the vegetative form, which grows anaerobically, and infection takes place. It is the moist, contaminated umbilical stump or the traumatized wound that provides suitable conditions for infection to take place.

The replication of the organism is not important, but the (exo)toxin that is produced has a profound effect out of all proportion to the initial infection. This exotoxin has a high affinity for nervous tissue and as little as 0.1 mg is sufficient to kill a person. Toxin is absorbed along the nerves, reaching the spinal cord, where the generalized features of the disease are produced.

Incubation period is 4–21 days, but most cases occur within 14 days. There is a relationship between incubation period and severity, with an incubation period of less than 9 days having a mortality of 60% and a period more than 9 days 25% mortality. This is due to the dose of the toxin.

Period of communicability. Not transmitted from person to person directly or indirectly.

Occurrence and distribution. Tetanus occurs worldwide, with higher rates in Africa, Asia (especially South-east Asia) and the Western Pacific. Neonatal tetanus is a serious problem in Africa, especially where birth practices are rudimentary. There is an association with agricultural areas where animal excreta is commonly used for fertilizing the soil, as a fuel, or as a plaster on the walls of houses. Domestic animals either share the same house as their owners or live in such close proximity that their faeces contaminate the surrounding soil.

Control and prevention. The aim should always be to prevent tetanus with vaccination and good hygiene practices, especially with the newborn.

The most effective way of preventing neonatal tetanus is the vaccination of all women of childbearing age. The policy is to give all women a lifetime total of five doses of tetanus toxoid. This is preferable to waiting until the woman becomes pregnant because many women do not attend antenatal clinic, especially those likely to use traditional applications to the umbilical cord stump. The effectiveness of various strategies is shown in Fig. 10.5. Women should therefore be given their first dose of tetanus toxoid at first contact or as early as possible during pregnancy. The second is given 4 weeks later and the third 6–12 months after the previous dose or during the next pregnancy. Doses four and five are given at yearly intervals. Where a woman has a certificate to say that she has received vaccination as a child then she only needs to have two doses during the first

pregnancy and one more before or during the second pregnancy.

Infants are given tetanus toxoid as part of their childhood vaccination programme in the form of DTP at 6, 10 and 14 weeks of age. An additional booster dose of DTP is given at 1 to 6 years of age and tetanus plus diphtheria as an adolescent. Adults who have not been vaccinated before should be given two doses of adsorbed tetanus toxoid (0.5 ml), separated by 4 weeks, and a third dose of 1 ml 6 months later. Booster doses every 10 years will maintain a high level of immunity.

In the event of a person being injured and presenting with a contaminated wound that could produce tetanus, the following action should be taken after cleaning out the wound and then giving penicillin:

- If the person has been fully vaccinated in the past a booster dose of toxoid is required only if this was more than 10 years ago.
- If there is no record of tetanus vaccination or protection is in doubt, then give the first dose of tetanus toxoid, plus 250 units of human tetanus immune globulin or 1500 units of equine tetanus

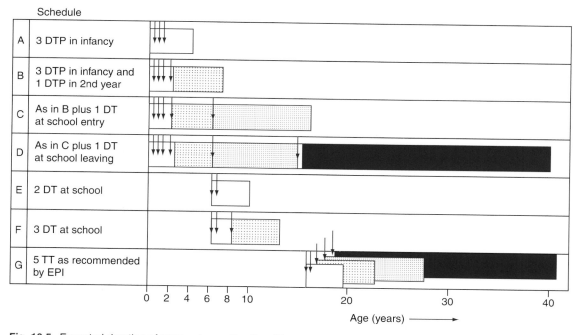

Fig. 10.5. Expected duration of tetanus immunity after different vaccination schedules. DTP, diphtheria, tetanus and pertussis; DT, diphtheria and tetanus; TT, tetanus toxoid; EPI, WHO Expanded Programme of Immunization. (Reproduced by permission of the World Health Organization, Geneva.)

antitoxin, following a test dose. Instruct the person to return at 4 weeks and then 6 months afterwards to complete the course of vaccination.

Good birth practices are important in preventing neonatal tetanus and several countries have developed systems for contacting traditional birth attendants and giving them courses of instruction. Prepacked sterilized blades for cutting the cord can be given, and iodine, spirit or similar antiseptic provided to apply to the cord stump. Where there is no system of traditional birth attendants, but delivery takes place in the home by a mother or other female relative, then an instruction sheet in the local language can be given to the pregnant woman when she attends for antenatal clinic or at any other contact with the health services.

Treatment. Tetanus is a self-limiting disease and if the patient can be kept alive for 3 weeks, then complete recovery should take place, but keeping the patient alive for this period of time is the problem. It is the toxin that is causing the symptoms and once this is fixed in the nerves, only support can be given to maintain respiration, urinary output and nutrient intake. The patient is sedated to reduce the spasms and in all ways expertly nursed. The contaminated wound must be cleaned and excised, antitoxin or immunoglobulin administered and penicillin given to kill any remaining organisms. Sadly, the mortality of tetanus is high, 40% in adults and 90% in neonates, so the objective should always be to try to prevent it.

Surveillance. The World Health Organization (WHO) has set out to eliminate maternal and neonatal tetanus (it can never be eradicated because *C. tetani* will always remain in the environment) as a health problem through intensified vaccination, the promotion of clean delivery practices and a programme of school vaccination. High-risk areas need to be identified from a knowledge of the birth practices, lack of health facilities or preponderance of cases. All children at school entry should be required to bring their vaccination certificates with them and if these are not adequate receive a course of tetanus toxoid. The target date has had to be revised, but Togo was declared free in 2006, India, Egypt and Mali in 2007, Zambia in 2008 and Burundi and Comoros in 2011.

Summary

- Several helminths require soil for the infective stage to develop whereas the tetanus bacillus lives in soil contaminated by animal excreta.
- Infection is acquired either by eating the soil, as a contaminant of food or water, or by penetrating the skin (hookworms, *Strongyloides*) or via a wound (tetanus).
- Personal hygiene and the prevention of soil contamination are preventive methods in the helminth infections, while clean delivery and vaccination prevent tetanus.

Further Reading

Chiodini, P.L., Moody, D.H. and Manser, D.W. (2001) *Atlas of Medical Helminthology and Protozoology*, 4th edn. Churchill Livingstone, Edinburgh, UK.

Muller, M. (2001) *Worms and Human Disease*, 2nd edn. CAB International, Wallingford, UK.

Pasvol, G. and Peters, W. (2006) *Atlas of Tropical Medicine and Parasitology*. Mosby-Wolfe, London.

11 Diseases of Water Contact

Water is an important medium for the transmission of disease processes. Normally, it is through drinking water which has become polluted by faecal material that infection is transmitted, or where it is used to wash food and the food subsequently eaten. Water also serves as a medium for fish or other organisms to live in; these may carry a parasitic stage that is transmitted when they are eaten (as covered in Chapters 8 and 9). This chapter describes one important disease that is still a problem (schistosomiasis) and one that is almost eradicated (guinea-worm disease, or dracunculiasis); both are transmitted by contact with water in which the intermediate stages are free living. Until its transmission cycle has been worked out Buruli ulcer is also included here, as contact with water seems to be its main epidemiological feature. Minimizing water contact with these infections is therefore the best method of control, if it can be applied.

11.1 Schistosomiasis

Organism. The main parasites are *Schistosoma haematobium*, *S. mansoni* and *S. japonicum*. Other species, such as *S. intercalatum* and *S. mekongi*, do occur, but they are only important in well-defined areas and their epidemiology and control are similar to those of one of the three main types.

Clinical features. Infection normally starts in childhood, often with very few signs of the disease until adulthood. Passing blood in the urine is one of the first signs of *S. haematobium* disease, but because it is so common in the local area it is generally ignored; boys thinking it quite normal that they should have period bleeding like girls do. Infection and egg output increases up to about 15 years of age and then declines; individuals vary in their response, some persons acquiring heavy infections and developing severe pathological changes,

while others have only minor symptoms. The more serious manifestations are liver fibrosis, portal hypertension and obstructive urinary problems, the pathology depending upon the species of parasite and the number of eggs deposited in the tissues; *S. mansoni* and *S. japonicum* infections lead to intestinal and liver damage, while *S. haematobium* infection leads to bladder complications, including bladder cancer.

Diagnosis is made by finding the characteristic eggs (Fig. 9.1), in *S. haematobium* in the urine, and in *S. mansoni* and *S. japonicum* in the faeces or from a rectal snip. Urine samples are best collected between 11.00 and 15.00 when egg output is at a maximum. Leaving the urine to stand, centrifuging it, or passing it through a filter increases the chance of finding eggs. While qualitative diagnosis is required in the individual case, quantitative estimates are more valuable in epidemiological investigations. In *S. haematobium*, the simplest method is to pass 10 ml of urine through a filter in a Millipore holder. The paper or membrane is taken out, dried and stained with ninhydrin and the eggs counted directly. Immunological methods, IFAT (immunofluorescence antibody test) and ELISA, have also been developed for schistosomiasis, but they only indicate recent or past infection, so eggs must be looked for to confirm the diagnosis. However, these tests are useful in epidemiological surveys for rapidly defining the extent of the infected area.

Pathology is related to the number of worms, which can be measured by the number of eggs produced. In *S. haematobium*, the production of 50 eggs/ml of urine or above is regarded as the level of severe pathology and much of present-day control strategy is aimed at reducing the egg count to below this level.

Transmission. Infection results from cercariae directly piercing the skin of a person when they go into the water. On penetrating the subcutaneous layer of the host, the cercaria becomes a schistosomule, migrates to the lungs and finally develops into an adult in the portal vessels of the liver. Both male and female worms are required, so pairing takes place prior to migration to the final destination in the mesenteric or vesical plexus. Adult worms can live 20–30 years, but are active egg producers for 3–8 years, although some have produced viable eggs for over 30 years. The egg output/day in *S. haematobium* is some 20–250, in *S. mansoni* 100–300 and in *S. japonicum* 1500–3500. It is this massive output of eggs in *S. japonicum* that leads to the more rapidly developing and severe pathology of infection with this parasite.

Less than 50% of eggs manage to pass through the bladder or intestinal wall to develop further, the remainder being trapped in the tissue. On reaching water, a temperature of 10–30°C and the presence of light induce hatching. Miracidia actively search out a snail using geotactic and phototactic behaviour, homing in on a chemical substance 'miraxone', inadvertently liberated by the snail. The miracidium must penetrate a snail within 8–12 h, their chance of success decreasing with age. Some 40% of snails are infected at a distance of 5 m in still water, but where the water is moving similar infection rates can occur at a far greater distance. Normally, infection occurs in water flowing at 10 cm/s or less. Even after the rigours of the journey, when miracidia have entered the correct species of snail, many are inactivated and only a small proportion develop into sporocysts. This is determined by the part of the snail entered and immunity to reinfection developed by the snail.

Cercariae are stimulated by light to emerge from the snail when the ambient temperature is between 10 and 30°C. Cercarial emergence increases as daylight penetrates the watery environment, producing a peak for *S. mansoni* at 12 noon and for *S. haematobium* in the mid-to-late afternoon. With *S. japonicum*, the stimulus produced by light is delayed and maximal cercarial liberation occurs at 23.00 h. The number of cercariae issuing from a snail can be immense, in the order of 1000–3000/day, but this depends upon the species and relative size of the snail. Where more than one miracidium has penetrated a snail there is depression of cercarial production; this may also occur if the snail is host to other trematode infections. Cercarial output is greatest in *S. mansoni*, less in *S. haematobium* and least of all in *S. japonicum*. Cercariae

survive for 24 h, but their greatest chance of penetrating the host is when they are young. When cercariae enter within 2 h of release only 30% die, but this rises to 50% at 8 h and 85% at 24 h.

The snail intermediate hosts are species specific, *Bulinus* spp. in *S. haematobium*, *Biomphalaria* spp. in *S. mansoni* and *Oncomelania* spp. in *S. japonicum*. They are illustrated in Fig. 11.1. They can adapt to a wide range of habitats, from natural waterways to temporary ponds and cultivated rice fields. Whenever there is sufficient organic matter on which to feed, snails will be found. Within a body of water, distribution may be quite irregular with dense colonies in some places and complete absence in others. Various factors which may influence snail colonization, are:

- Electrolyte concentration. Snails demand a minimum calcium concentration, and cannot tolerate high salt content or a low pH.
- Light is not required by the snail, and they can often survive in near total darkness.
- Rainfall may herald the end of the dry season and provide water in which snail populations can increase, but if the rainfall is too heavy it may flush out the snails, resulting in a subsequent decrease. Snail populations may therefore follow a seasonal pattern.
- Temperature rise encourages expansion of the population up to a maximum of approximately 30°C.
- Density is a limiting factor and results in reduced growth.
- Aestivation or the ability of snails to survive out of the water for weeks or months allows populations of snails to continue from one season to another, possibly also transferring immature infections of *S. haematobium* and *S. mansoni*. The snail host of *S. japonicum* can survive conditions of desiccation best of all.

Snails are capable of self-fertilization, although cross-fertilization is more common. Their reproductive capacity is phenomenal and a single snail can produce a colony within 40 days and be infective in 60. When conditions are optimal, many species of snails will double their population in 2–3 weeks. In measuring the age of snail populations, size of snails is a useful indicator. A large number of small samples from several different areas are preferable to a few large samples in estimating the numbers and density in watercourses. Infection rates in snails are generally low, only some

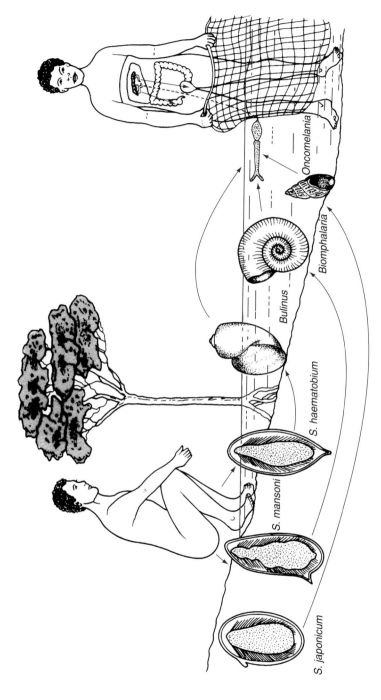

Fig. 11.1. Schistosomiasis life cycles and species.

S. japonicum

S. mansoni

S. haematobium

Oncomelania

Bulinus

Biomphalaria

1–2% of the colony being infective, but even so, this level is sufficient to account for high prevalence rates in the human population.

Humans contaminate water either by urinating or defecating into or near watercourses. Egg output is variable between individuals and at different times in their lives; a few individuals have heavy infections and egg outputs, while the majority have light infections. In areas of high endemicity, children between 5 and 14 years are responsible for over 50% of the contamination. As the infection rate declines, then older age groups become more important.

People are infected by collecting water, washing (both clothes and the person), in their occupations (such as fishing) or during recreation. Children are most commonly infected when they play in the water, while in adults it is when they carry out their domestic duties or occupations. Infection is generally due to repeated water contact over a long period of time, but can occur from a single immersion if it coincides with a large number of cercariae in the water.

Animals such as water buffalo, cattle, pigs, dogs, cats and horses can also serve as reservoirs of *S. japonicum*, but they are less important than humans as sources of infection.

Incubation period. 2–6 weeks.

Period of communicability. 10–20 years.

Occurrence and distribution. *S. haematobium* and *S. mansoni* were originally diseases of Africa, where they are widely distributed, but with the massive exodus of slaves that took place in the 17th and 18th centuries this legacy was carried with them. The East African slave trade carried *S. mansoni* to the Arabian peninsula, and *S. haematobium* to the Yemen and Iraq. The Western trade was solely in *S. mansoni*, which found a suitable snail host in South America and the Caribbean. *S. japonicum* probably originated in China, where it has been discovered in mummified bodies, but is also found in the Philippines, Taiwan and Sulawesi in Indonesia (Fig. 11.2). No cases have been found in Japan since 1978. A separate species, *S. intercalatum*, pathogenically similar to *S. mansoni*, is found in the Congo, Cameroon, Central African Republic (CAR), Chad, Gabon and São Tomé. *S. mekongi* is restricted to the Mekong River basin in Laos, Thailand and Cambodia. Other localized species are *S. malayensis* in Peninsular Malaysia and *S. mattheei* in southern Africa.

Control, prevention and treatment. There are two approaches to the control of schistosomiasis:

- Reduce the transmission of the parasite.
- Reduce the level of infection in individuals.

The first attempts to control the parasite while the second aims at minimizing the pathological effects. The various methods of control are:

Reduce contamination of the environment. Humans pollute the environment by urinating or defecating into bodies of water. This can be minimized by encouraging the use of latrines. Unfortunately, it is very difficult to get everybody in a family or community to always use a latrine and the few non-users will be sufficient to maintain a level of pollution (see Section 2.4.2). There is also the longevity of the adult worms, meaning that prevalence rates will remain static in the community for a considerable period of time.

Reduction of the snail intermediate host. The snail is a vulnerable link in the life cycle of the parasite and can be attacked in an effort to break transmission. The various methods that can be used are:

- predators;
- biological control;
- water management and engineering; and
- molluscicides.

Various kinds of fish (*Tilapia* and *Gambusia* particularly) are natural predators, but they will only reduce snails to a certain level unless they have an additional source of food when there are few snails left. Snails, especially of the *Marisa* and *Helisoma* genera, compete for food supplies and *Marisa* will even prey on eggs and juveniles of *Biomphalaria*. Another approach to biological control is the sterile male technique, but as many snails are hermaphrodite, this is only suitable with *Oncomelania*.

Where foci of infection consist of small and temporary ponds these can be drained or filled (by controlled tipping of household refuse). Where canals and irrigation systems are responsible, then a concrete lining, increasing the rate of flow and any method to reduce vegetation can discourage snail habitation. Unfortunately, these methods are rarely effective on their own and need to be combined with a molluscicides, niclosamide (Bayluscide), which can be administered as a liquid, which is suitable for treating moving water, or as granules in

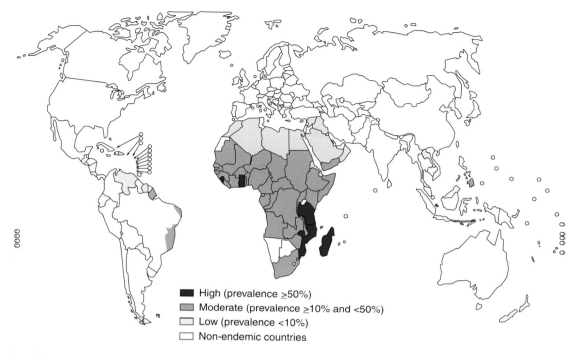

High (prevalence ≥50%)
Moderate (prevalence ≥10% and <50%)
Low (prevalence <10%)
Non-endemic countries

Fig. 11.2. Global distribution of schistosomiasis, 2009. (Reproduced by permission of the World Health Organization, Geneva.)

lakes and ponds. Continuous application is required to have a sustained effect on the snail population. This method has the disadvantage of killing fish and is expensive. Cheaper preparations, such as copper sulfate, are still in limited use and naturally occurring plant preparations such as Endod (*Phytolacca dodecandra*) have shown promise. However, the remarkable recovery of snail populations once control methods are removed, and the cost of molluscicides, make snail reduction a less effective approach to schistosomiasis control.

Reduction of water contact. Preventing water contact can be highly effective in the individual. Various ways of encouraging this are:

- Health education, especially in schoolchildren, but this is often ineffective unless an alternative, e.g. swimming pool, is provided.
- Providing places to wash has been disappointingly ineffective for the cost involved.
- Where areas of absent or minimal transmission occur in occupational or recreational bodies of water, people can be encouraged to use these, rather than the heavily infected parts.

- Wearing rubber boots when wading through water, or if accidental exposure occurs then rubbing vigorously with a towel and applying 70% alcohol.
- Drinking water can be treated with iodine or chlorine, or if left to stand for at least 48 h cercarial die-off will be complete.

Reduction of human infection by mass chemotherapy. Praziquantel (PZQ) single dose mass drug administration at 40mg/kg is now the method of choice. A suitable target population is schoolchildren between 5 and 15 years of age, where mass therapy is used. Alternatively, only the positive cases, or those with heavy infections, are treated following a simple diagnostic procedure. Individual treatment, based on worm-load estimation, aims at disease control by reducing morbidity. It permits limited resources to be more widely spread and attempts the less ambitious target of disease reduction rather than transmission reduction.

The antimalarial drug artemethur is also valuable in the control of schistosomiasis and could be

---

used in areas where there is no malaria, such as China, southern Brazil and South-west Asia. It can be used in combination with praziquantel.

Reduction of the animal reservoir. Animal reservoirs are responsible for maintaining *S. japonicum*. In order of importance these are dogs, cows, pigs, rats and water buffalo. As most of these are domestic animals, proper animal management can reduce contamination of the environment. Vaccination of domestic animals could be used. Baboons and monkeys have been shown to be reservoirs of *S. mansoni* and could play a part in maintaining infection. There is little prospect of controlling these animals.

Vaccination. There are difficulties in preparing a vaccine because the schistosome is able to absorb host antigen and mask its presence, but several vaccines are under trial. A 28 kD *S. haematobium* GST (glutathione-S-transferase) vaccine is showing some promise, while *S. mansoni* antigens have also been tried, but no vaccine has shown more than partial protection. Another approach is to reduce egg production in female worms, with which some success has been achieved in *S. japonicum*.

Strategies for schistosomiasis control. Various different approaches to the control of schistosomiasis have been tried depending on the resources and nature of the disease, as follows:

- The raising of economic standards by the provision of water supplies, sanitation, environmental engineering and water management has been shown to be effective on a long-term basis in countries such as Japan and China.
- In well-controlled irrigation schemes, molluscicciding on its own may be effective. Where discipline and motivation of the population are less certain, then a double approach of mass chemotherapy and reduction of water contact is more effective.
- When resources are meagre and the greatest benefit for limited finance is required, then treatment of high worm load cases is the method of choice.

Surveillance. Effectiveness of control strategies can be measured by:

- change in incidence rate;
- a shift in peak prevalence to an older age group;
- reduction in geometric mean egg output; and
- greater awareness of socio-economic values, e.g. the use of water supplies and sanitation facilities.

11.2 Guinea Worm

Dracunculus medinensis, the largest of the nematode worms to attack humans, used to be a serious problem in India, Pakistan, southern Iran, most of West Africa and the Sudan, infecting some 80 million people. It is spread by spilt water washing larvae back into an unprotected well or by infected people using walk-in wells. The World Health Organization (WHO) launched an eradication programme to make all wells safe with a surrounding wall and concrete apron so as to prevent spilt water from washing back into the well. Walk-in wells were converted into lift wells or alternative water supplies provided. By these simple strategies, *Dracunculus* infection has been eradicated from most of the area. In 2011, only 1058 cases of dracunculiasis were recorded. This has been the most successful eradication programme to use such a simple strategy (Fig. 11.3).

11.3 Buruli Ulcer

Organism. *Mycobacterium ulcerans* is found in the exudate of the Buruli ulcer. The organism produces a unique toxin, mycolactone, which causes necrosis of tissues.

Clinical features. There is at first just a small papule surrounded by shiny skin, but this soon breaks down to reveal a large necrotic ulcer with undermined edges. Tissue damage may be extensive, involving bone and other structures. Some 60% of lesions are on the lower limbs, 30% on the upper limbs and 10% on the rest of the body. Disabling contractures can result and squamous cell carcinoma is a longer term complication.

Diagnosis is made on clinical grounds and from a stained smear of the exudates, using Ziehl–Neelsen stain for acid-fast bacilli. Specimens can also be taken by fine needle aspiration or punch biopsy. The early detection of mycolatone will allow a better method of diagnosis. Culture of the organism at 30–33°C can also be made, but this takes 6–8 weeks. A PCR has been developed that takes 2 days.

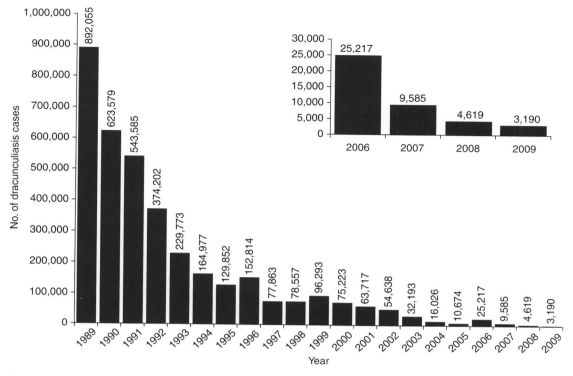

Fig. 11.3. Annual number of dracunculiasis cases reported worldwide, 1989–2009. (Reproduced by permission of the World Health Organization, Geneva.)

Transmission. The method of transmission has not been elucidated, but there are presumed to be environmental factors due to the relationship with rivers and wetlands. Bacteria may be associated with insects, snails or water plants. *M. ulcerans* has been found in the salivary glands of biting water insects, but it is thought that this is just part of the water environment in which the organism thrives rather than being a means of transmission. Focal outbreaks have followed migrations and movements of people, such as those due to floods or dam construction. In Australia, koalas and possums are found naturally infected. Infection may be transmitted from these animals to humans by mosquitoes.

Incubation period. Unknown.

Occurrence and distribution. Four countries in West Africa, Benin, Côte d'Ivoire, Ghana and Togo, have an increasing incidence, but other countries in Africa, and Central and South America, Australia and New Guinea also have cases (see Fig. 11.4). Children and women living near rivers or wetlands in a rural situation are predominantly affected. There has been a progressive increase in cases and more attention is being given to working out the transmission and how to control the infection.

Control and prevention. Health education in areas of high endemicity, with the provision of facilities for treating lesions as soon as they occur, has reduced the period of debility and the severity of the deformities.

Treatment. Treat with rifampicin and streptomycin/alizarin for 8 weeks. The earlier treatment is started the more effective it will be. Surgical excision of the ulcer and skin grafting may be necessary in the advanced case, which also benefits from antibiotic treatment to reduce the size of the ulcer.

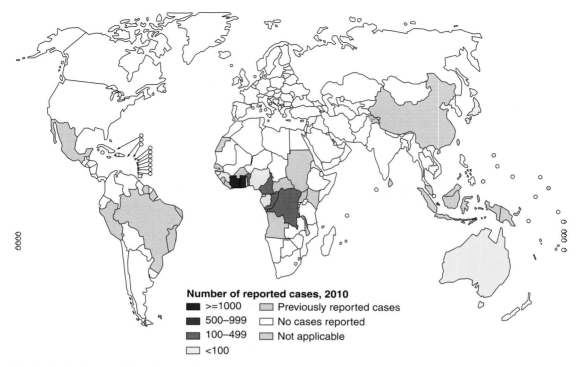

Number of reported cases, 2010

■ >=1000   ▨ Previously reported cases
■ 500–999   ▢ No cases reported
▨ 100–499   ▨ Not applicable
▢ <100

Fig. 11.4. Distribution of Buruli ulcer worldwide, 2010 (Reproduced by permission of the World Health Organization, Geneva).

Surveillance. WHO is collecting information on Buruli ulcer using forms BU01 and BU02 available on www.who.int/buruli/control/en/, from which more information can be obtained.

Summary

- Infection with schistosomiasis is due to cercariae in water, which have developed in an intermediate host snail, penetrating the exposed skin.
- Water becomes contaminated by faeces or urine so effective sanitation, the reduction of snails and preventing water contact are methods of control in schistosomiasis. The most effective method is mass treatment, administering praziquantal to schoolchildren or selectively to those with serious pathology.
- Guinea worm has been effectively controlled by mechanical methods to make water collection

safe, leading to its eradication from many countries.
- A water-involved method of transmission is indicated in Buruli ulcer, but this has not been fully worked out.

Further Reading

Mahmoud, A. (2001) *Schistosomiasis, Tropical Medicine: Science and Practice – Tropical Medicine 3*. Imperial College Press, London.

Web resources

Schistosomiasis Control Initiative (SCI), Imperial College London. Available at: www3.imperial.ac.uk/schisto (accessed 1 March 2012).

WHO Buruli ulcer [information], World Health Organization, Geneva, Switzerland. Available at: www.who.int/buruli/en/ (accessed 1 March 2012).

12 Skin Infections

The skin is a common site for several communicable diseases, presenting with rashes of various kinds. Infection is often transmitted from person to person directly by skin contact or by other means, especially the airborne route. Control is by the avoidance of contact with infected individuals and, where available, the use of vaccines.

Some skin infections, tropical ulcers and those due to scabies and lice have been covered in Chapter 7 as they share common methods of control. Typhoid often has an accompanying skin rash but is more appropriately covered with other faecal–oral disease in Chapter 8. Meningococcal meningitis often presents with a petechial rash and is covered in Chapter 13. Many of the arbovirus diseases present with skin rashes but as their method of transmission is by vectors they are covered in Chapters 15 and 16.

12.1 Chickenpox/Shingles (Varicella)

Organism. Herpesvirus varicella-zoster virus (VZV).

Clinical features. A generally mild disease, chickenpox is a common infection of children. Illness commences with fever followed by a characteristic skin rash of macules, papules, vesicles, pustules and dried crusts. The lesions occur in groups, appearing over several days, so pocks of different stages will be seen at the same time. In chickenpox the rash is distributed centrally, appearing on the chest and abdomen and sparsely on the feet and hands.

The majority of people contract the disease in childhood when it is an inconvenience rather than a life-threatening condition, but if this has not occurred and they subsequently develop the illness as adults it can be very serious. This is a particular problem in island and isolated communities, where varicella can be a fatal disease in the elderly. Pregnant women who contract the disease in late pregnancy or shortly after delivery are at risk of severe generalized chickenpox with a 30% mortality. Neonates who develop chickenpox within 10 days of birth are also liable to a serious generalized infection. Chickenpox in early pregnancy may result in congenital malformations. Death results from generalized viraemia, pneumonia, haemorrhagic complications, encephalitis or cardiomyopathy.

The virus remains latent in the body, lodged in nerve bundles, and in later life, especially during a debilitating disease (such as human immunodeficiency virus (HIV) infection), the identical virus (VZV) causes shingles. This presents as a vesicular rash with erythema in a well-defined area of skin supplied by the affected dorsal root ganglia. Pain and paraesthesia occur along the course of the affected nerve.

Diagnosis is on clinical criteria, especially the central distribution of the rash and the presence of lesions at different stages, which differentiate it from smallpox. Vesicular fluid can be taken to confirm the diagnosis with PCR or immunofluorescence. Any case of a pox rash that dies or has an unusual distribution should be a smallpox suspect (see Section 19.3) and be reported (see Section 5.3).

Transmission. The infection is transmitted by fluid from the vesicles. This can occur in the pharynx before the main rash, when transmission is by droplets; otherwise spread is by direct skin contact, airborne dispersion of vesicle fluid or through articles soiled by discharges.

Incubation period is from 2 to 3 weeks.

Period of communicability is from 3 days before the onset of the rash to 6 days after its first appearance.

Occurrence and distribution. Chickenpox occurs worldwide in epidemic form, often spreading serially (Section 2.2) from one place to another. A disease of children in temperate regions, it is more commonly found in adults in the tropics.

Control and prevention. One attack of chickenpox confers lifelong immunity, so it is preferable for children to have the disease rather than be protected and run the risk of developing it as adults. Special groups such as neonates, pregnant women and the sick should be protected by preventing cases of chickenpox from coming into contact with them. In hospital, cases of chickenpox should be isolated.

A live attenuated varicella virus vaccine has been developed, but is not widely available. It is useful for vaccinating high-risk groups, such as women of childbearing age who have not had chickenpox and the immunocompromised. There is a risk in using vaccination by shifting the age of developing naturally acquired chickenpox to older age groups where the disease is more serious, so it is unlikely to become part of the routine childhood vaccination programme. However, where a child over 13 has not had chickenpox then vaccination with two doses given 4–8 weeks apart can be considered.

Treatment. Acyclovir and vidarabine can be used to treat adults, children with serious disease and older persons with shingles. Human varicella-zoster immunoglobulin (VZIG) is available in some centres and can be used within 10 days of exposure for contacts liable to develop severe disease, such as pregnant women, neonates and the immunosuppressed.

Surveillance. Outbreaks should be reported so that susceptible individuals can be protected and given vaccination if available. Any suspect case of smallpox must be reported to the World Health Organization (WHO) (Section 5.3).

12.2 Measles

Organism. Measles virus is a member of the Paramyxoviridae family of viruses.

Clinical features. Measles normally commences with a prodromal fever, cough, conjunctivitis and small spots (Koplik's spots) most easily seen inside the mouth. The characteristic blotchy rash begins on the third to seventh day of the illness, generally on the face, but soon spreads to the whole body.

In developing countries, measles is a serious disease and accounts for a considerable amount of mortality and morbidity in the childhood population. It has a particularly severe effect on the nutritional status of the child so the healthy child will lose weight and the malnourished child will become critically ill. The peak of infection is between 1 and 2 years of age, at the very time when breast milk alone is an inadequate source of food and weaning foods may not yet have been introduced. The association of nutritional change and measles can be, and often is, a lethal combination.

There are a number of reasons for the nutritional depletion produced by measles. Any disease process puts extra demands on the body, increasing catabolism. Fever and the desquamation of all epithelial surfaces demands protein replacement, which is handicapped by a sore mouth, often secondarily infected by *Candida*, preventing the child from sucking properly, so that even breast milk is not taken. Then from the other end, diarrhoea, which is such a common feature of measles in developing countries, discharges further the body reserves. But perhaps the greatest weight loss is due to immunosuppression, much of this taking place after the child has recovered from the acute attack.

The disease process attacks all epithelial surfaces, producing most of its complications in the respiratory tract. Pneumonia is the commonest complication, while laryngotracheobronchitis is serious, with a high mortality. Acute respiratory infections (ARIs, see Section 13.2) are one of the leading causes of childhood ill health, and the sequelae of measles responsible for a large component of this problem. If the acute pneumonia does not kill, the damage done makes the child more susceptible to further attacks of respiratory infection when the measles has long gone.

The effects on the eye can cause blindness. Corneal lesions result from epithelial damage, which can lead to ulceration, secondary infection and scarring. In severe cases, perforation or total disorganization of the eye can occur. These severe effects only result if there is concomitant Vitamin A deficiency, so giving Vitamin A to all measles cases is effective. Measles, by its nutritional and direct effects, has been regarded as the most important cause of blindness in a number of tropical countries.

Measles is an important cause of otitis media. It can also result in encephalitis, either the acute form or a late slow-onset sclerosing panencephalitis, which is always fatal.

Diagnosis is on clinical criteria, but measles IgM can be found in the saliva with immunological tests.

Transmission. Although the main feature of measles is the skin rash, it is transmitted by the airborne route, from nasal and pharyngeal secretions. This can be by articles contaminated with secretions, such as cloth or clothing used to wipe a running nose, as well as by respiratory droplets produced in a coughing bout. Virus can remain active in droplets in the air or on surfaces for up to 2 h.

Measles is the most contagious of all infectious diseases and no age is spared. In the Fijian outbreak in the 1870s, adults as well as children succumbed, so that whole families were affected at the same time, deprivation and starvation resulting in a high death rate. Now that adults have experienced measles as children, the age of infection is getting younger. This is explained by greater contact of communities due to improvement of communication, while the intense social contact at a very young age (babies carried on their mothers' backs) gives maximum opportunity for early transmissions.

Incubation period. 10–14 days.

Period of communicability is from 1 day before the first signs of infection until 4 days after the rash starts (or 4 days before to 4 days after the rash begins).

Occurrence and distribution. Measles has been a severe infection in Western Countries for a considerable period of time, producing mortality in poor and slum populations similar to that now seen in developing countries. Introduced with European exploration, it caused devastating epidemics, particularly in island communities, some of which never recovered their former population numbers. However, in many developing countries, in which it is a major problem, there is evidence that measles has been present for several 100 years, the pattern having changed from sporadic epidemics with all ages involved to one of endemicity in which the under 5 year olds are predominantly affected.

Control and prevention of measles is by vaccination. As measles is such an infectious disease, it can be reckoned that every child will develop it. Some 10% will either have such a mild infection or be partially protected by maternal antibodies as to appear not to have been infected. A further 10–20% will not have measles until the following year owing to the epidemic effect, so the expected number of cases of measles can be calculated from the birth rate minus 25%. If the birth rate in a developing country is 50/1000 then 75% of this means that 37.5 cases of measles/1000 can be expected each year, which represents 37,500 cases in an administrative unit of a million people. Calculations like these can be used to estimate the number of children to be vaccinated and hence the vaccine requirements.

At least 80% of susceptibles will need to be vaccinated to produce control of the disease, but a lower target may be acceptable in more isolated communities. This target will need to be achieved every year in rural areas, but as much as every 6 months in urban areas. Measles vaccine is 90% effective if the cold chain is not broken.

Maternal antibodies protect the newborn infant for the first 6 months of life, but thereafter the child becomes readily susceptible to infection with a peak around 1 year. The seroconversion rate is some 76% at age 6 months, 88% at 9 months and 100% at 12 months. Giving measles vaccination at 1 year would produce the best conversion, but by that time in developing countries some 50% will already have had the disease. Giving it at 6 months will be before all but a few have had the disease, but the seroconversion rate is so poor that not many will be protected. The best compromise is a first vaccination at 9 months, with a second vaccination at 12–18 months. In conditions of high infectivity, such as during an epidemic, admission to hospital or in a refugee camp, or in areas of high HIV prevalence (or if the infant has HIV), then reducing the age of vaccination to 6 months is justified. In this case, two further vaccinations should be given, the second between 12 and 15 months.

In developed countries, vaccination is given at 12–13 months so the time taken to reduce the incidence in the population will be less, as shown in Fig. 12.1. The greater the coverage the more rapidly this is achieved. For example, 60% coverage will theoretically take 12 years to reduce the

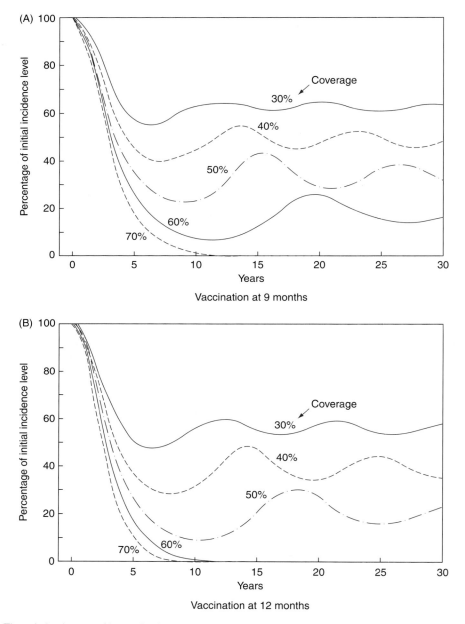

Fig. 12.1. The relative impact of immunization programmes on measles incidence in the age group 0–19 years, according to age at vaccination and population coverage. (Reproduced by permission from Cvetanović, B., Grab, B. and Dixon, H. (1982) *Bulletin of the World Health Organization* 60(3), 405–422.)

incidence to zero if vaccination is given at 12 months, but will never be achieved with vaccination at 9 months. However, 70% coverage will achieve zero incidence with vaccination given at 9 months;

this is being achieved by an increasing number of developing countries.

Effective measles vaccination coverage will not only reduce the number of children developing the disease in an epidemic, but will have the secondary benefit of raising the age of developing the disease, as can be seen in Fig.12.2. Epidemics had occurred in the Namanyere area of Tanzania regularly every second year until 1978, when there was only a minor increase, the main epidemic being delayed until 1979. This meant that children born in 1977 who could have expected to become infected in their second year of life (1978) had had their measles put off until 1979 when they were beyond the age of maximum mortality.

The chances of a susceptible child developing measles when admitted to hospital are very high as it is already sick with another complaint. It is fortunate that measles vaccine can produce protective immunity quicker than the wild virus (about 8 days for the vaccine and 10 for the disease), so as long as the child is vaccinated within 48 h of admission, it will be protected. Because of the severity of disease in the debilitated child, there are very few contraindications and the malnourished and those with minor infections should all be vaccinated. HIV infection is not a contraindication as the child is more likely to die from measles than from any complications of receiving a live vaccine.

As vaccination coverage is increasing, a potential problem could arise because less maternal antibody is produced by mothers who have acquired their immunity from vaccination rather than by having measles. This means that infants of a younger age will become susceptible, so vaccination may need to be given earlier if coverage is not complete.

Measles vaccine is conveniently combined with rubella (MR) or both with rubella and mumps (MMR) in countries intending to vaccinate against these diseases. Despite adverse publicity given to the MMR vaccine, no complications have been confirmed and the vaccine should continue to be used. However, MMR or MR should only be used in countries with a high vaccination coverage (over 80%) or else there is a danger of shifting the age of developing rubella, and hence congenital rubella syndrome (CRS), to women of childbearing age (see Section 12.3).

Because of the effectiveness of measles vaccination, there is the very real hope that measles can be eliminated as a public health problem. A measles elimination programme has therefore been launched by WHO, and in 2010 the region of the Americas had eliminated measles. Measles deaths have been reduced by 78% from an estimated 733,000 in 2000 to 164,000 in 2008, three out of four of these deaths being in India.

Treatment. There is no specific treatment, but supportive therapy with fluids and easily digested foods needs to be given. Vitamin A supplementation should be given to all children with measles. Complications may require additional treatment, such as antibiotics for bacterial chest infections.

Surveillance. All cases of measles should be recorded and monthly totals charted to indicate

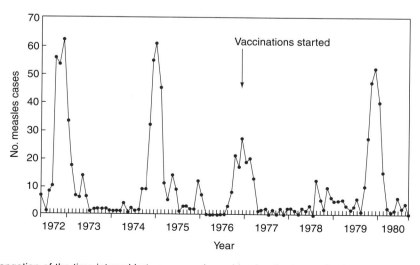

Fig. 12.2. Prolongation of the time interval between measles epidemics due to vaccination in Namanyere, Tanzania.

epidemics and estimate when new epidemics will occur (Fig. 12.2). Measles has a seasonal pattern, which can vary markedly from country to country (Fig. 1.9.) so this needs to be determined to work out the best time to supplement routine vaccination programmes. If measles cases are focal then this may indicate gaps in vaccination coverage (Fig. 3.2). As all children should be vaccinated an estimate of vaccine coverage can be made by comparing the number of new vaccinations with the number of children born.

12.3 Rubella

Organism. Rubella virus, a member of the Togaviridae family of viruses.

Clinical features. Infection in the adult is generally mild, presenting with a maculopapular rash of short duration, fever, conjunctivitis and cervical lymphadenopathy. Some 20–50% of infections are subclinical. However, if the woman is pregnant, especially in the first 10 weeks of pregnancy, her developing infant will suffer from CRS. The congenital defects are more gross the earlier in pregnancy infection is acquired, resulting in stillbirth in the first few weeks. Otherwise, a range of congenital defects can result in ophthalmic complications (cataracts, glaucoma, microphthalmia, pigmentary retinopathy and chorioretinitis), auditory complications (deafness), cardiac complications (patent ductus arteriosus, pulmonary artery stenosis and ventricular septal defects) and microcephaly. In addition, infants are more likely to suffer from meningoencephalitis, hepatitis and thrombocytopenia. Milder defects will develop between the 11 and 16th weeks, and after the 20th week of pregnancy there is no further risk.

Diagnosis is by detecting IgM from serum or saliva, and is important if infection in a pregnant woman is suspected.

Transmission. The virus is transmitted in droplets from the nasopharynx by the airborne route or by direct contact. Most infections are acquired from children and adults during an outbreak, but infants with CRS can produce virus from pharyngeal secretions and urine for up to 1 year so are a potent source of infection.

Incubation period. 15–20 days.

Period of communicability. From 7 days before the onset of the rash to 4 days after. CRS infants continue to shed virus for up to 12 months.

Occurrence and distribution. There is a worldwide distribution, but the importance of rubella in developing countries has not been appreciated until comparatively recently. It occurs in epidemic form, probably because of the number of susceptibles in the population, with children becoming infected at 2–8 years of age in urban areas and 6–12 years in rural areas.

Control and prevention. The objective is to prevent CRS by vaccination of children and adults. Although adolescent girls and women of childbearing age are the target population, just vaccination of this group will never eliminate rubella so all children of both sexes should ideally be vaccinated. However, if the vaccination programme is far from complete the effect will be to postpone the age of infection to older and more dangerous ages in women likely to become pregnant. Developing countries therefore need to decide between protecting adolescent girls and women of childbearing age only, with no attempt to eliminate rubella, or to vaccinate all children aged 9–15 months as part of the routine childhood vaccination programme. If the vaccination programme is considered sufficiently efficient to embark on the latter strategy, then an extra campaign to target all women and girls over 12 should be run at the same time for the first few years of introducing rubella vaccination.

If a policy of childhood vaccination is adopted then rubella vaccine is best administered with measles vaccine as MR, or in combination with measles and mumps as MMR (see Sections 12.2 and 12.4).

Surveillance. An estimate of the level of CRS can be obtained from hospital records and MCH (maternal and child health) records of deaf and blind infants. Measles vaccination records and numbers of cases of measles are good indicators of the efficiency of the childhood vaccination programme in deciding which strategy of rubella vaccination to introduce.

12.4 Mumps

Organism. Mumps virus is a member of the Paramyxoviridae family of viruses.

Clinical features. Mumps is not a true skin infection, but is included here as it shares a common means of control with measles and rubella. It is an infection of the salivary glands, producing enlargement and pain in the parotid gland, but can lead to orchitis, mastitis, meningitis, pancreatitis and acute respiratory symptoms (see Section 13.2). Commonly an infection of children 2–5 years of age, the serious manifestations are more likely in adults, especially males.

Diagnosis is made on clinical grounds, but serological confirmation can be made with mumps-specific IgM, a rise in IgG, or culture of saliva or urine.

Transmission. The virus is transmitted via direct contact or by droplets spread by the airborne route. Any contact of saliva, such as sharing of cutlery, wiping the mouth with a common cloth or kissing, can result in transmission.

Incubation period. 14–24 days.

Period of communicability. 6 days before to 6 days after the start of parotitis.

Occurrence and distribution. Mumps is probably more common than realized, with up to 85% of the population found to have been infected by the time they are adults, although few will have manifested the disease. With such a high proportion of the population meeting the virus there is a relatively high risk of complications and cost–benefit studies have shown that vaccination produces substantial economic savings.

Control and prevention. The reason for including mumps in the routine childhood vaccination programme is similar to that for rubella (Section 12.3). Where there is an efficient programme with the majority of children being vaccinated then it is advantageous to include it with measles and rubella as the MMR vaccine. However, if less than 80% of children are vaccinated than this could result in an epidemiological shift to older age groups, increasing the likelihood of complications. If mumps vaccination is included then a second opportunity, either by the routine programme or by catch-up campaigns, should be given, unless coverage is over 90%.

Treatment. Oral hygiene and the relief of symptoms. Cases should be isolated.

Surveillance. Comparing the number of children born with those that complete their childhood vaccinations or are vaccinated against measles will give an estimate of the efficiency of the vaccination programme and whether mumps vaccination should be added.

12.5 Streptococcal Skin Infections

Organism. Streptococcus pyogenes, group A.

Clinical features. Streptococcal infections of the skin can present as pyoderma, impetigo, erysipelas or scarlet fever. Pyoderma and impetigo are superficial skin infections with vesicles, pustules and crusts. Erysipelas is a red, tender, oedematous cellulitis of the infected limb or part of the body, originating from the point of infection, with moderate fever. Scarlet fever presents as a generalized rash that blanches on pressure, with high fever, strawberry tongue and flushing of the cheeks. In some cases there is an appreciable mortality, or else the disease can result in otitis media, glomerulonephritis or acute rheumatic fever (Section 13.10). Although not a skin infection, streptococci can also cause puerperal fever due to post-delivery infection of the female genital tract (see Section 18.3.3).

Diagnosis. The characteristic features of the infection, especially with scarlet fever, can be diagnostic, with confirmation by culture of the organism from the point of infection or the pharynx on to blood agar.

Transmission is mainly by the respiratory route or direct contact with the skin lesion (in impetigo). Flies can transfer the organism and are a major means of infecting scratches and wounds in tropical countries. The organism can be carried in the nose, pharynx, anus and vagina, or in chronic skin lesions, and is an important cause of hospital infections.

Incubation period. 1–3 days.

Period of communicability. 10–21 days or until a chronic infection has been treated.

Occurrence and distribution. Worldwide, predominantly in children, but scarlet fever is more common in temperate regions. Infected skin lesions either due to streptococci or staphylococci are very common in tropical regions.

Control and prevention. Treat all cases promptly and dress infected lesions in a sterile manner. Any person with an infected lesion should not be involved in operations or hospital duties until healed. Personal hygiene, especially the washing of hands after defecation and the discouragement of nose picking should be advocated. Use of proper latrines and the control of flies are longer term preventive measures.

Treatment. Benzathine penicillin G intramuscular, or penicillin G or V orally.

Surveillance. Scarlet fever and puerperal fever are notifiable diseases in some countries.

12.6 Leprosy

Organism. Mycobacterium leprae.

Clinical features. Leprosy more dramatically than any other disease illustrates the conflict between the infecting organism and the host. *M. leprae* is widespread in the environment, yet only a small proportion of people ever show clinical symptoms of the disease, and the few that contact the disease respond in different ways to the challenge.

The generation time from inoculation to multiplication of a stable number of *M. leprae* is only 18–24 days, but the development of the disease will take anything from 7 months to in excess of 7 years (mean 3–6 years). The first lesion is described as indeterminate (Fig. 12.3), because at this early stage it is impossible to decide to which place in the spectrum of disease it will develop. There is either a single ill-defined, slightly hypopigmented macule, commonly seen on the face, trunk or exterior surfaces, or there may be a small anaesthetic patch. The lesion will then develop into a lepromatous or tuberculoid type, or oscillate in the transitional state of borderline leprosy between these two extremes.

Lepromatous leprosy (LL) reflects the complete breakdown of the host's immune responses and the maximum infection with *M. leprae*. In the early stages, signs of disease may be very few but a skin smear will reveal large numbers of mycobacteria (multi-bacillary). Early signs that have been described but rarely observed are oedema of the legs and nasal symptoms of stuffiness, crust formation and blood-stained discharge. These are unlikely to be recognized as leprosy and it is generally not until the more obvious skin lesions become apparent that the diagnosis is made.

Leprosy lesions favour the cooler parts of the body so the buttocks, trunk, exposed limbs and face are the more likely sites. Lesions may be macules, papules or nodules, with or without a colour change, and often show lack of sweating when the patient becomes hot. The signs of nerve damage do not appear until much later in lepromatous leprosy, with a concurrent thickening of the skin of the forehead, loss of eyebrows and damage to the cartilage of the nose. The eyes are also attacked with an infiltrative keratitis, iritis and eventually blindness.

Tuberculoid leprosy (TT) is at the opposite end of the spectrum, showing the full response of cell-mediated immunity to the attacking organism (Fig.12.3). *M. leprae* has a predilection for nervous tissue and it is within this nervous tissue that the cell-mediated response takes place, causing early damage to the nerves. The tuberculoid patient therefore tends to present early with signs of weakness or loss of sensation. Palpation of the nerves will often demonstrate a thickening with loss of sensation or motor power in the distribution of the affected nerve. The ulnar nerve as it bends over the medial epicondyle at the elbow, or the lateral popliteal nerve where it curves round the neck of the fibula, are good places to palpate nerves for thickening. Dermal lesions are not raised, often appearing as apparently normal areas of skin, but lacking sensation or sweating when the patient exercises. Occasionally though, lesions are well defined and scaly with raised edges, but quite different from the succulent macules and papules of lepromatous leprosy. Loss of sensation should be demonstrated with a pin as well as with light touch. A skin smear in tuberculoid leprosy is nearly always free of bacilli (pauci-bacillary), so the diagnosis depends upon the detection of nerve damage.

Borderline leprosy, as its name suggests, is on the border between the two extremes of lepromatous and tuberculoid leprosy. True borderline (BB) leprosy is uncommon, with the disease tending to progress to either the lepromatous (BL) or tuberculoid (BT) part of the spectrum. Signs therefore vary between the two extremes with features of each, but predominating in the features of one or the other. Borderline leprosy is common, but its instability leads to reaction and nerve damage, which can often be severe.

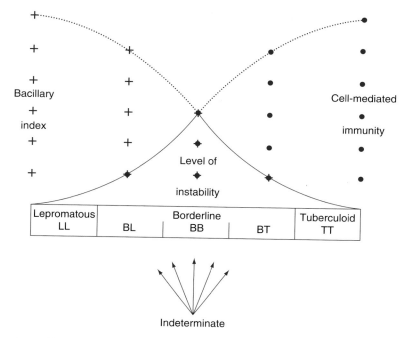

Fig. 12.3. The spectrum of leprosy, illustrating the proportion of bacilli present, the cell-mediated immune response and the level of instability in the different forms of the disease.

Where the host response is adequate and cell-mediated immunity high the disease tends towards the tuberculoid end of the spectrum; where response is low the disease tends to lepromatous leprosy. Simultaneous HIV infection will shift the host response from tuberculoid towards lepromatous. Otherwise, the host response can vary over the course of the illness, producing reactions, which can either be upgrading (towards tuberculoid leprosy) or downgrading (towards the lepromatous). These are type 1 reactions. The nearer the case is to the centre of the spectrum the more severe the reaction. Type 1 reactions may affect all tissues, or skin and nerves only, or produce a generalized systemic reaction.

A different type of reaction (type 2) is found in lepromatous and borderline lepromatous cases and is associated with massive destruction of bacilli. Immune complexes are formed in the tissues and these lead to an increased reaction in existing lesions. The characteristic finding is erythema nodosum leprosum, which appears on the skin as painful red nodules, commonly on the face and exterior surfaces.

Diagnosis. A skin smear is made from every suspected case of leprosy, collecting dermal tissue without drawing blood. A negative smear does not mean that a case is not leprosy, as tuberculoid cases rarely have mycobacteria. Smears are stained with Ziehl–Neelsen stain and the number of mycobacteria counted to give the *bacillary index.*

6+	Over 1000 bacilli in an average field
5+	100 to 1000 bacilli in an average field
4+	10 to 100 bacilli in an average field
3+	1 to 10 bacilli in an average field
2+	1 to 10 bacilli in 10 fields
1+	1 to 10 bacilli in 100 fields

Mycobacteria can also be obtained from nasal scrapings of the inferior turbinate. A skin biopsy is taken from tuberculoid and borderline patients, or a nerve biopsy where there is no skin lesion.

Transmission. After a long period of uncertainty it has finally been shown that leprosy is transmitted via droplets from the nose and mouth during close and frequent contact. Large numbers of bacilli are found in the nasal discharges of lepromatous cases, and these are able to survive for 2–7 days outside the body. Individuals vary in their susceptibility and it is possible that repeated doses of bacilli, or a large infective dose, are required to produce disease.

Incubation period. 1–20 years.

Period of communicability. Possibly 1 month to 20–30 years. Treatment with rifampicin renders the patient non-infectious after 3 days.

Occurrence and distribution. Leprosy is found mainly in the tropical regions of the world, with poor socio-economic conditions probably a major factor. Lepromatous leprosy is more common in Asia and tuberculoid in Africa. This differing susceptibility might help to explain the response to BCG (Bacillus Calmette–Guérin) vaccination (see Section 13.1) in these two peoples. BCG given at birth can produce a hypersensitivity and change the cell-mediated immunity from negative to positive, but some people appear to have no natural immunity and remain always susceptible to the lepromatous form of the disease. BCG protected over 80% of school children in Uganda, but only 40% of children under 5 years of age in Myanmar.

Leprosy can occur in an epidemic as well as an endemic pattern, but owing to the incredibly protracted life history of the disease, the epidemic form is rarely seen. Between 1921 and 1925 there was an epidemic on the Pacific island of Nauru; 30% of the population was infected and the disease was notably non-focal. All ages were susceptible, with most people developing tuberculoid (BT–TT) leprosy which healed spontaneously.

It has been estimated that up to 5% of people are susceptible to lepromatous leprosy and contact with a lepromatous case increases the risk of infection. Children and young adults are more commonly affected, but the children of leprosy patients do not develop lepromatous leprosy any more frequently than the general population. It would seem that leprosy is very similar to tuberculosis (TB) in that the organism is more common than realized, asymptomatic infections may occur, but only those that are susceptible will develop the disease.

Due to active control measures and multi-drug therapy there has been a marked reduction of leprosy in the world, with less than 213,000 people infected in 2010. Foci of high endemicity remain in Angola, Brazil, Central African Republic (CAR),

Democratic Republic of Congo (DRC), India, Madagascar, Mozambique, Nepal and Tanzania.

Control and prevention. The immediate control is a reduction of the leprosy reservoir by case finding, treatment and follow-up, especially of those with the lepromatous form of the disease. A small proportion of cases will present themselves, but an active search must be made for others, concentrating on selective groups. Schoolchildren should receive priority, as they are likely to contain a quarter of all cases and a higher proportion of new ones. Also, contacts of any case should be examined at frequent intervals, as leprosy is more common in those people that have prolonged contact with a leprosy case. All new cases are treated by multiple drug therapy (see below).

BCG vaccination induces hypersensitivity and increased resistance to developing leprosy in some ethnic groups, so is valuable in the prevention of leprosy as well as TB (Section 13.1). *M. leprae*-based vaccines are under trial in several countries, with promising results. The long-term reduction of disease will require an improvement in general hygiene, better housing and less overcrowding.

Treatment is determined by the bacillary index of the case.

1. High risk (multi-bacillary) LL and BL cases: A three-drug regime consisting of rifampicin 600 mg once a month supervised, dapsone 100 mg daily self-administered, clofazamine 300 mg once a month supervised, then 50 mg daily self-administered. Treatment should be continued for a minimum of 12 months.
2. Non-bacillary cases, BT or TT: Rifampicin 600 mg once a month supervised, plus dapsone 100 mg daily self-administered, for 6 months or six monthly doses within a 9 month period.
3. Non-bacillary single skin lesion: Single dose of rifampicin 600 mg, ofloxacin 400 mg and minocycline 100 mg.

All patients with positive skin smears at the start of treatment should have repeat skin smears at 6 and 12 months. Clofazamine has the advantage of being anti-inflammatory as well as bacteriostatic so can be used in the treatment of reactions at a dose of 100 mg three times a week. Steroids and thalidomide are useful in the treatment of reactions.

Part of any leprosy programme is the development of a rehabilitation service. This not only encourages leprosy patients to present themselves for treatment, but helps to return them as participating members of the community. Much can be done from limited resources, such as making sandals out of old tyres and pieces of wood. The elements of rehabilitation are to protect anaesthetic limbs, actively treat sores and ulcers, and provide support (including surgery) to restore function. The eyes are also damaged in leprosy and supportive treatment can do much to prevent blindness from developing.

Surveillance. Dedicated leprosy field workers have been found to be of considerable value in detecting new cases and following up cases under treatment, otherwise a system within the existing health service should be developed. Combining leprosy and TB surveillance is a useful economy.

Initially, whole populations should be screened in areas of high endemicity, then concentration should be on examining schoolchildren and all contacts of cases. All cases should be registered, often managed as a combined programme with TB. Section 13.1 on TB follow-up and registration is equally applicable to both diseases.

Summary

- A number of infections present with skin rashes; they are mainly transmitted by droplets or contact with contaminated surfaces and articles.
- Reduction in contact and personal hygiene are important, but measles, mumps and rubella are all prevented by vaccination.
- Leprosy is a decreasing problem in the world as a result of active searching and a well-managed treatment regime.

Further Reading

Grosset, J.H. (1998) *WHO Expert Committee on Leprosy. Seventh Report-Technical Report Series No. 874*, World Health Organization, Geneva.

World Health Organization (2005) *The Current Evidence for the Burden of Group A Streptococcal Disease*. Discussion Papers on Child Health, No. WHO/FCH/CAH/05.07. WHO Ref. No. WHO/FCH/CAH/05.07; WHO/IVB/05.12. WHO, Geneva.

Web resources

WHO leprosy elimination home page. Available at: www.who.int/lep/en (accessed 2 March 2012).

13 Respiratory Diseases and Other Airborne-transmitted Infections

The vulnerable respiratory apparatus is easily invaded by microorganisms. Breathing is continuous and as respiratory gases are wafted in and out infecting organisms find free passage to deep inside the body. The site of entry is commonly the nasopharynx, but entry can also occur through the oropharynx and the conjunctiva. The lachrymal glands drain into the nasopharynx and experimental studies have shown that this is often a more certain method of infection than directly through the nose. The respiratory system also includes connections to the middle ear, the sinuses and the gastrointestinal tract.

The ciliated lining and mucus-secreting cells of the respiratory tract can act as non-specific host defence mechanisms entrapping microorganisms and passing them to the exterior. In attempting to expel these secretions from the body by coughing or spitting, organisms may be transmitted to another host. The lymphoid tissues, especially the tonsils and adenoids, guard the respiratory apparatus, but sometimes may themselves become foci of infection.

Respiratory infections are transmitted by direct contact during coughing and sneezing, and generally the closer the contact the greater the chance of spread. Droplets are also sprayed on to surfaces and contact with these by hands and fingers can be just as important a method of infection. As contact between human beings is a necessary part of life, control becomes more difficult and non-specific. Even so, the respiratory diseases are an enigma, the voluminous quantities of expelled organisms are sufficient to infect entire populations, yet only some individuals manifest disease. It is the infective dose and the host response that determine whether infection will occur. Environmental factors that increase the infective dose (e.g. overcrowding) or reduce the host resistance (e.g. malnutrition or concomitant infections) can have a marked effect.

This chapter includes airborne-transmitted infections that present as diseases of the respiratory system and also diseases of other systems of the body that are transmitted by the airborne route. Most of the skin infections, covered in Chapter 12, are also transmitted by the airborne route.

13.1 Tuberculosis

One of the major diseases in the world, tuberculosis (TB) is a considerable problem in developing countries. Not only are a proportion of the population infected with a debilitating and often fatal disease, but the period of infectiousness is prolonged (approximately 5 years in an untreated case), permitting transmission to many other persons. Indeed, in a number of countries an endemic balance has been achieved whereby the number of cases that resolve spontaneously, are cured by medical treatment, or die, are replaced by an equal number of new cases entering the TB pool. Infection with human immunodeficiency virus (HIV) has added to the likelihood of people developing TB, so it is increasing in sub-Saharan Africa. Worldwide, 8 million persons develop TB every year and 2 million die from it. It is estimated that 13.17 million people are co-infected with both HIV and TB.

Organism. *Mycobacterium tuberculosis*, but infection can also be caused by *M. bovis* (from cattle) or *M. africanum*. There are many mycobacteria occurring naturally in nature, including *M. avium*, *M. intracellulare* and *M. scrofulaceum*, that can sensitize the individual and interfere with the BCG (Bacillus Calmette–Guérin) vaccination against TB. In endemic countries, *M. tuberculosis* is widespread, and a quarter to a third of people in developing countries will develop the disease.

Clinical features. A productive cough with weight loss, fever and anaemia are the most important signs of TB. Any chronic cough persisting for 3 weeks or more, especially if there is also weight loss and anaemia, should be regarded as a possible case of TB, and sputum smears taken. Haemoptysis is an important diagnostic sign; there may be streaking of the sputum with blood or coughing up of fresh blood. A difficulty arises with the HIV-positive person as in this case a chronic cough is not a good indicator of TB; rather, night sweats lasting for more than 3 weeks, combined with a cough or fever of any duration, should be used instead.

TB infects people over a spectrum of severity depending on the host response, the dose of organisms and the length of time. The first sign of infection is the primary complex in which the organism is localized to an area of the lung, with a corresponding enlargement of the hilar lymph nodes. In the majority of people, this heals completely or with a residual scar, and the person develops immunity to further challenge. If healing does not occur, then the focus extends to cause glandular enlargement, pleural effusion or cavity formation. The third phase of the disease results from complications of the regional nodes. These may be obstructive, leading to collapse and consolidation, cause erosion and bronchial destruction or spread locally. The final stage is one of bloodstream spread, disseminating bacilli to all parts of the body where they may produce tuberculous meningitis or miliary infection. Longer term complications are those of bones, joints, the renal tract, skin and many other rare sites. These features are illustrated in Fig. 13.1.

The risk of developing local and disseminated lesions decreases over a period of 2 years. In the majority of cases, if the disease is going to progress, it will do so within 12 months of infection or 6 months from the development of the primary complex. By the end of 2 years, 90% of complications will have occurred. Bone and other late complications make up a very small proportion beyond this time.

Diagnosis. TB is spread by droplet infection, so sputum-positive cases transmit the disease much more efficiently than those whose sputum is negative on microscopy. The risk to the community is therefore from pulmonary TB and the emphasis should be on finding these cases by taking a sputum smear, ideally confirmed by culture. The comparative costs of diagnostic techniques are:

Smear	0.02
Culture	0.20
Sensitivity	0.40
Full plate X-ray	1.00

Fifty sputum smears can be made for the equivalent cost of one X-ray and this comparative cost should be considered when diagnosing cases in the community. Anybody presenting to the health services with a cough for 3 weeks or more should be asked to produce some sputum and a smear made; this is dried and treated with Ziehl–Neelsen stain for acid fast bacilli. X-ray examination has a high sensitivity so is of more value in countries with a low incidence of TB and plentiful resources, but sputum microbiology is still necessary to confirm the diagnosis and provide cultures for drug-susceptibility testing.

A fully automated DNA test, the nucleic acid amplification test (NAAT), which simultaneously detects positive cases and rifampicin drug resistance is set to revolutionize the diagnosis of TB. It is more sensitive than ordinary sputum smears, which depend upon the accuracy of the microscopist, and gives results within 100 min, so suspected cases can be diagnosed and started on treatment much more rapidly. The test is particularly useful for detecting TB in the person with HIV as well as the multi-drug-resistant case.

When a new case is diagnosed, a simpler form of search is made in the house and surrounding households. Any contacts of the case, such as family or friends, are examined to see if anybody has a productive cough or clinical signs, and a smear made. Contacts should be given BCG. Chemoprophylaxis is given to children under 6 years old and to contacts positive for HIV, and followed up at regular intervals. Follow-up information can all be included in the national registration system.

Transmission is by the airborne route with coughing and spitting the main methods of disseminating the organism. Many people meet the tubercle bacillus in early life, acquire resistance and are quite unaware of ever having come into contact with it. A proportion, approximately 5%, will manifest the disease in varying levels of severity. This might be nothing more than an enlargement of the primary focus with a few systemic effects, and resolve spontaneously, while other cases may have respiratory symptoms or progress rapidly to bloodstream spread, presenting as a case of miliary infection or tuberculous meningitis. The type and severity of the disease is determined by the host response, but why one person should develop TB and another not cannot generally be determined.

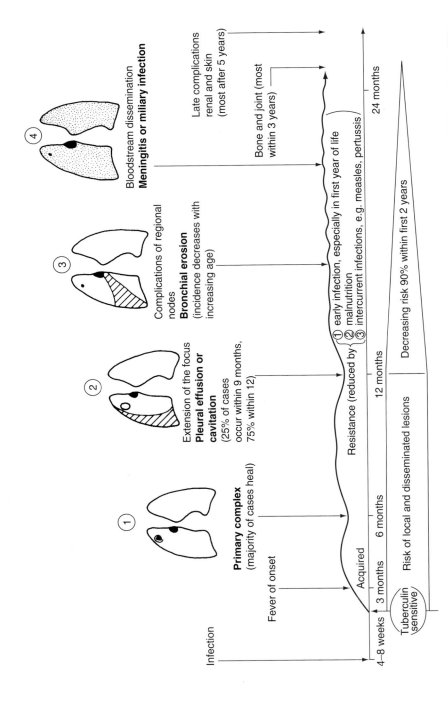

Fig. 13.1. The evolution of untreated primary tuberculosis. (Modified figure. Reproduced by permission from Miller, F.J.W. (1982) *Tuberculosis in Children*. Churchill Livingstone, Edinburgh, UK.)

There is some evidence that susceptibility may be genetically determined as people who have suffered from TB, even if adequately cured, are more likely to develop a new infection a second time. Some families are particularly susceptible, as with the famous literary family the Brontës, in which first the mother died from TB, followed by nearly all the children, yet the father never succumbed to the disease. The dose of bacilli might also be important because young children in close contact with an active case more commonly develop severe TB (miliary or meningitis). Factors that are known to reduce resistance are:

- young age, especially the first year of life;
- pregnancy;
- malnutrition;
- intercurrent infections such as measles, whooping cough and streptococcal infection;
- HIV infection; and
- occupations or environments that damage the lung (mining, dust, smoke).

As well as variation among individuals, there are also considerable differences in the susceptibility of populations. This can be measured by the annual TB infection rate, which compares the tuberculin reaction of non-vaccinated subjects of the same age every 5 years. With BCG vaccination at birth, this can no longer be done, but data obtained before this became a universal policy is still valid. Another method of estimating incidence is from TB notifications, as shown in Fig. 13.2.

Environmental factors are also significant in infection, and the population density is as important as its susceptibility. The dose of bacilli that the individual will meet is increased by continued contact over a period of time. This dose/time factor is more likely to be found in conditions of poverty and overcrowding. If the dose is sufficiently large and maintained for long enough, even the defences of the immunologically competent individual may be broken down.

The risk of infection is greatest in the young and rises again in the old, so overcrowding increases the opportunity for infection to be acquired at a younger age. As the young mix extensively they will also have a greater opportunity to pass on the infection. At the other end of life, the elderly often form persistent foci in a community – a potent source of infection to the young.

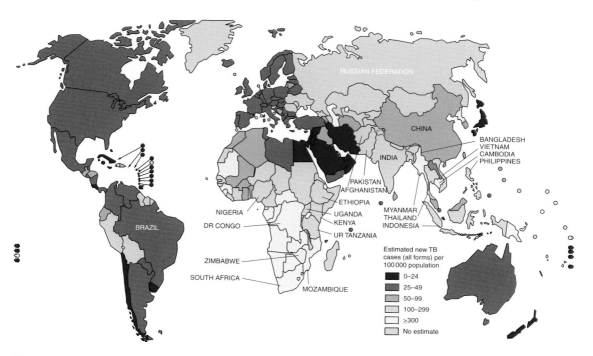

Fig. 13.2. Estimated TB (tuberculosis) incidence rates, 2010. Note key: the lighter the colour, the higher the incidence. (Reproduced by permission of the World Health Organization, Geneva.)

HIV infection has changed the epidemiology and presentation of TB, especially in Africa, leading to more lower lobe and extrapulmonary disease. (There are estimated to be more than 20 million persons worldwide with dual TB and HIV, the majority of these in Africa.) Reduced host response has increased susceptibility and allowed reactivation or reinfection to take place, as well as increasing the likelihood of new infection from a contact or case. However, there is evidence to suggest that HIV/TB patients are less infectious than those with just TB. Conversely, TB patients are more likely to rapidly progress to full-blown acquired immunodeficiency syndrome (AIDS) when infected with the HIV virus. Initially, HIV-infected TB patients commonly present with pulmonary infection similar to the HIV-negative case, but as the disease progresses extrapulmonary TB predominates and other manifestations of HIV disease such as chronic diarrhoea, generalized lymphadenopathy, oral thrush and Kaposi's sarcoma become more common. All HIV-positive cases should therefore be investigated for TB and all TB cases tested for HIV. Despite the increase in extrapulmonary TB, it is still the sputum-positive case that is responsible for transmission of infection and this must remain the priority in searching for cases.

Consumption of unpasteurized milk may result in bovine TB in humans where the disease is present in the animal population. This presents with enlargement and suppuration of the cervical lymph nodes rather than pulmonary disease. It is now less common than formerly with the testing of cattle and pasteurization of milk, but in developing countries where cattle and their produce are an important part of the diet, such as in Central and South America, bovine TB is still found.

Incubation period. The period between infection and development of the primary complex is 4–12 weeks.

Period of communicability. A new, untreated case of TB will normally produce organisms for 12–18 months, but in those that develop a low-grade infection with a chronic cough, infection can continue for a considerable period of time (about 5 years). Once treatment has started, the person becomes non-infectious in about 2 weeks.

Occurrence and distribution. TB may well be one of the most ancient of human diseases, having been detected in bones submerged off the coast of Israel dating to 9000 years ago. It is found worldwide (Fig. 13.2) at various levels of severity. In 2008, there were estimated to be 9.6 million to 13 million cases of TB with 1.3 million deaths. There were an additional 0.52 million deaths from TB in HIV-positive persons. The majority of TB is found in the WHO South-east Asian Region (34%), Africa Region (30%) and Western Pacific Region (21%). In 2008, India and China had an estimated 35% of the total TB cases in the world.

Countries of low TB prevalence are defined as those where less than 10% of children under 15 have a positive tuberculin test. These are largely the countries of Western Europe and North America. TB is, however, increasing in Eastern Europe and the former USSR. Nearly the whole of the tropical world has a high prevalence rate, with some countries experiencing over 50% of the under 15 year olds tuberculin positive. Also, urban areas have higher rates than rural areas. There are high rates in Africa and parts of South America. Asia, India, Myanmar, Thailand and Indonesia all have high tuberculin-positive rates too. In the Americas, the indigenous peoples have a much higher TB rate than the non-indigenous. There is a high susceptibility in Pacific Islands in which TB was an unknown disease until the arrival of explorers, who introduced the disease.

Control and prevention. There are four main strategies for the control and prevention of TB, in the following order of priority:

- search and contact tracing for new cases;
- adequate treatment of all cases, especially the sputum positive;
- improvement of social and living conditions; and
- BCG vaccination.

Vaccination by BCG induces cell-mediated immunity to the mycobacteria but does not generate humoral immunity, as do other vaccines. BCG vaccination therefore alerts the body's defences rather than inducing antibody formation. After a BCG vaccination, a primary infection will still take place, but the progressive or disseminated infection will be reduced. BCG protects against miliary and meningitis infection, the worst kinds of childhood TB, but does not have much effect on adult cases, which are generally the source of infection.

The effectiveness of BCG varies considerably in different countries. In Europe there is a good response, while in India it is marginal. This is thought to be due to atypical mycobacteria circulating in the environment, so BCG should be given in developing countries at birth or as soon after as possible. In developed countries, BCG is given selectively to high-risk groups, such as immigrants. BCG should not be given to children who are known to be HIV positive, even if they are asymptomatic, nor to pregnant women.

BCG is a freeze-dried vaccine given intradermally. Other methods, such as multiple puncture, jet injection or scarification have been found to be not so satisfactory. The vaccine is sensitive to heat and light so must be carefully protected.

Sputum smear examination is a very simple technique for screening populations, especially where there has recently been a case of TB. All contacts of a case should have several sputum smears taken, concentrating on the young and elderly.

TB is particularly a disease of poor social conditions and overcrowding, as shown by the remarkable decline of the infection in industrialized countries prior to the advent of chemotherapy. The disease was as bad, if not worse, in Europe at the turn of the century than in many developing countries now, but showed a progressive and continuous reduction of cases as living conditions improved. As standards increased, there was a demand for improved housing with fewer people sharing the same room, so that overcrowding declined. Personal hygiene improved and such practices as spitting disappeared almost completely. (See Fig. 13.3.)

Treatment and prophylaxis. The functions of chemotherapy can be summarized as follows:

- Treat individual cases to reduce morbidity and mortality.
- Reduce the number and period of infectious cases.
- Provide a method of disease reduction in developing countries where the raising of social standards would take some time to achieve.
- Prevent the emergence of resistant strains.

A newly diagnosed case of TB should be treated with a four-drug regime for 2 months, consisting of:

Isoniazid	300 mg daily
Rifampicin	10 mg/kg up to 600 mg daily
Pyrazinamide	35 mg/kg up to 2 g daily
Ethambutol	25 mg/kg daily

After the 2 month period, isoniazid and rifampicin only are taken daily for a further 4 months. In areas of known isoniazid resistance, then a three-drug

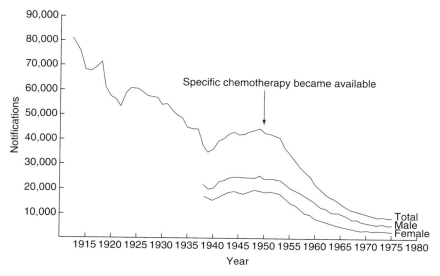

Fig. 13.3. The decline of tuberculosis (TB) in England and Wales 1912–1975. (From DHSS (1977) *Annual Report of the Chief Medical Officer, Department of Health and Social Security for 1976*, Her Majesty's Stationary Office, London. Crown copyright, reproduced with the permission of the Controller of HMSO.)

regime of isoniazid, rifampicin and ethambutol is taken for the 4 month period. In cases of miliary or meningitis TB or bone/joint disease treatment should continue for 9–12 months.

In a case where retreatment is required or drug resistance is suspected then streptomycin at 15 mg/kg daily is added to the four-drug regime for 2 months, then the four-drug regime is continued for a further month, and isoniazid, rifampicin and ethambutol for 5 months. Once the drug susceptibility test (DST) result is known the regime can be modified accordingly.

Early and adequate treatment is essential if drug resistance is not to develop. Sadly, there are now many cases of multi-drug-resistant TB (MDR-TB), resistant to both isoniazid and rifampicin. A link with HIV infection has shown the development of MDR-TB to occur twice as often in patients with both TB and HIV. These cases will need to be put on MDR regimes, which include more drugs, are expensive and need to be taken for a longer period.

A more serious problem has been the development of extensively drug-resistant TB (XDR-TB), a virtually untreatable form of TB. This is particularly prevalent in Eastern Europe, Russia and Central Asia. Considerable expenditure and strict control will be required to contain this problem.

Prophylaxis with daily isoniazid (300 mg) for 6 months can be given to close contacts under 35 years of age and people with HIV, and to babies (5 mg/kg) born to mothers who develop TB shortly before or after delivery.

The World Health Organization's (WHO's) Stop-TB strategy (also known by the 'brand name' DOTS – Directly Observed Therapy, Short-course) includes political and financial commitment, standardized diagnosis, treatment, and adherence support and monitoring. Until recently, this strategy recommended that all cases should have directly observed therapy (DOT) to ensure adherence. However, evidence from randomized trials has shown that DOT (as opposed to self-administration) does not improve cure rates. For all patients, WHO recommends good education on the diagnosis of TB and importance of treatment adherence. Patients should choose a treatment supporter, who is someone who is accessible, concerned and reliable, such as a family member or community health worker/volunteer. The treatment supporter encourages the patient when they are feeling demotivated, and to keep follow-up appointments and take the right tablets for the full course of treatment, until cured.

Surveillance. A system to follow up all diagnosed cases of TB discharged from a hospital or health centre is required on the following lines:

- Register the case with a central registry on diagnosis.
- When the patient is discharged, inform the registry, the nearest clinic to the person's home and the supervising doctor.
- The clinic ensures the patient receives regular follow-up treatment or goes and finds them if they default.
- The supervising doctor visits on a regular basis to check the clinic records and make sure that the registered patients are receiving treatment.
- When the full course of treatment is completed and the doctor is satisfied that the patient is cured, the Central Registry is notified.

Reminders and double checks can be built into the system, such as the central registry sending out quarterly checks on each patient.

The sophistication of the system depends upon the resources of the country, but lack of resources is never an excuse not to have a system at all. To not follow up a partially treated patient is a waste of expensive hospital treatment, encourages the development of resistant organisms and increases the risk to the community. Follow-up is always cheaper than re-diagnosis and treatment.

Evaluation of TB control programmes is by measuring the proportion of new smear-positive cases that are cured or are certified to have completed treatment. The WHO target is 85%. Other useful indicators are:

- annual rate of new TB cases diagnosed;
- rate of sputum-positive cases diagnosed;
- proportion of children under 5 years of age diagnosed;
- proportion of miliary and meningeal TB;
- rate of sputum smears examined;
- rate of BCG scars, on survey;
- relapse rate; and
- rate lost to follow up.

A decrease in the proportion of children under 5 years of age diagnosed and of those with miliary and meningeal TB will indicate improvement; however, this will need to be confirmed by a sputum smear survey. Nursing staff should be taught to always give the BCG vaccination in the same place, normally the deltoid area of the left arm, so that touring staff, schoolteachers, etc. can rapidly examine a group of children.

Not only is the standard treatment regime for TB likely to use gatifloxin instead of ethambutol, allowing for a reduction in the length of treatment to 4 months, but new diagnostic techniques are also likely to be introduced over the next few years. In order to facilitate these changes, WHO has established a Stop TB Partnership to prepare countries for the introduction of these new tools in order to minimize the delay between licensure, availability and adoption.

13.2 Acute Respiratory Infections (ARIs)

The acute respiratory infections (ARIs) are the commonest causes of ill health in the world. WHO has estimated that there are 14–15 million deaths a year in children under 5 years of age and that a third of these are due to ARIs, yet despite their importance they are a poorly defined group of diseases. They include the common cold, influenza, pneumonia, bronchitis and a number of other infections. They can be separated by clinical criteria, but it is the differing response of the individual to the organism/s that determines the clinical severity and management. A mild infection from an upper respiratory tract infection in one person may develop in another to a life-threatening attack of pneumonia. It is, therefore, not only the organism that determines the disease, but also the patient's response to that organism.

Organisms. A number of different organisms produce infection, including *Streptococcus pneumoniae, Haemophilus influenzae, Mycoplasma pneumoniae,* influenza, rhinoviruses, adenoviruses, metapneumovirus and respiratory syncytial virus (RSV). The most important of these are *S. pneumoniae* or the pneumococcus, *H. influenzae* bacteria, and RSV and parainfluenza viruses. As well as there being a wide range of viruses, each species may have a number of serotypes, with new ones appearing from time to time. The host defends him or herself by producing an appropriate immune response, but because of the large number of serotypes this is a continuous process. Infection will cause illness in some people but not in others who have developed an immune response either to the specific organism or to an antigenically similar serotype. New antigenic mutations, as occur in influenza, can cause epidemic or pandemic spread

because no prior contact with the new variant has been made.

Clinical features. ARIs are divided into upper respiratory and lower respiratory, the former producing a runny nose, sneezing and headache, while the main symptoms of lower respiratory infection are a cough, shortness of breath and inward drawing of the bony structure of the lower chest wall during inspiration, which is called chest indrawing. Both are generally accompanied by fever. The main pathological feature is pneumonia, which can either be lobar or bronchial. In lobar pneumonia one or more well-defined lobes of the lung are involved whereas in bronchial pneumonia the condition is widespread. The causes of pneumonia are listed in Table 13.1.

Diagnosis. Identifying the organism by culture of the sputum can be attempted where facilities permit, but in most developing countries ARI will be diagnosed on clinical criteria.

Transmission is by coughing out a large number of organisms in an aerosol of droplets, which are either breathed in, enter via the conjunctiva, or land on surfaces and subsequently enter mucous membranes from fingers. (See further under influenza, Section 13.3.) Susceptibility and response is determined by host factors, some of which are:

- *Age.* Young children develop obstructive diseases such as croup (laryngotracheobronchitis) and bronchiolitis. Tonsillitis is commonest at school age, whereas influenza and pneumonia are important causes of death in the elderly. In young children, mortality is inversely related to age.
- *Portal of entry.* Volunteers have been more easily infected by some organisms applied to the conjunctiva than through the nasopharynx.
- *Nutrition.* Low birth weight and malnourished children have a higher morbidity and mortality. Certain nutritional deficiencies, such as lack of Vitamin A and zinc, contribute to the development of a more severe disease and higher death rate. Breastfeeding appears to have a protective effect.
- *Socio-economic.* ARI is a disease of poverty with higher incidence in lower socio-economic groups and those that live in urban slums. Higher rates of lower respiratory disease have

Table 13.1. The causes of pneumonia.

Organism	Clinical indicators	Occurrence
Streptococcus pneumoniae	Fever, cough, rusty sputum	Infants, elderly
Haemophilus influenzae	Slow onset, purulent sputum	Secondary infection
Influenza A and B	Fever, muscle pains	Epidemic
Morbillivirus	Measles	Seasonal epidemics
RSV (respiratory syncytial virus)	Wheezing, croup	Seasonal winter peak
Adenoviruses	Sore throat, conjunctivitis	Children, winter months
Metapneumovirus	Asthma, bronchiolitis	Children
Coronavirus-SARS (severe acute respiratory syndrome)	Respiratory distress	Close contact, animals?
Parainfluenza	Croup, wheezing	Children, immunodeficient
Mycobacterium tuberculosis	Cough, haemoptysis, weight loss	Close contact
Mycoplasma pneumoniae	Slow onset, malaise	Epidemic, young adults
Chlamydia pneumoniae	Slow onset, malaise	Young adults
Chlamydia psittaci	Fever, unproductive cough	Associated with birds
Staphylococcus aureus, Streptococcus pyogenes, Klebsiella pneumoniae	Abscess formation	Secondary infection, particularly of influenza
Legionella pneumophilia	Increasing fever, anorexia	Air conditioners, males
Coxiella burnetti	Fever, weight loss	Associated with sheep
Pneumocystis jiroveci	Progressive dyspnoea	Immunosuppressed, HIV
Nocardia asteroides	Chronic, disseminated	Immunosuppressed, HIV
Cryptoccus neoformans	Mycosis, disseminated	Immunosuppressed, HIV
Coccidioides immitis	Disseminated abscesses	Airborne from soil
Histoplasma capsulatum	Cavitation, emphysema	Airborne from soil

been found with increasing family size. Much of the reason for this increase appears to be due to increased contact and agglomeration, as shown in children attending day-care facilities or school, where infection occurs irrespective of social class.

- *Air pollution.* A correlation with domestic air pollution has been shown in South Africa and Nepal. Passive smoking may affect pulmonary function and make the child more susceptible to infection as well as influence the child to become a smoker.
- *Climate.* More respiratory infections are found in the cooler parts of the world or in the higher altitude regions of the tropics. There is a distinct seasonal effect in many countries, with more respiratory infections in the winter. However, cold alone is not a causative factor. The 'cold' derives its name from the belief that becoming chilled or standing in a draught is responsible, but when volunteers are subjected to these stresses and inoculated with rhinoviruses, they develop no more 'colds' than controls. In the tropics, respiratory infections occur more commonly with the rains.

- *Other infections.* Any infection that causes damage to the respiratory mucosa will allow a mild infecting organism to progress to more serious consequences. The most important of these diseases is measles, post-measles pneumonia being particularly common.

Incubation period. This varies with the organism, but in most cases is 1–3 days.

Period of communicability. Variable; for the entire period of any respiratory symptoms.

Occurrence and distribution. Worldwide, the most important cause of death in children in developing countries.

Treatment. The first line of action is to assess the severity of illness and give treatment. This is supportive therapy for mild infections and the active administration of antibiotics to the severe case. The mild infection is best treated at home and kept away from sources of other infection, which may cause more serious disease, while the severe case requires early treatment to prevent complications and death. In children, the respiratory rate and chest indrawing are used to decide management:

- Mild cases with a respiratory rate of less than 40 breaths/min in children 2–12 months old, and 50 breaths/min in children 1–5 years old, are treated at home with supportive therapy. The mother should be encouraged to nurse her child, giving it plenty of fluids (breastfeeding or from a cup), regular feeding, cleaning the nose, maintaining the child at a comfortable temperature and avoiding contact with others.
- Moderate cases with a respiratory rate over 40 breaths/min in under 1 year olds and 50 breaths/min in children 1–5 years old, but with no chest indrawing, should be given antibiotics (oral co-trimoxazole (4 mg/kg twice daily); oral amoxycillin (15 mg/kg three times a day); or intramuscular penicillin G) and nursed at home.
- Severe cases with chest indrawing, cyanosis or cases too sick to feed must be admitted as inpatients and given active support as well as treatment with antibiotics.

Control and prevention. The first step in management of a child with ARI is to separate the mild from the moderate and to treat the moderate and severe. The essence is speed and active treatment. This can easily be taught at primary health-care level. The mother can be educated on the management of her child with a mild infection and when to refer it. It is the delay in referral and treatment that will allow a moderate case to become severe and the severe case to die.

The village health worker can identify and treat the mild or moderate case of ARI using simple diagnostic criteria and a standard treatment protocol. Measuring the respiratory rate and knowing which action to take are the most important aspects. Training and supervision of primary health-care workers is a priority in the management of ARI.

Preventive actions that can be undertaken are:

- *Reduce contact.* Acute respiratory infections are just as common in industrialized countries as they are in developing countries, but infant deaths from respiratory infections in the former have declined. The reason would appear to be due to smaller families and greater birth intervals, permitting increased individual care of

children and better nutrition. The child is reared at home and does not need to be carried around where it is exposed at a very young age to infecting organisms.

- *Good nutrition.* Well-nourished children are in a stronger position to defend themselves against any infection. Encourage breastfeeding especially during early stages of illness. Providing additional nutritional support to children with measles can prevent them developing post-measles pneumonia.
- *Health education.* Teach people to cough away from others, cover the mouth when coughing, not to spit or smoke and provide proper ventilation for smoke and fumes.
- *Vaccination of childhood infections.* The danger of developing pneumonia after measles is a serious problem, so prevention of measles will reduce the severe forms of ARI. Indeed, measles vaccination is perhaps the single most effective preventive method (Section 12.2). The routine childhood vaccination programme offers protection from pertussis, diphtheria, *H. influenzae* and the pneumococcus, as well as TB.
- *Other vaccines.* Influenza vaccine is prepared annually according to the expected strain of influenza and should be given to those at risk (e.g. immunocompromised and those with chronic respiratory infections) if facilities allow. Vaccines against RSV, parainfluenza and the adenoviruses are in preparation.

Surveillance. Measles generally occurs in seasonal epidemics, which can be forecasted and top-up vaccination given (Section 12.2). Influenza occurs annually or in pandemics with warning given of strain of organism and vaccine composition, allowing sufficient time for persons at risk to be protected.

13.3 Influenza

Organism. There are three types of influenza virus, A, B and C. The surface of the virus is coated with haemagglutinin (H antigen with 16 subtypes) and an enzyme, neuraminidase (N antigen with nine subtypes). The virus is designated as A(H1N1), A(H2N2) … A(H3N2), etc. with, in addition, the site of isolation, culture number and year, e.g. A/Beijing/262/95(H1N1). Influenza A is the least stable, with antigenic shift of the H and N antigens, influenza B is more stable and influenza C is the most stable with low pathogenicity (producing mainly subclinical infection). Antigenic drift in both A and B viruses produces new strains and is responsible for the frequent epidemics that occur at regular intervals.

Clinical features. Influenza presents with fever, malaise, muscle aches and upper respiratory symptoms of sudden onset. Headache, anorexia and sore throat are common features. The uncomplicated illness lasts about 5 days.

There is initially a dry cough, but this can be severe or secondary infection can ensue, predominantly with *Streptococcus pneumoniae, Staphylococcus aureus* or *Haemophilus influenzae,* and this is the main cause of mortality. Other than pneumonia or acute bronchitis, infection can lead to otitis media in children and cardiac damage in adults. Reye's syndrome in children and encephalitis in adults are serious although uncommon complications.

Influenza is a serious infection in the elderly, with high death rates. When a major antigenic shift occurs as it did in 1957 (the Asian flu pandemic) then all ages are susceptible and the number of deaths can be considerable.

In developing countries, influenza can be a more serious infection; the 2002 epidemic in Madagascar had a 3% case fatality rate, the majority of deaths being in young children. Also, a common sequela of influenza is pneumonia, a major cause of death in children in developing countries.

Influenza B tends to be a childhood infection, so that once immunity has been built up protection has been acquired to the more stable virus. Infection in childhood also produces some cross immunity, but reinfection with both A and B does occur.

Subclinical infection occurs frequently, boosting the pre-existing immunological memory. Previous exposure to strains within the same subtype will to a certain extent lessen the clinical impact of closely related strains, reducing the viral load and infectiousness. On a community-wide basis this cross-reactive herd immunity will lessen the severity of the epidemic.

Diagnosis is on clinical grounds, taking care to differentiate influenza (occurring seasonally or in epidemics) from other causes of respiratory infections, especially the common cold. Direct immunofluorescence (DIF), ELISA or RNA amplification can be used to make the diagnosis, with PCR now the method of choice in influenza-detection laboratories. Virus can be isolated from pharyngeal or nasal secretions and cultured in specialist centres.

Transmission is by respiratory droplets through sneezing or coughing, but can also be by direct contact with mucus- or droplet-contaminated surfaces. The amount of virus shed is correlated with the severity of symptoms and fever, peaking in the early course of the disease, although pre-symptomatic and asymptomatic transmission can also occur. Children and immunocompromised individuals shed virus for longer periods and in higher titres.

Droplets are comparatively large sized (>5 μm) and can be projected up to 3 m but are more likely not projected further than 1 m. They infect people directly when they settle on the mucous membrane of the nose or mouth (and possibly the conjunctiva) or indirectly when they land on surfaces. Airborne transmission can also occur from smaller particles derived from dried out droplets that become aerosolized. These result in aerosols of particles in dust from contaminated surfaces but are more likely from medical procedures such as manual ventilation, suction and bronchoscopy. Aerosol transmission might also occur in systems where air is recycled, such as in aircraft. However, long-distance transmission does not occur.

Contact transmission is probably more important than previously thought, with virus remaining for long periods of time on hard non-porous surfaces. This is then transferred by hand to the individual or from person to person, infection taking place through mucous membranes.

Influenza is highly infectious and spreads throughout whole communities, potentiated by overcrowding and frequent social contact, such as at the workplace or in markets.

The natural reservoir of influenza is in birds, particularly aquatic species (ducks and geese), while the pig is important because it is susceptible to infection both from birds and humans, so new mixed infections can develop. The close association of humans with domestic birds and animals, particularly in south China, is thought to be where most new variants have arisen (see further in Section 19.2).

Incubation period is 1–5 days with a mean of 2 days.

Period of communicability is 2 days before onset of symptoms to 5 days after.

Occurrence and distribution. Influenza A is responsible for pandemics and regular seasonal outbreaks and influenza B for smaller localized outbreaks, while influenza C produces mild infections. In the tropics, epidemics tend to occur in the rainy season, while in temperate climates influenza is nearly always a disease of the winter months. Pandemics have occurred in 1889, 1918, 1957, 1968, 1977 and 2010 (swine flu). Several epidemics of avian flu A(H5N1) since 1997, and especially in 2006 and 2007, caused considerable concern because of the number of human cases (382), and the high fatality (241 deaths) that also occurred. Fortunately, there was no evidence of a major antigenic shift in A(H5N1) to suggest that humans would now be susceptible, with only some limited occurrences of human-to-human transmission. (See further in Sections 19.1 and 19.2.) Another form of avian influenza, A(H9N2), has been responsible for several mild human cases.

In 2010, A(H1N1) swine flu, which had originated in Mexico in 2009, reached pandemic proportions with cases in all parts of the world, but fortunately was not as severe as had been anticipated. It predominantly affected younger age groups, and pregnant women had a four times greater risk of developing severe disease than the general population. (See further in Sections 18.2 and 19.2.) The pandemic continued into 2011 in the northern hemisphere, but with a death rate little different from that expected from seasonal flu.

Seasonal influenza epidemics in the years immediately following a pandemic tend to be relatively severe.

Control and prevention. As influenza is so infectious, the majority of the population becomes infected during an epidemic, but any reduction of social contact, particularly in crowded places, can reduce this likelihood. Spitting should be outlawed and people encouraged not to cough directly at other people. Infected persons should stay at home and not go to a health centre or hospital.

People should be advised to cough into tissues, which are disposed of immediately. Antiviral-impregnated tissues have been found to be valuable in the reduction of some upper respiratory infections.

Hand washing and regular cleaning of surfaces with ordinary cleaning products are now considered to be major methods of reducing transmission.

Fluid-repellent surgical masks will offer some protection when in close contact with an infectious case, as long as the mask is not handled and droplets then transferred to mucous membranes. Infected persons should be encouraged to wear masks when in contact with people.

Influenza vaccine is available for protecting at-risk persons, such as people over 65, those with chronic chest or kidney disease and the immunocompromised. The difficulty of producing a vaccine is that a new one has to be made each year containing the expected composition of antigenic subunits. The WHO collaboration centres, with reference laboratories throughout the world, provide advance warning to assist countries producing vaccine, but new techniques such as virus manipulation to anticipate natural change in the virus could allow banks of virus to be kept in store. At present, WHO recommends the inclusion of an A(H1N1) and A(H3N2) subtype and a single B virus, but each year different strains will be required.

The use of vaccines in a pandemic situation to protect the population in an unaffected country or area is a distinct possibility, concentrating on school-aged children, as they have the highest transmission rates. This would be particularly important in highly lethal forms of the virus such as A(H5N1), where people coming into close contact with poultry would be the target population. The development of new vaccines may provide protection for longer periods of time and allow the possibility of vaccinating populations against influenza outbreaks.

Pneumococcal vaccination programmes (see Section 13.8) will do much to reduce secondary infection and serious disease to develop.

Treatment. There is no treatment, but antiviral agents will reduce the duration of fever and severity of symptoms and can be stockpiled when there is risk of an epidemic. Neuramidase inhibitors such as oseltamivir (Tamiflu®) and zanamivir, or the less useful M-2 channel blockers such as amantidine and rimantidine, can be used. They can also be given prophylactically, but widespread use has resulted in the development of resistance. Antivirals are particularly valuable in reducing the development of secondary infection in vulnerable people, but antibiotics might also be required. In individual cases, antibiotic sensitivity should first be determined, but in epidemic situations stockpiles might need to be kept of doxycycline, co-amoxiclav (amoxicillin + clavulanate) or ciprofloxacin.

Surveillance. Sentinel reporting centres with an agreed case definition probably provide a better idea of the influenza situation than collecting data of variable quality from every clinic and hospital. This can be compared with laboratory-confirmed cases where facilities permit.

WHO reports on the global situation in the *Weekly Epidemiological Record* (WER) from a worldwide network of reporting centres. More detailed information can be obtained from the Flu Net web site which provides up-to-date information from the Global Influenza Surveillance Network (GISN) and other national reference laboratories. Data are provided on virus subtypes and their global movement in the form of maps and graphs.

13.4 Whooping Cough (Pertussis)

Organism. *Bordetella pertussis*. *B. parapertussis* produces a milder disease.

Clinical features. Illness commences with upper respiratory symptoms, fever and a cough, which becomes paroxysmal with the characteristic whoop, or sometimes ends in vomiting. The classic 'whooping' disease is not seen in children under 3 months of age, when instead they have attacks of cyanosis and stop breathing. Whooping cough is a serious disease if it occurs at a young age, the severity being inversely proportional to age. A mild infection in the older child, it becomes an important cause of death in the very young.

Diagnosis is mainly on clinical criteria, but culture of the organism from a nose or throat swab can be attempted, although the organism is difficult to grow. Serology is useful.

Transmission is via airborne spread of droplets particularly during the early stage of illness. Older children and adults may have such a mild infection that their importance as a source of infection is not realized. Vaccinated individuals can have subclinical infection in which organisms are disseminated.

Incubation period is 7–10 days.

Period of communicability is 4 weeks from the first symptoms, being most infectious in the first week, before the paroxysms start.

Occurrence and distribution. Whooping cough is a serious disease in tropical countries, contributing to high rates of infant mortality. Vaccination programmes have markedly reduced the disease in the temperate regions of the world, but where the vaccination programme has decreased or been abandoned it has rapidly returned as a major health problem.

Where the young infant is always carried around by its mother there is an increased opportunity for exposure, coming into close contact with other children who might be infectious.

Control and prevention. Isolation of cases, especially of young children and infants, should be instituted. Infective children should be kept from school, markets and any place where young children are likely to congregate. Known contacts of a case of whooping cough (e.g. in the extended family of a case) should be given a booster vaccination if they have been vaccinated before, otherwise they should receive prophylactic erythromycin and vaccine.

The median age for the disease is 2 years, but because of its severity vaccination should be started at 1–2 months. Three doses of vaccine are given, normally combined with tetanus and diphtheria as triple vaccine. Antibodies to pertussis decrease rapidly, even after a three-dose course, and WHO now recommends a booster dose between 1 and 6 years, ideally around 2 years.

Treatment. Erythromycin is only effective when given in the first week of the disease. Fluid loss is an important cause of mortality so mothers should be encouraged to give extra fluids and breastfeed immediately after a coughing bout.

Surveillance. In many countries whooping cough is a notifiable disease.

13.5 Diphtheria

Organism. *Corynebacterium diphtheriae* and, rarely, *C. ulcerans*.

Clinical features. Diphtheria produces both local and systemic effects. The organism can infect the tonsils, pharynx, larynx, nose or skin, forming a pale grey membrane and local inflammation. Symptoms are fever, sore throat and enlarged cervical lymph nodes in the pharyngeal form, blood-stained discharge in the nasal form and skin ulcers in the cutaneous form. The inflammatory reaction produced in the respiratory tract can lead to swelling of the neck and respiratory obstruction. From the primary site, exotoxin is produced which can cause myocarditis or neuropathy, especially cranial nerve palsies.

Diagnosis. Throat, nose or skin swab of the exudate. A culture of the organism should be sent to a reference laboratory if possible.

Transmission. Diphtheria can be transmitted by:

- airborne transmission of droplets;
- direct contact with lesions and exudates;
- indirect contact through articles soiled with discharges; and
- ingestion of contaminated milk.

In a non-immunized population there is a high incidence of carriers and a low incidence of cases in a ratio of approximately 19:1. Between 6% and 40% of children are infected each year so that by 5 years old some 75% have been infected and by 15 years old nearly all. This means that by 15 years of age the majority of children have developed immunity, either through a subclinical infection or one in which clinical symptoms were revealed.

Incubation period is 2–5 days.

Period of communicability. About 2 weeks.

Occurrence and distribution. Commonly a disease of children, diphtheria can occur in non-immunized adults with serious results. Outbreaks of the disease are seen, but it is probably a much more frequent disease than realized, as subclinical transmission through skin, and possibly nasal lesions, maintains immunity. This was probably the situation in many tropical countries, but now universal childhood vaccination programmes are protecting young children. A breakdown of these programmes, or remaining pockets of unvaccinated adults, leads to serious disease.

Control and prevention. Diphtheria is prevented by vaccination of all children with three doses of diphtheria toxoid. This is normally combined with pertussis and tetanus as a triple vaccine (DTP), commencing in the first or second month of life. A booster dose should be given between 1 and 6 years of age. As with polio and rubella vaccination, diphtheria immunization shifts the likelihood of disease

to an older and more dangerous age so complete coverage of all children is imperative. Adults visiting an endemic country from one in which the vaccination status is good should have an adult type booster Td (tetanus and diphtheria) in which the concentration of toxoid is reduced. Ideally, adults, particularly travellers, should have booster doses of Td every 10 years. This applies equally to adults living in countries with a poor vaccination coverage. In the event of an outbreak, previously vaccinated contacts should be given a dose of Td and those not vaccinated should be given Td and an antibiotic (erythromycin or penicillin).

Treatment. If diphtheria antitoxin is available it should be given to cases following a test dose for hypersensitivity. Erythromycin or procaine penicillin G should be used for specific treatment.

Surveillance. Diphtheria is a notifiable disease in most countries.

13.6 Meningococcal Meningitis

Organism. Neisseria meningitidis. Twelve serogroups have been identified, but of these A, B, C and Y are the most important in producing disease, while A and C and W135 predominate in epidemics. See also Table 13.2.

Clinical features. There is a sudden onset of fever with severe headache, vomiting, neck stiffness and progressive loss of consciousness. A petechial rash, which does not blanch, is an important sign in pale skins, but is not seen on black skins. Infants show floppiness and high-pitched crying, while children may present with convulsions.

Normally the diagnosis is easy to make from the rigidity of the neck stiffness and the history, but in the infant it can be more difficult. The other main cause of high fever, headache and vomiting in tropical countries is cerebral malaria, from which the disease must be differentiated.

Diagnosis is by lumbar puncture, but should not delay early treatment, which can be given straightaway. A Gram stain is only reliable in some 50% of cases, so culture should be attempted wherever possible and data on antibiotic sensitivity obtained. Blood should also be taken for culture and PCR. Smears from petechiae can also be examined by Gram stain. Group-specific meningococcal

Table 13.2. The causes of meningitis.

Organism	Clinical indicators	Occurrence
Neisseria meningitidis	Fever, headache, rash	Epidemic, African meningitis belt, children and adults
Haemophilus influenzae	Fever, vomiting, lethargy	Infants
Streptococcus pneumoniae	Fever, purulent cerebrospinal fluid (CSF)	Infants, elderly
Mycobacterium tuberculosis	Fever, cough, haemoptysis	Children, young adults
Staphylococci	Secondary infection	Unsterilized instruments
Escherichia coli	Floppy infant, not feeding	Following delivery
Group B streptococci	Floppy infant, not feeding	Following delivery
Listeria monocytogenes	Neonates, following birth	Infection in the mother from domestic animals or cheese
Campylobacter jejuni	Diarrhoeal illness	All ages (see Section 9.2)
Echoviruses	Clear CSF, rash	Epidemic and seasonal
Coxsackieviruses	Clear CSF, rash	Epidemic and seasonal
Arboviruses	Clear CSF, encephalitis	Epidemic (see Section 15.2)
Influenza A or B	Reye's syndrome	Children given salicylates
Herpes zoster	Reye's syndrome	Children given salicylates
Epstein–Barr (EB) virus	Infectious mononucleosis	Young adults
Mumps virus	Parotid swelling, encephalitis	(See Section 12.4)
Rubella virus	Rash, encephalitis	Neonates (see Section 12.3)
Polio virus	Flaccid paralysis	Children (see Section 8.11)
Herpes simplex types 1 and 2	Primary sore or genital infection	Neonates, children or adults
Treponema pallidum	Secondary or latent syphilis	Adults (see Section 14.1)
Cryptococcus neoformans	Fungal infection	Tropics, males
Leptospira interrogans	Fever, myalgia, rash	Infection from rat urine
Lymphocytic choriomeningitis virus	Influenza-like symptoms	Associated with mice
Bacillus anthracis	Anthrax	From cattle
Brucella sp.	Brucellosis	From domestic animals
Yesinia pestis	Plague	During a plague epidemic
Angiostrongylus cantonensis	Nematode worm	Eating snails and slugs
Borrelia burgdorferi	Lyme disease	Deer ticks (see Section 16.8)
Negleria and *Acanthamoeba*	Amoebic meningoencephalitis	Swimming pools, immunocompromised

polysaccharides can be identified in the cerebrospinal fluid (CSF) using latex agglutination and, where there are the facilities, specific DNA can be detected.

Transmission is by airborne spread of droplets and from direct contact with secretions from the nose or throat. The organism is found commensally living in the nasopharynx, so other factors must also be responsible for meningitis to occur.

Epidemic meningitis was first studied in cooler climates and an association found with overcrowding, especially in military institutions. The organism, when introduced into an overcrowded environment, produced both cases and carriers (nasal). As the number of carriers increased, the number of cases of meningitis did so likewise.

In the African (Sahel) region epidemics occur in the cool dry season when cold nights encourage people to sleep indoors, often in overcrowded situations (Fig. 13.4). This is also the time of the year when the dry dust-laden wind the Harmattan blows, which dries out the respiratory mucosa, and is the time of the year when upper respiratory infections are more common too. Movements of people take place as a result of pilgrimages and traditional markets potentiate the transfer of infection.

The organism inhabits the nasal mucosa within which it is anatomically very close to the meninges, although these are separated by formidable barriers of bone and membrane. The generally accepted theory is that the organism passes from this site into the bloodstream, crosses the blood–brain barrier and enters the CSF.

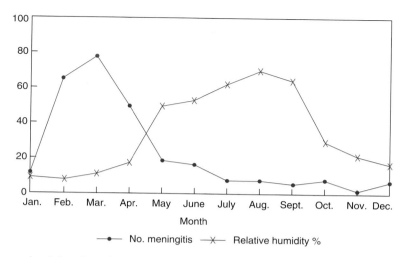

Fig. 13.4. The seasonal variation of meningococcal meningitis in relation to relative humidity in the Sahel region of Africa.

Difficult though the direct route may seem, it has been shown that minute passages through the bone of the skull do occur and transmission of organisms along this route is a possibility as well. Furthermore, if organisms are introduced directly into the subarachnoid space, infection will only occur if a critical level is exceeded (10^3 organisms in dogs), suggesting that this route could frequently be invaded, but only when there is excessive infection does meningitis develop.

Incubation period. 2–10 days; mean 4 days.

Period of communicability. Once effective treatment has started the patient ceases to be infective within 24 h, but any carrier will continue to produce organisms for between 2 weeks and 10 months.

Occurrence and distribution. Meningococcal meningitis occurs in epidemics, especially in the Sahel part of Africa in a band stretching from Senegal to Ethiopia. The epidemics are markedly seasonal, occurring in the early, coolest part of the year when the relative humidity is at its lowest. With the arrival of the rains the epidemic abates (Fig. 13.4). The amount of rainfall (1100 mm) delineates the southern boundary of the meningitis belt, and the northern boundary is the desert. Within this area, major epidemics, mainly of group A, occur at 7–14 year intervals, with lesser ones in between.

As well as the meningitis epidemic belt in Africa, there have also been epidemics of group A organisms in India and Nepal, and of group B in the Americas, Europe and Pacific Island nations. More recently, W-135 epidemics have been associated with the annual Hajj, either with the main gathering in Saudi Arabia or from pilgrims returning to their home countries.

Epidemic meningitis is commonest in the age group 5–15 years, with males more frequently affected than females. Only about 1 in 500 persons infected with the organism will develop meningitis. Large, poor families, and other conditions where there is overcrowding, such as at religious and social gatherings, and in refugee camps and labour lines, make meningitis more likely.

Control and prevention. Overcrowding encourages the transfer of the infecting organism and the carrier state, as well as increasing the dose of bacteria that may be transmitted, so all efforts should be made to reduce overcrowding. It may be necessary to close schools and reduce collections of people, such as markets and religious gatherings, if an epidemic has started or appears likely to do so. In the long term, improvement of housing and family planning will have an effect.

Chemoprophylaxis should be given to close contacts, such as all family members, school friends and anyone sharing in a large communal sleeping place (such as a dormitory). Rifampicin 10 mg/kg twice daily for 2 days or, if still sensitive to sulfonamides, sulfadiazine 150 mg/kg for 2 days can be used. Chemoprophylaxis is not recommended in large epidemics.

There are several vaccines containing either A and C, or A, C, Y and W-135. Unfortunately, the very young and those with acute malaria develop reduced immunity. There is also a genetic variation, with some ethnic groups having a poor response. Due to these different factors, duration of immunity is variable, from 3 years or less in young children, and must be measured for each community when formulating a vaccination programme. Vaccine can be used to immunize those most at risk, concentrating on the 2–20 year age group, and household contacts of cases. When there is an epidemic, mass vaccination should be given to communities in the affected area, including vaccinating children below 2 years of age. It has been suggested that an incidence of 15 cases per 100,000 in a well-defined population for 2 consecutive weeks heralds the beginning of an epidemic and the need to start mass vaccination. Everyone attending the Hajj must be vaccinated with ACYW135 vaccine.

A conjugated C vaccine has been found to be effective in all age groups, especially young children, and in several countries this vaccine is included in the national childhood vaccination programme (see Section 3.2.2). If an epidemic is found to be due to a group C organism then this vaccine should be used. A combined A and C polysaccharide vaccine can be given as a single injection to children over 2 years of age to provide several years of protection.

A conjugate vaccine for meningitis A (MenAfriVacc) recently developed in India is more effective than the polysaccharide vaccine. A campaign is now in operation to target 20 million children in Burkina Faso, Mali and Niger.

WHO has established an International Coordinating Group (ICG) on Vaccine Provision for Epidemic Meningitis Control to provide access to vaccines and treatment. It also encourages a two-pronged strategy of epidemic preparedness (improved surveillance and case finding) and epidemic response (stockpiling of vaccines and epidemic management strategy).

Treatment may need to be organised on a massive scale when an epidemic occurs by using dispensers, schoolteachers or other educated people to care for isolated communities. Temporary treatment centres (schools, churches, warehouses, etc.) may need to be set up, rather than bringing people into hospital. Benzyl penicillin, ampicillin or chloramphenicol should be used, but in many countries resistance to these antibiotics will require the use of ceftriaxone or one of the cephalosporins. If the organism is unknown, chloramphenicol is used. In epidemics, long-acting chloramphenicol in oil preparations, given as a single injection avoids the problem of repeat injections. Dehydration is common and intravenous fluids may be required initially, followed by frequent drinks administered by an attending adult.

Surveillance. The regular epidemics that occur in Africa can be forecast and a state of preparedness put into action. Increased surveillance should be undertaken at this time using case detection and increased searches by laboratories. When a case of meningitis is detected, all contacts should be examined with nasopharyngeal swabs. Subtyping of the organism can assist in mapping out epidemics.

13.7 *Haemophilus influenzae* (Meningitis and Pneumonia)

Organism. *Haemophilus influenzae*, commonly serotype b (Hib).

Clinical features. *H. influenzae* can cause a range of illnesses, the most important being meningitis and pneumonia. In meningitis, there is fever, vomiting, neck stiffness and a rigid back in older children; in infants there is a bulging fontanelle. *H. influenzae* is a common cause of secondary infection in measles and other respiratory infections, resulting in pneumonia (see Section 13.2). Other infections are conjunctivitis in the newborn, otitis media, epiglottitis, cellulitis, septic arthritis, osteomyelitis, empyema and pericarditis.

Diagnosis. The CSF is often purulent, but this can occur in other causes of meningitis (see Table 13.2.), so cultures of the CSF or blood should be made. Serological tests are also of value.

Transmission. Airborne transmission of droplets and direct contact with nasopharyngeal secretions. The organism is carried asymptomatically in the nose of carriers who are often the source of infection to infants.

Incubation period. 2–4 days.

Period of communicability. Chronic nasal infection can remain for a prolonged period.

Occurrence and distribution. H. influenzae used to be the commonest cause of meningitis in infants and young children under 5 years old, mainly 4–18 months of age. At present it is still a serious problem in some developing countries, but with the advent of universal Hib vaccination the incidence is likely to decline considerably, as it has done in developed countries.

Control and prevention. Routine vaccination of all children with Hib vaccine is now recommended. Vaccine should be given at the same time as DTP vaccine or as a combination vaccine (DTP/Hib). Countries might decide to give a booster dose at 12–15 months, but in most developing countries *H. influenzae* infection occurs before this age. Where vaccination programmes are starting or catch-up vaccination of adults and children over 18 months is to be given then a single dose of vaccine is sufficient. Hib can safely be given at the same time as meningococcal vaccine.

In the event of an outbreak of several cases of meningitis, vaccination should be given to all children aged under 5 years within the area. Contacts of all ages in households or close communities where there are unvaccinated children should be given prophylaxis with rifampicin. (See also Section 13.6.)

Treatment is with ampicillin or chloramphenicol.

Surveillance. All family and contacts of a case of meningitis should be investigated by nose swabs. Children under 5 years of age that have been in contact with a case should be followed up and treatment started if they develop early signs, such as fever.

13.8 Pneumococcal Disease

The pneumococcus causes a variety of diseases, including ARI (Section 13.2), pneumonia (Table 13.1), meningitis (Table 13.2) and otitis media (Section 13.9), which are more conveniently covered elsewhere, but in view of the availability of a vaccine, pneumococcal disease will also be discussed here.

Organism. Streptococcus pneumoniae, the pneumococcus.

Clinical features. S. pneumoniae is the commonest cause of ARIs and pneumonia, presenting with a cough, fever and rusty coloured sputum (from bloodstaining). Both bronchopneumonia and lobar pneumonia result, leading to a high mortality in infants and the elderly. S. pneumoniae is also the commonest cause of otitis media, causing fever and pain in the ear. If untreated, this can lead to bacteraemia and fulminant meningitis, with a high fatality rate. There is a high fever and lethargy, and the patient rapidly descends into a coma. S. pneumoniae is also a common cause of conjunctivitis.

Diagnosis is by culture of sputum, blood, eye discharges or CSF. A Gram stain will show the characteristic blue-staining diplococci, providing a rapid diagnosis, but culture should also be done.

Transmission is normally airborne spread of droplets during sneezing or coughing from infected persons or healthy carriers. Some 25% of people carry S. pneumoniae in the nasopharynx, although these might not all be disease-producing serotypes. Transmission can also be by direct contact or through articles soiled with secretions, such as handkerchiefs or cloths used to wipe the eye in conjunctivitis.

Incubation period. 1–3 days.

Period of communicability is as long as secretions are produced in the clinical case, but the importance of healthy carriers is unclear, with some possibly responsible for producing infection in the young or elderly over considerable periods of time. Adequate treatment should render the case or carrier non-infectious within 2 days.

Occurrence and distribution. Worldwide distribution, especially in developing countries, with ARI a major cause of mortality in children. It is one of the commonest causes of terminal pneumonia in the elderly in the developed world. Overcrowding and deprived socio-economic conditions favour disease. Miners and people living in smoke-filled huts, such as in Papua New Guinea, have an increased incidence.

Control and prevention. Active management and treatment of cases of ARI and pneumonia should be implemented as covered in Section 13.2 above, and for otitis media in Section 13.9 below. Family planning and the reduction of overcrowding will reduce the situation in which the infection commonly spreads. Smoking should be discouraged and houses designed so that smoke is taken away from inside the house. Hand washing and the careful disposal of discharges from the nose, throat and the infected eye should be practised.

The pneumococcal conjugate vaccine (PCV) has been shown to be highly efficacious against invasive pneumococcal disease but only moderately efficacious against otitis media. The vaccine is now included in the routine childhood vaccination programmes in many countries including, where funds permit, in developing countries. Priority should be given to countries with a high prevalence of HIV, and in other conditions that increase the risk of pneumococcal disease, such as sickle-cell disease.

PCV is most conveniently given at the same time as DTP vaccination, but when first introduced a single catch-up dose may be given to unvaccinated children at 12–24 months and to high-risk children at 2–5 years of age.

The childhood vaccination programme has produced considerable herd immunity, protecting unvaccinated children and people over 65 years of age. However, several of the serotypes used in the vaccine have been replaced by other serotypes. So far this has not been a problem except with otitis media, which in one study showed an increase.

Treatment. Penicillin G or erythromycin are effective in the majority of cases, but where resistant strains are found or the child is seriously ill, co-trimoxazole, amoxicillin or ampicillin should be used.

Surveillance. See Section 13.2 (ARI) and Section 13.9 (otitis media).

13.9 Otitis Media

Acute ear infections are a common problem in children and are responsible for considerable morbidity (Table I.1). Acute middle-ear infection, or otitis media, is the main disease, but this can lead to chronic otitis media or mastoiditis (chronic infection of the bony air cells below the ear) or meningitis.

The ear is joined to the nasopharynx by the Eustachian tube through which infecting organisms pass, so ear infections are generally associated with respiratory infections.

Organism. *Streptococcus pneumoniae* and *Haemophilus influenzae* are the most common causative organisms, but various viruses may initiate infection, and *Pseudomonas aeruginosa* and *Staphylococcus aureus* are common in the discharges of chronic otitis media.

Clinical features. Fever and pain in the ear are the main presenting symptoms, but in the young child crying and irritability will be more prominent. The eardrum is red and bulges outwards, rapidly leading to perforation and the appearance of pus. There will be deafness in the ear until the perforation has healed, or permanent deafness if the condition remains untreated.

Diagnosis is on clinical grounds and the infecting organism can be cultured if the ear drum has ruptured.

Transmission is secondary to an upper respiratory infection such as a sore throat or tonsillitis.

Incubation period. 1–4 days.

Period of communicability. Not normally transmitted from person to person except as an upper respiratory infection.

Occurrence and distribution. This is a very common condition throughout the world and many children develop ear infections during the course of their childhood. Where the drum has ruptured then deafness will result, leading to problems at school, so what started off as a seemingly insignificant problem can lead to poor development and disability throughout the life of the individual. Otitis media and deafness occurring in the first 2–3 years of life can interfere with spoken language acquisition, leading to difficulties in communication, understanding and a barrier to education.

There is a particularly high level of otitis media in Australian aboriginals and the Inuit people of the Arctic, with Pacific Islanders and native North Americans next in order of magnitude. This may be due to these people having larger Eustachian tubes which offer lower resistance to the passage of organisms.

Control and prevention. Upper respiratory infections should be adequately treated and the eardrum always examined for redness and bulging.

The same risk factors as cause ARI (Section 13.2) predispose to otitis media, so relevant preventive action can be instituted.

The childhood vaccinations of measles, Hib and PCV should reduce the incidence of respiratory infections and hence of otitis media, but replacement serotypes of *S. pneumoniae* may result in an increase due to this organism.

The child with deafness should be examined and, if found to have a discharging ear, treated as below. If the eardrum does not heal then corrective surgery can be performed.

Treatment. In acute otitis media penicillin G or erythromycin given systemically for 5 days may be sufficient, but if there is poor response or perforation has occurred then co-trimoxazole twice a day or amoxicillin three times a day for 5 days should be used. In the chronically discharging ear it is imperative to dry the ear out with wicking, and the mother can be taught to do that. Clean tissue paper is twisted into a point and placed in the ear, replacing it as soon as it becomes wet and repeating until the ear remains dry. The child should not swim or water be allowed to enter the ear when washing. Boric acid in spirit ear drops can be instilled to help in drying the ear.

Surveillance. Surveys of deaf and partially deaf children will give an indication of the amount of otitis media leading to perforation of the eardrum. Where finances permit, this is best done by tympanometry, but a simple test using the spoken voice can give a rough estimate:

- Responds to a whisper – no deafness.
- Responds only to the normal voice – moderate hearing impairment.
- Responds only to a loud voice – severe deafness.

13.10 Acute Rheumatic Fever

Organism. Group A β-haemolytic streptococcus (GAβHS). The M-protein in the wall of the streptococcus is responsible for its virulence, and certain predominant serotypes, 1, 3, 5, 6, 14, 18, 19, 24, 27 and 29 have a much greater rheumatogenic potential.

Clinical features. Acute rheumatic fever (ARF) is a delayed non-suppurative sequel of upper respiratory tract infection or scarlet fever with GAβHS. ARF is important because it can lead to rheumatic heart disease (RHD), the resulting cardiac damage producing considerable morbidity and mortality.

Diagnosis of ARF is based on major and minor clinical criteria and a rising serum antibody titre of a recent streptococcal infection by the antistreptolysin-O titre (ASOT), antihyaluronidase or anti-DNAase B test.

Transmission. ARF results from an interaction of the bacterial agent, human host and environment. The GAβHS is transmitted from person to person through relatively large droplets, up to a distance of 3 m. ARF develops at a fairly constant rate of 3% following untreated epidemics of streptococcal pharyngitis. The attack rate is much lower (<1%) following endemic or sporadic streptococcal infections. Healthy primary schoolchildren are commonly found to be carriers of GAβHS. Cutaneous streptococcal infection is a frequent precursor of acute nephritis, but has not been shown to cause ARF. Scarlet fever, however, is associated with ARF.

Why only a small percentage of the youthful population develop ARF remains an enigma. ARF patients, as a group, show a higher antibody level to group A streptococcal antigens, suggesting that repeated exposure to GAβHS may precipitate illness. Susceptibility is due to the immunological status of the host, including both humoral and cell-mediated immunity, with a 2% familial incidence of ARF. A larger proportion of children born to rheumatic parents contract the disease. The carditis of RHD might be the result of an autoimmune mechanism developing between group A streptococcal somatic components and myocardial and valvular components.

Incubation period of the initial streptococcal infection is 1–3 days and for ARF it is 19 days.

Period of communicability. 10–21 days of an acute, untreated streptococcal infection.

Occurrence and distribution. ARF/RHD is the commonest form of heart disease in children and young adults in most tropical and developing countries. The peak incidence is 5–15 years, but both primary and recurrent cases can occur in adults. There is neither a sex predilection nor a racial predisposition.

ARF is a disease of lower socio-economic groups, particularly those massed in the densely populated areas of urban metropolitan centres. It is widespread with a high incidence in South Asia, Pacific Islands, North and South Africa and urban Latin America. It has been estimated that RHD causes 25–40% of all cardiovascular disease in the developing world. A quarter of a million deaths in the world every year are estimated to be due to RHD.

Control and prevention. There is no permanent cure for RHD and the cumulative expense of repeated hospitalization for supportive medical care is a considerable drain on the meagre health resources of developing countries. The only reasonable solution is prevention of rheumatic fever. ARF is now a rare condition in developed countries due to improved housing, reduction of overcrowding and the provision of adequate health services, so this should be the long-term aim.

Prevention of the first attack (primary prevention) is by proper identification and antibiotic treatment of streptococcal infections. The individual who has suffered an attack of ARF is inordinately susceptible to recurrences following subsequent streptococcal infection and needs protection (secondary prevention). While primary prevention is preferable, the incidence of ARF as a sequel of streptococcal sore throat is never greater than 3%, even in epidemics. A vast number of infections would need to be treated in order to achieve any meaningful reduction of the total number of sore throats, and streptococci are responsible for only 10–20% of them.

Most cases of severe RHD would be prevented by adequate prevention of recurrences of ARF. No matter how mild the first attack of ARF, secondary prevention with intramuscular long-acting benzathine penicillin G 1.2 million units should be given at monthly intervals. Penicillin V or sulfadiazine may be used for oral prophylaxis. Regular taking of prophylaxis is essential and compliance is a major problem. Patients with no evidence of cardiac involvement should receive prophylaxis for a minimum of 5 years after the last attack of ARF, while those with carditis should continue until they are 25 years old. Prophylaxis should be continued with penicillin in the pregnant woman.

The emphasis of a prevention programme should be on health education, early diagnosis and treatment of sore throats, and the provision of treatment facilities at primary level.

Surveillance. In developing strategies, baseline data on streptococcal epidemiology and ARF/RHD prevalence in high-risk groups should be collected. A fully established programme centre would operate a central register, coordinate case-finding surveys, run a system of secondary prophylaxis (especially follow up) and promote health education. Community control of ARF and RHD is viable only if it is firmly based on existing health services, which are an integral part of the primary health-care activities in the country. It is especially relevant to school health services, by screening children and supporting those on secondary prophylaxis.

Summary

- Infections of the respiratory system are the most important cause of morbidity and mortality in the world.
- Although numerous organisms are responsible for producing infection, it is the response of the host that determines the severity of the disease.
- The main method of transmission is by droplets, either coughed directly on to another person or on to surfaces from which they are inadvertently transferred to mucous membranes.
- Additional factors such as age (the young and the old), overcrowding, malnutrition, smoking and other concurrent infections increase the frequency and severity of infection.
- Epidemic infections, particularly influenza, have a seasonality during the rainy season in the tropics and during the cooler months in northern climates.
- Meningitis, otitis media and rheumatic fever are also due to infection acquired by the respiratory route.
- Many of the respiratory infections are prevented by vaccination, which is the main method of immediate control, but established personal hygiene habits, the raising of living standards and the control of family size are long-term preventive measures.

Further Reading

Van-Tam, J. and Sellwood, C. (2010) *Introduction to Pandemic Influenza.* CAB International, Wallingford, UK.

World Health Organization (2004) *Rheumatic Fever and Rheumatic Heart Disease: Report of a WHO Expert Consultation, Geneva, 29 October–1 November 2001.* WHO Technical Report Series 923. WHO, Geneva.

World Health Organization (2005) *The Current Evidence for the Burden of Group A Streptococcal Disease*. Discussion Papers on Child Health, No. WHO/FCH/CAH/05.07. WHO Ref. No. WHO/FCH/CAH/05.07; WHO/IVB/05.12. WHO, Geneva.

World Health Organization (2010) *Treatment of Tuberculosis: Guidelines*, 4th edn. Document No. WHO/HTM/TB/2009.420, WHO, Geneva.

Web resources

FluNet: international flu network of virological data. Available at: www.who.int/flunet (accessed 5 March 2012).

Influenza: WHO influenza home page. Available at: www.who.int/csr/disease/influenza/en/ (accessed 5 March 2012).

Tuberculosis (TB): WHO tuberculosis home page. Available at: www.who.int/tb/en (accessed 5 March 2012).

14 Diseases Transmitted via Body Fluids

External mechanisms, food, water or organisms taking advantage of the respiratory apparatus have been the main routes of transmitting infection covered in the previous chapters, but a large group of other diseases includes infections transmitted from one human to another by the physiological fluids of the body: blood, serum, saliva, seminal fluid, etc. These are the diseases of very close contact, direct from person to person, with sexual transmission accounting for the largest number of persons affected. They are, therefore, social diseases, determined by the habits and attitudes of people, and it is only by effecting changes in these values that any permanent improvement will occur.

14.1 Venereal Syphilis

Organism. Treponema pallidum subspecies *pallidum.*

Clinical features. The primary lesion of syphilis is the chancre (a painless ulcer with a serous discharge), which is normally found on the genitalia of males and females, but can occur in the mouth, on the breast or in the anorectal region. A regional lymph node often enlarges to form a bubo. The primary lesion heals spontaneously after a few weeks, but 6 weeks to 6 months later the signs of secondary syphilis appear. These may take several forms, but the commonest are a maculopapular rash with mucocutaneous condylomata around the genitalia and anus. As the infection is systemic, a generalized lymphadenopathy and splenomegaly can occur, often accompanied by fever. Following the period of secondary syphilis, there is a latent phase after which the destructive cardiovascular (aortic aneurysm) and central nervous system (CNS) symptoms (meningitis, paresis or tabes dorsalis) occur, often many years later. Should a woman be pregnant while she has syphilis then her fetus may be seriously affected. If she is pregnant during early syphilis, then the child will probably be stillborn, while during the later stages of disease the child is likely to suffer from congenital defects (deafness, sabre tibia, Hutchinson teeth and CNS involvement).

Diagnosis is made by finding *T. p. pallidum* in the serous exudate from a chancre or by gland puncture. This can be examined by dark ground microscopy or immunofluorescent staining. Serological tests can assist in the diagnosis or be used in epidemiological studies. The rapid plasma reagin (RPR) assay is a sensitive test, while specific assays such as the fluorescent treponemal antibody absorbed (FTA-Abs) test or *T. pallidum* haemagglutination antibody (TPHA) test are more difficult and expensive to perform. Cross reaction between the treponemas of yaws, pinta and endemic syphilis negate the differential diagnosis of these diseases. All patients with syphilis should be encouraged to have a HIV (human immunodeficiency virus) test, because of the high frequency of dual infection.

Transmission. Syphilis is transmitted by direct contact with an infectious lesion or its discharge during sexual intercourse. Transmission can also occur congenitally or from blood transfusion, if the donor is in the early stages of syphilis. Kissing can more rarely transmit the spirochete.

Because of the almost identical nature of the *T. pallidum* of endemic syphilis and venereal syphilis, it has been considered that venereal syphilis developed from the more benign endemic form. Once a venereal method of transmission had been developed, the disease was able to extend its boundaries from the tropics to the Arctic.

Infection with *T. p. endemicum* confers immunity to venereal syphilis and infection with *T. p. pallidum* gives immunity to the other treponemal infections and from contracting venereal syphilis again, but this is reduced by HIV infection. There is also some innate resistance or inadequacy of the transmission mechanism, as only some 30% of contacts of a known infected source become infected.

Incubation period. 9–90 days (usually 3 weeks).

Period of communicability. Up to 1 year after the primary lesion first appears.

Occurrence and distribution. The venereal diseases are totally cosmopolitan, taking no account of climate, ethnic group or social class; wherever sexual contact occurs there the venereal diseases can occur also. It is estimated that there are some 12 million cases in the world today, with a large proportion of these in the tropics. The highest incidence is in the 20–24 year age group, followed by those aged 25–29.

Syphilis is predominantly a disease of urban areas and in conditions of sexual imbalance, such as mines, military establishments and among seamen. With the rapid urbanization that has occurred in the developing world, and large movements of migrant labour, syphilis has been on the increase in the tropics. When migrant workers return home they bring venereal disease back with them and their wives become infected.

The main reservoir of infection is generally in commercial sex workers or deserted women forced into prostitution to support their children. Owing to the prolonged incubation period, the hidden site of the primary lesion within the vagina, and the latent period of the disease, syphilis is either not suspected or purposely hidden. A large number of contacting males can therefore be infected by a single female.

Control and prevention. Contact tracing and the adequate treatment of all cases is the main method of control, but in developing countries this is largely an impossible task. In restricted communities, such as mines or plantations, it can be used to considerable value, but in the vast, sprawling urban slums, where people come and go and addresses are not known, it is a hopeless task. The prohibition of commercial sex workers only drives the practice underground and is generally not acceptable in developing countries where they form a recognized segment of society in many cultures. A preferable answer is to try and examine known commercial sex workers at regular intervals and encourage them to bring in others for check-ups.

A commercial sex worker aware of the damage that can be caused by the disease, once converted, can be a greater proponent of health education than any trained worker.

Health education should start at school, encouraging delay of first sexual experience and the benefits of a monogamous relationship. Programmes should also be targeted at high-risk groups, such as miners, truck drivers and the commercial sex industry, encouraging safe sex and the use of condoms. The likelihood of contracting a sexually transmitted infection is proportional to the number of sexual partners.

Diagnostic and treatment facilities need to be widely available on a walk-in basis. It is preferable to provide special clinics as well as the routine health services. Unfortunately, many private practitioners, often not even medically qualified, offer inadequate treatment, so encouraging resistant organisms to develop as syphilis is often contracted at the same time as other sexually transmitted infections (STIs).

All pregnant women should be tested for syphilis, preferably both in early and late pregnancy. All blood donors should also be screened. (See also Box 14.1.)

Treatment is with benzathine penicillin 2.4 million units as a single dose (but often given intramuscularly at two different sites). Alternatively, tetracycline 500 mg four times a day or doxycycline 100 mg twice daily, both for 14 days, can be given, especially in the patient allergic to penicillin who is not pregnant.

Surveillance. Antenatal and family planning clinics provide an important opportunity to examine a large number of women and also to prevent cases of congenital syphilis. Routine RPRs should be performed and all positive cases fully investigated and treated.

14.2 Gonorrhoea

Organism. Gonorrhoea is a bacterial disease caused by *Neisseria gonorrhoeae* (the gonococcus).

Clinical features. In the male, infection commences as a mucoid urethral secretion, which soon changes to a profuse, purulent discharge (as opposed to nongonococcal urethritis where the discharge is scanty, white, mucoid or serous). The discharge is best seen first thing in the morning (dewdrop) and a smear should be made from this before the patient urinates. The main symptom is pain on micturition, but the degree of discomfort is very variable. In the female, the infection generally passes unnoticed, but may present with urethritis or acute salpingitis. It is this latter presentation of the disease that can lead, in an acute or chronic form of pelvic inflammatory disease, to sterility in the female. This is a serious problem in the unmarried woman and a cause of divorce in the married. In the male, untreated or improperly treated infection can result in urethral stricture, while generalized symptoms of arthritis, dermatitis or meningitis can rarely occur in either sex. In the pregnant woman, there is a danger of the newborn infant developing gonococcal conjunctivitis at the time of delivery. The discovery of this infection in the newborn infant may be the manner in which the infection is found in the woman.

Diagnosis. Due to the similarity in presentation of gonococcal and non-gonococcal urethritis, the emphasis is on making a diagnosis from a urethral discharge. A smear should be made and stained with Gram stain, the finding of Gram-negative intracellular diplococci indicating gonococcal infection. Where facilities permit, the discharge should be cultured, but as the organism is very sensitive it must be inoculated on to a culture plate or placed in transport medium (less satisfactory) as soon as possible. Urine can be tested by PCR to give a positive diagnosis but culture should also be undertaken for surveillance and drug sensitivity.

Transmission is by sexual intercourse or by contact with the infected mucous exudate. *N. gonorrhoeae* is unable to penetrate stratified epithelium, but has a predilection for mucous membranes, where it produces an accumulation of polymorphonuclear leucocytes and outpouring of serum to give the characteristic discharge.

Important factors in the transmission of gonorrhoea are:

- the short incubation period;
- the often asymptomatic disease in women (estimated to be 80%);
- promiscuous sexual intercourse;
- urbanization and changing social values;
- use of contraceptives; and
- inadequate treatment.

The combination of a short incubation period and promiscuous sexual activity means that a large number of people can become infected in rapid succession. As women are often largely unaware of their infection they provide a continuous reservoir of the disease. Urbanization changes the social balance that occurs in the village, traditional values and taboos are lost and promiscuity develops. Contraceptives allow increased opportunity for sexual intercourse although the condom provides limited protection. The contraceptive pill, by reducing the acidity of genital secretions, removes some of the natural defences, while the intrauterine contraceptive device encourages mechanical spread to the uterus and tubes. Improper treatment, both by doctors and quacks, usually with grossly inadequate doses of antibiotics, has led to chronic infections and the development of resistant organisms.

Incubation period is 2–7 days (average 3 days).

Period of communicability can be months in untreated cases, especially in hidden infections in women.

Occurrence and distribution. The number of cases of gonorrhoea in the world today is estimated to be some 62 million. Underreporting, illegal treatment and the protection of contacts make any standard method of contact tracing and case treatment quite inadequate in most developing countries. Gonorrhoea is not so much found as a reservoir in commercial sex workers as more widely distributed among the promiscuous under-25s.

Control and prevention. Where possible, cases presenting at STI clinics should be encouraged to bring their partners (or provide information so that they can be traced) for counselling and treatment. Alternatively, contact cards can be sent anonymously to all contacts of a case, recommending them to present at a clinic. Condoms can be given out at the same time as a person comes to a clinic. Health education concentrating on the dangers of sexually transmitted diseases is the main preventive action (see also under syphilis, Section 14.1 above, and Box 14.1). The eyes of babies, as they are being born, should be wiped and a 1% aqueous solution of silver nitrate instilled (Section 7.7).

Treatment, which used to be a simple matter with penicillin, is now fraught with problems of resistance – not only to this antibiotic, but also to many others that have subsequently been tried. Any recommended treatment regime may be ineffective in certain parts of the world and local expertise must be consulted to develop routines that are compatible with the resistance patterns and available resources. Recommended regimens are:

- ciprofloxacin 500 mg as a single oral dose (but not in pregnant women or children), or
- azithromycin 2 g orally as a single dose, or
- ceftriaxone 125 mg by single intramuscular injection, or
- cefixime 400 mg as a single oral dose, or
- spectinomycin 2 g by single intramuscular injection.

Patients diagnosed with gonorrhoea often have *Chlamydia* infection as well so treatment for this condition should be combined as a routine (see Section 14.3 below).

Surveillance. Strains of the gonococcus resistant to the standard treatment regime in the country are likely to be imported from time to time, so sensitivity should be regularly tested and the treatment regime modified accordingly.

14.3 Chlamydia

Organism. Chlamydia trachomatis.

Clinical features. Chlamydial infection presents as a urethritis in the male and as a cervical discharge in the female and is often indistinguishable from or present at the same time as gonorrhoea. The discharge can be purulent but is more likely to be mucoid with symptoms of burning on micturition. In the female, there may be oedema of the cervix and bleeding, but in 70% of sexually active women the infection is asymptomatic. This is a serious problem as it can lead to salpingitis and pelvic inflammatory disease. Asymptomatic males serve as carriers, spreading the infection, but suffering few complications.

Diagnosis may be indicated if *N. gonorrhoeae* cannot be found in the smear or culture of the discharge. It can be confirmed by the nucleic acid amplification test (NAAT), ligase chain reaction, enzyme immunoassay (EIA) or by direct immunofluorescence. A rapid test has been developed based on the recognition of lipopolysaccharide markers which gives results within 30 minutes.

Either self-collected vaginal swabs can be used or else those obtained in clinics. A urine test is effective in men. Due to its ease and low cost it is hoped that this method may become available for use in developing countries.

Transmission is by sexual intercourse, while contaminated hands can lead to conjunctival infection. Babies born to mothers with infection of their genital tract can develop chlamydia ophthalmia neonatorum. *C. trachomatis* is a risk factor for HIV infection in the female.

Incubation period. Uncertain, but probably 7–14 days.

Period of communicability. This is as long as active infection is present, which could be weeks to months in the undiagnosed case.

Occurrence and distribution. Worldwide distribution among the sexually active. Probably one of the commonest STIs, but because it so often goes undiagnosed the full burden of infection remains unknown.

Control and prevention. The same as for gonorrhoea and syphilis.

Treatment is with azithromycin 1 g orally in a single dose, doxycycline 100 mg orally twice daily for 7 days, erythromycin 500 mg orally four times a day for 7 days or tetracycline 500 mg orally four times daily for 7 days. Sexual intercourse must be avoided until both partners are free of signs. Erythromycin is the recommended treatment if the patient is pregnant, but amoxycillin can also be used. All cases of gonorrhoea should be treated for chlamydia unless it has been confirmed to be absent by full laboratory tests.

Surveillance. Several sexually transmitted infections can occur together so any discharge, urethritis or pelvic pain may indicate possible syphilis and gonorrhoea, which should always be looked for.

14.4 Trichomonas and Non-gonococcal Urethritis

Organism. A number of organisms have been found to be responsible for urethritis not caused by the gonococcus or *Chlamydia trachomatis*, and these include *Trichomonas vaginalis*, *Ureaplasma urealyticum* and *Mycoplasma hominis*.

Clinical features. A low-grade urethritis with mucoid rather than purulent discharge in the male, in which intracellular diplococci are not found in the smear, suggests a non-gonococcal urethritis (NGU). Infection is a low-grade discharge in the female and is often asymptomatic in the male. Often the first sign is a staining of the underclothes in the female or the presence of fishy smell in the male. The infection is often asymptomatic or ignored so that a reservoir of infection can occur if simultaneous treatment to both sexual partners is not given. In areas where gonococcal urethritis is common, the prevalence of NGU is also high so treatment should be given for both conditions.

Diagnosis. Both a dry and wet smear (mixed with 2–3 drops of saline) and a culture should be made. The absence of intracellular diplococci indicates an NGU. Motile *T. vaginalis* may be found in a wet preparation. Where facilities permit, confirmation can be made by PCR.

Transmission is by sexual intercourse. *T. vaginalis* is a risk factor for HIV infection in the female.

Incubation period is 5–20 days, average 7 days.

Period of communicability. In the asymptomatic case, infection can continue for a considerable period of time.

Occurrence and distribution. NGU is more common than gonorrhoea and is found all over the world, with high levels where people have multiple partners.

Control and prevention is the same as for gonorrhoea and syphilis (see above).

Treatment for *Trichomonas* infection is with metronidazole 2g orally or tinidazole 2g orally in a single dose. Sexual intercourse must be avoided until both partners are free of signs.

Surveillance. Several sexually transmitted infections can occur together so NGU is an indicator of possible syphilis and gonorrhoea, which should always be looked for.

14.5 Lymphogranuloma Venereum

Organism. *Chlamydia trachomatis* immunotypes L1, L2 and L3, which are different from the immunotypes causing trachoma and genital infection.

Clinical features. Lymphogranuloma venereum is a chronic infection presenting as a small painless papule, vesicle or ulcer on the genitalia that often goes unnoticed, lymphadenitis being the clinical sign. The lymph nodes become grossly enlarged and generally suppurate with fistulas and fibrosis developing, especially in the rectal area if treatment is delayed.

Diagnosis is by finding the organism in lymph node aspirate with immunofluorescence, PCR or a DNA probe. A fourfold rise of the complement fixation test is also indicative of infection.

Transmission. Although sexual intercourse is considered to be the main means of transmission, infection can also happen by direct contact with open lesions.

Incubation period. 3–30 days.

Period of communicability is for as long as there are active lesions, which may be for several years.

Occurrence and distribution. Although it occurs worldwide, lymphogranuloma venereum is commoner in the tropics, especially in sub-Saharan Africa and parts of Asia.

Control and prevention. Treatment should be commenced as soon as the diagnosis has been made, the patient being advised to refrain from sexual intercourse and close contact with others until all lesions have healed. Other methods of control are the same as for syphilis and gonorrhoea above.

Treatment is with doxycycline 100mg daily for 14 days, erythromycin 500mg four times daily for 14 days or tetracycline 500mg four times daily for 14 days.

14.6 Granuloma Inguinale (Donovanosis)

Organism. *Klebsiella granulomatis*.

Clinical features. Granuloma inguinale is a chronic, progressive, ulcerating disease of the anogenital area without regional lymphadenopathy. An initial lesion on the genitalia becomes eroded and ulcerated, with new nodules forming at the margins as the lesion extends into the inguinal and anal regions. The lesions readily bleed on contact and ulceration can continue to produce extensive destruction. Carcinoma of the vulva has been reported to be associated with granuloma inguinale.

Diagnosis is made from smears or scrapings of the lesions stained with Giemsa, in which intracellular rod shaped organisms (Donovan bodies) are found.

Transmission. The disease is transmitted by direct contact with lesions either via sexual intercourse or other methods. It is frequently associated with anal intercourse.

Incubation period. 1–16 weeks.

Period of communicability is while open lesions are present, which can be for a considerable period of time in the untreated patient.

Occurrence and distribution. The disease is found mainly in the tropical regions of the world, especially in southern India and New Guinea and among the aboriginal people of Australia. It is less commonly found in Africa and people of African origin, such as in the Caribbean and the northern part of South America. It is a disease of the sexually active 20–40 year age group, in males more than females, but children under 5 years of age also contract the disease (presumably from contact with their parents).

Control and prevention. Control is the same as for syphilis and gonorrhoea described above. Care should be taken to prevent transmission from open lesions to others and other parts of the body.

Treatment is with azithromycin 1g orally on the first day followed by 500mg daily for a maximum of 14 days, doxycycline 100mg twice daily for 14 days, erythromycin 500mg orally four times a day for 14 days, or tetracycline 500mg four times daily for 14 days.

Surveillance. As with all sexually transmitted diseases it is possible that more than one STI is present.

14.7   Chancroid

Organism. Haemophilus ducreyi.

Clinical features. The acute venereal infection commences with a papule which then ulcerates to form a soft chancre on the external genitalia. This is accompanied by a painful regional lymphadenopathy, which is often unilateral. The chancre has an indurated base which differentiates it from syphilis. Chancroid is a predisposing cause of HIV infection, with which it is frequently associated.

Diagnosis. The organism can be identified with Gram stain from the exudate of lesions, but this is often difficult owing to secondary infection. Otherwise, culture on to a selective medium can be made.

Transmission is by sexual intercourse or by direct contact with lesions.

Incubation period is 3–14 days.

Period of communicability is as long as lesions continue to discharge, which can be months in the untreated case.

Occurrence and distribution. Predominantly found in the tropical regions of the world where it is common in men who probably obtain their infection from a commercial sex worker.

Control and prevention. See syphilis above. The wider availability of condoms has led to a decrease in chancroid.

Treatment. Chancroid can be treated with one of the following regimes:

- azithromycin 1g orally as a single dose, or
- ceftriaxone 250mg intramuscularly as a single dose, or
- ciprofloxacin 500mg orally twice daily for 3 days, or
- erythromycin 500mg orally 4 times daily for 7 days.

14.8   Genital Herpes

Organism. Herpesvirus simplex type 2 (HSV-2); less commonly type 1 (HSV-1).

Clinical features. Painful vesicles develop on the genitalia or surrounding area of both females and males, and these can subsequently ulcerate. Healing occurs after initial infection, only for the vesicles to recur at frequent intervals, often precipitated by stress or menstruation. Infection of the neonate can occur during delivery, resulting in encephalitis, liver damage or lesions in the eye, mouth or skin. Infection with HSV-2 carries an increased risk of developing HIV infection.

Diagnosis is made on clinical presentation and by scrapings of the lesions, in which characteristic multinucleated giant cells with intranuclear bodies are seen on microscopy. Confirmation can be made by fluorescence antibody testing, isolation of the virus or PCR.

Transmission is by sexual intercourse or direct contact, such as orogenital, or to the infant during delivery.

Incubation period. 2–12 days.

Period of communicability is 2–7 weeks during the initial clinical infection and 5 days during a recurrence.

Occurrence and distribution. A worldwide and increasing problem among the sexually active. As the infection is difficult to treat there is a recurrent reservoir of infection with each clinical attack, and if one of these should occur during delivery, then neonatal death or disability will result. There is some suggestion that infection with HSV-1, normally as mouth ulcers in childhood, has some protective effect on acquiring HSV-2 infection. Decreasing natural infection of HSV-1 in many developed countries may help to explain the increase in HSV-2 infection.

Control and prevention. The same as with gonorrhoea and syphilis (see above). Infected persons should be warned of the increased risk of developing HIV infection. Several vaccines are under trial but the development of immunity is severely reduced in those persons with a previous infection of HSV-1.

Treatment. There is no cure but acyclovir 200 mg orally five times daily for 7 days or acyclovir 400 mg orally three times a day for 7 days, or other analogues, will reduce the formation of new lesions, pain and the period of healing, but not recurrent attacks. Treatment can be given with each episode, helping to reduce the duration, the number of outbreaks and, possibly, viral shedding.

Surveillance. Any case of genital herpes should be tested for HIV infection.

14.9 Human Papillomavirus (HPV)

Organism. Human papillomavirus (HPV). There are many different types, with types 6–11 being associated with genital warts and types 16, 18, 31, 33 and 35 producing cervical dysphasia, which can lead to cancer of the cervix. Types 16 and 18 are responsible for 70% of cancer cases.

Clinical features. The main clinical presentation is genital warts on the external genitalia or within the vagina, but a large proportion of infected persons show no clinical signs. When cellular immunity is depressed, condylomata acuminata, large fleshy growths in moist areas of the perineum, develop. However, the most serious consequence of HPV infection is the development of carcinoma, particularly of the cervix, but the anus and penis can also be involved. It is being more commonly recognized that oropharyngeal squamous cell carcinoma can develop from oral sex.

Diagnosis. Clinical diagnosis can be made if genital warts are present. Cervical smears stained by the Papanicolau method can detect precancerous changes and are routinely performed as a screening test in many countries.

Transmission is by sexual intercourse, but direct contact, as with other warts, is possible. Unprotected intercourse will lead to transmission of the oncogenic type 80% of the time.

Incubation period. 1–3 months, but can be as long as 20 months.

Period of communicability. Probably for a considerable period of time as cancer of the cervix appears to be associated with the cumulative number of sexual encounters.

Occurrence and distribution. It has been estimated that between 9 and 13% of the world population is infected with HPV, which is some 630 million people. Some 70% of these infections are subclinical with only a proportion developing genital warts and some 28–40 million the pre-malignant condition. There are 0.5 million cases of cervical cancer every year in the world. The prevalence of chronic persistent infection is about 15% in developing countries and 7% in developed countries. Some 80% of the worldwide incidence of cervical cancer is in developing countries.

Control and prevention. The usual methods of reducing STIs, such as delaying the age of first intercourse, monogamous relationships and the use of condoms will all assist in decreasing the likelihood of developing HPV infection. The promotion of cervical smear testing in developed countries has allowed detection of precancer and early cervical cancer amenable to surgical treatment, but few if any developing countries are able to afford such a service.

There are two vaccines to prevent HPV infection: a quadrivalent (HPV types 6, 11, 16 and 18) vaccine which can be given to girls from age 9 years and a bivalent (HPV types 16 and 18) vaccine which can be given to girls from age 10 years. The target population is girls of 9–13 years, and the vaccine is administered in three doses and ideally given as part of the school health programme. A catch-up vaccination may also be considered for older girls and young women when a vaccine programme is started. Protection lasts for at least 5 years but programmes have not been running for long enough to decide when booster doses need to be given.

Treatment. Treatment of the warts is by cryotherapy, podophyllin, immune modulators (e.g. imiquod) or with trichloroacetic acid. Cone biopsy of the cervix can reduce the precancerous condition, but more extensive surgery will be required when cancer has developed.

Surveillance. Cytological services for screening women at regular intervals have been shown to be cost-effective in reducing cervical cancer and should be set up wherever resources permit.

14.10   Human Immunodeficiency Virus (HIV)

Organism. Human immunodeficiency virus (HIV), either type 1 (HIV-1) or type 2 (HIV-2), HIV-1 being more pathogenic.

Clinical features. HIV infection leads to a disruption of specific T-lymphocytes that bear the CD4

receptor (CD4+). This leads to a disruption of the cell-mediated immune mechanisms, resulting in an increased susceptibility to opportunistic infections. The breakdown of the body's defence system and the range of symptoms produced is called acquired immunodeficiency syndrome (AIDS). Presentation is generally by the symptoms of the opportunistic infection so can be many and varied.

Primary infection 2–4 weeks after exposure presents as an acute febrile illness often with lymphadenopathy, pharyngitis, maculopapular rash, orogenital ulcers and meningoencephalitis. A transient lymphopenia may develop with low CD4 count. If the primary infection is mild or ignored there follows a dormant period for several months, after which symptoms of an opportunistic infection occur. The opportunistic infections found are listed below under the account of clinical staging, with details of the sections (in parentheses) where more information will be found in the text.

Any process that stresses the immune mechanism, such as repeat infections, will accelerate progression to AIDS. Tuberculosis (TB) and leprosy are affected by the disruption of the immune process. In any person with TB who contracts HIV, the infection will progress more rapidly, while tuberculoid leprosy cases can convert to lepromatous leprosy. It has been suspected that there is an interaction between HIV and malaria, and this has now been shown to be the case. In a survey in just one district of Kenya, there have been almost 1 million excess malaria cases and 8.5 thousand excess HIV cases since the HIV epidemic first started in the 1980s over a period until measurements ceased in 2006.

Diagnosis and case definition. The World Health Organization (WHO) case definition for HIV infection is:

Adults and children 18 months or older:
Positive HIV antibody testing (rapid or laboratory-based EIA). This is confirmed by a second HIV antibody test (again a rapid or laboratory-based EIA) that relies on different antigens or different operating characteristics.

and/or

Positive virology test for HIV or its components (HIV-RNA or HIV-DNA or ultra-sensitive HIV p24 antigen), confirmed by the results of a second virological test obtained from a separate determination.

Children younger than 18 months:

Positive virological test for HIV or its components (HIV-RNA or HIV-DNA or ultra-sensitive HIV p24 antigen), confirmed by the results of a second virological test obtained from a separate determination taken more than 4 weeks after birth.

Positive HIV antibody testing is not recommended for definitive or confirmatory diagnosis of HIV infection in children until 18 months of age.

The case definition for advanced HIV, including AIDS (for reporting) is:

Clinical criteria of advanced HIV in adults and children with confirmed HIV infection:

Presumptive or definitive diagnosis of any clinical stage 3 (advanced) or stage 4 (severe) symptoms (see below);

and/or

Immunological criteria for diagnosing advanced HIV in adults and children 5 years or older with confirmed HIV infection:

CD4 count less than 350 per mm^3 of blood in an HIV-infected adult or child;

and/or

Immunological criteria for diagnosing advanced HIV in a child younger than 5 years of age with confirmed HIV infection:

%CD4 <30 among those younger than 12 months; %CD4 <25 among those aged 12–35 months; %CD4 <20 among those aged 36–59 months.

WHO clinical staging of HIV/AIDS for adults and adolescents with confirmed HIV infection (cross references in parentheses not part of the definition but indicate where further information can be found):

Clinical stage 1

Asymptomatic
Persistent generalized lymphadenopathy

Clinical stage 2

Moderate unexplained weight loss; <10% of presumed or measured body weight
Recurrent respiratory tract infections; sinusitis, tonsillitis, otitis media (Section 13.9) and pharyngitis
Herpes zoster (as shingles, see Section 12.1)
Angular cheilitis

Recurrent oral ulceration
Papular pruritic eruptions
Seborrhoeic dermatitis
Intractable scabies not responding to treatment (Section 7.1)
Fungal nail infections

Clinical stage 3

Unexplained severe weight loss; >10% of presumed or measured body weight
Unexplained chronic diarrhoea for longer than 1 month
Unexplained persistent fever above 37.6°C, intermittent or constant, for longer than 1 month
Persistent oral candidiases
Oral hairy leukoplakia
Pulmonary TB (Section 13.1)
Severe bacterial infections, such as pneumonia (Table 13.1), empyema, pyomyositis, bone or joint infection, meningitis (Table 13.2) or bacteraemia
Acute necrotizing ulcerative stomatitis, gingivitis or periodontitis
Unexplained anaemia, haemoglobin <8 g/dl; neutropenia, neutrophils $<0.5 \times 10^9/l$; or chronic thrombocytopenia, thrombocytes (platelets) $<50 \times 10^9/l$

Clinical stage 4

HIV wasting syndrome
Pneumocystis jiroveci pneumonia (Table 13.1)
Recurrent severe bacterial pneumonia
Chronic herpes simplex infection; labial, genital or anorectal of more than 1 month's duration, or visceral at any site (Section 14.8)
Oesophageal candidiases, or of trachea, bronchi or lungs
Extrapulmonary tuberculosis (Section 13.1)
Kaposi's sarcoma (Section 1.1)
Cytomegalovirus retinitis or infection of other organs, excluding liver, spleen and lymph nodes
CNS toxoplasmosis (Section 17.5)
HIV encephalopathy
Extrapulmonary Cryptococcus, including meningitis (Tables 13.1 and 13.2)
Disseminated non-tuberculous mycobacterium infection
Progressive multimodal leukoencephalopathy
Chronic cryptosporidiosis, with diarrhoea (Section 8.3)
Chronic isosporiasis
Disseminated mycosis; coccidiomycosis or histoplasmosis
Recurrent septicaemia, including non-typhoidal *Salmonella* bacteraemia

Lymphoma; cerebral or B-cell non-Hodgkin's or other solid HIV-associated tumours (Section 1.1)

Invasive cervical carcinoma

Disseminated *Strongyloides* (Section 10.4)

Atypical disseminated leishmaniasis (Section 15.12)

Symptomatic HIV-associated nephropathy or symptomatic HIV-associated cardiomyopathy

Reactivation of American trypanosomiasis, meningo-encephalitis and/or myocarditis (Section 15.11)

(In children there are additional or modified criteria, particularly in clinical stages 2 and 3, whereas stages 1 and 4 are the same.)

Transmission is by:

- sexual contact with an infected person;
- inoculation with infected blood or blood products (including unsterile needles and syringes);
- from an infected mother to child before or during delivery, or for up to 2 years after if breastfed; and
- from tissue transplants (rare).

Unprotected sexual contact is the commonest method of transmission, both heterosexual and homosexual. The important epidemiological factor is the number of sexual contacts, so that prostitutes or promiscuous homosexuals with hundreds if not thousands of new contacts annually are at greatest risk. However, one contact with an infected person is able to produce infection. Anal intercourse carries a higher risk of infection than vaginal. There is no evidence of increased risk during menstruation. Circumcision is protective in the male, probably due to improved hygiene. There is an association with other STIs, particularly genital herpes simplex virus type 2 and ulcerating conditions such as chancroid. Other STIs may potentiate infection.

Transfusion of infected blood will almost always transmit HIV. Pooled blood, such as used for producing factor VIII for the treatment of haemophilia is particularly dangerous because it contains donations from many people, any of which could be infected. Syringes and needles, if they are not properly cleaned and sterilized, can contain small quantities of blood sufficient to transmit infection. This method may be responsible for many infections in developing countries and is an important way of transmitting infection among drug abusers. Transmission by needle stick injury can occur, but is uncommon.

The infected mother can pass on infection to her child. Infection can be transmitted congenitally, but it is more likely to occur from a mixing of the mother's and infant's blood at the time of delivery. HIV is found in breast milk, and accounts for almost 50% of children infected. The risk to the child is reduced by treating the HIV-positive mother with antiretroviral therapy. (See Section 18.1.7.)

Serological tests may not become positive for up to 3 months after the person becomes infected so it is possible for people to transmit infection before they are shown to be positive.

Incubation period. The time from infection to becoming HIV positive is 1–3 months. The development period for AIDS can range from 1 to 18 years, with a mean of 10 years. In perinatal infection, the incubation period is often shorter than 12 months.

Period of communicability. Infectiousness is highest during initial infection, probably extending throughout the life of the individual, and increasing again as immunity becomes suppressed. Other STIs, especially of the ulcerative kind, increase the likelihood of transmission. People treated with an effective antiviral therapy regime can achieve undetectable viral loads but the treatment has not been shown to completely eliminate the risk of transferring infection. Other precautionary measures should also be utilized.

Occurrence and distribution. There is worldwide occurrence (Fig. 14.1), with some 33 million people living with HIV in 2007. An estimated 4.1 million become newly infected with HIV each year and 2.8 million die from it. The worst affected area is sub-Saharan Africa, with South Africa showing no sign of any decline in its epidemic, whereas improvement has taken place in other parts of the continent. The considerable tragedy in Africa is that infection rates in young women are three times those in young men, indicating the gender inequality. Many women lack socio-economic independence, education and access to health information and health services, making it difficult for them to avoid exposure to the virus.

Infection has now spread to most other parts of the world, with prevalence increasing in China, Indonesia, Papua New Guinea and Vietnam, and signs of outbreaks in Pakistan and Bangladesh. There are estimated to be 8.3 million people with HIV in Asia, two-thirds of them in India. The annual number of new HIV cases diagnosed continues to

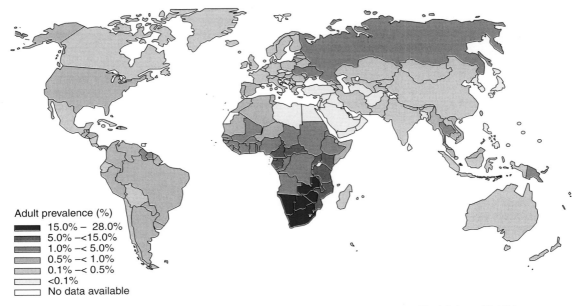

Adult prevalence (%)

- 15.0% − 28.0%
- 5.0% −<15.0%
- 1.0% −< 5.0%
- 0.5% −< 1.0%
- 0.1% −< 0.5%
- <0.1%
- No data available

Fig. 14.1. A global view of HIV infection in 2007, 33 million people (range: 30–36 million) living with HIV. (Reproduced by permission of the World Health Organization, Geneva.)

rise in Russia and the Ukraine, while the Caribbean remains the second most affected area in the world.

In East Africa, initial spread of infection was along transport routes, with lorry drivers making use of local bar girls at each of their stops; this has tended to be a common method of spread in other countries as well. In South Africa, HIV infection was introduced into the mining communities in which it spread rapidly via prostitutes. Sadly, many infections in developing countries have been caused by the use of poorly sterilized needles when people have attended clinics for other illnesses.

Parts of South America and some Caribbean islands have very high incidence rates due to the general attitude towards promiscuity. A worrying trend has been the unchanged incidence in Western countries, despite the availability of antiretroviral therapy (ART). It appears that the availability of treatment is reducing the fear of infection and allowing more risky behaviour to take place.

There has been a strong movement to increase the availability of ART in developing countries, although it is only reaching one in five people who need it. It is hoped that ART therapy will reduce the stigma of AIDS and allow preventive programmes to be more effective. Both preventive and

treatment strategies need to proceed at the same time because viral shedding can still continue in the treated person.

Four key populations have been identified for special attention as they tend to have higher rates of HIV than the general population, yet receive the least resources, these are:

- sex workers;
- men who have sex with men;
- injecting drug users; and
- prisoners.

In many countries, it is a vicious circle with sex workers and homosexuals being criminalized so that they end up in prison where the situation only gets worse. Many sex workers, prisoners and men who have sex with men also inject drugs, doubling their risk of infection.

HIV-1 is common in the Americas, Europe, Asia, Central and East Africa, whereas HIV-2 is found in West Africa or in people that acquired their infection.

Control and prevention. Methods of control and prevention are aimed at the three routes of transmission: sexual, via blood and perinatal. The search for a vaccine has been a major priority, using either a live attenuated vaccine or a live recombinant vaccine, but none has progressed beyond the trial stage. The problem with all the vaccine candidates so far developed is the rapid rate at which the HIV virus alters its antigenic make-up. So until a vaccine has been developed other control measures are required.

To prevent **sexual** spread:

- Limit the number of sexual partners, encouraging monogamous relationships.
- Avoid sexual contact with persons at high risk, such as commercial sex workers, bisexuals and homosexuals.
- Encourage male and female condom use with the addition of vaginal microbicides.
- Encourage programmes to circumcise males in high incidence areas.
- Provide adequate facilities for the detection and treatment of STIs.
- HIV testing and counselling to be made available both at special counselling centres and general clinics. Patients presenting with infections that are more common with HIV are counselled and offered HIV testing (called opt-in testing). However, where more than 1% of antenatal women are HIV positive, WHO recommends 'provider initiated HIV counselling and testing', whereby all patients regardless of their presenting illness are tested unless they decline (opt-out testing).
- General education for girls and sex education for both boys and girls.
- Lifestyle training (how to say 'no').

To prevent **blood** spread:

- Screen all blood for transfusions.
- Test donors before they give blood.
- Only use blood transfusions when essential.
- Discontinue paid blood donors.
- Use disposable syringes, needles, giving sets, lancets, etc. or ensure they are properly sterilized.
- Injecting drug users should be discouraged from sharing equipment, preferably using needle exchange schemes.
- Medical workers should wear gloves when dealing with possible infected blood, e.g. at delivery and in the laboratory.

To prevent **perinatal** spread:

- Encourage all mothers attending antenatal clinic to have an HIV test.

- Advise HIV-infected pregnant women about the risk to their infants and themselves during and after pregnancy.
- Promote good obstetric practice; reduce trauma and decide on the necessity of such procedures as artificial rupture of membranes and fetal scalp monitoring. Only cut the umbilical cord when it has stopped pulsating.
- Give priority antiretroviral therapy to HIV-positive pregnant women and to the newborn infant.
- Provide information on breastfeeding to allow each mother to decide on whether to breastfeed or artificially feed her newborn child.

Caesarean section should not be encouraged in developing countries as the risk to the mother in subsequent pregnancies is considerably increased, but it might be the strategy of choice in developed countries. A similar dilemma is with breastfeeding, which is responsible for much of the neonatal transmission, but to encourage bottle-feeding and leave the child more likely to die from diarrhoea due to contaminated bottles is not sound practice. (See further in Section 18.1.7.) WHO recommends that no change should be made in the vaccination programme to mothers and children even though they may be infected with AIDS, except in the HIV-positive child who should not be given BCG.

There have been several trials of vaccines against HIV, the most recent having a vaccine efficacy of 31.2% with no significant impact on viral load or CD4 counts, but this could be the basis for the development of more effective candidates.

AIDS is **not** spread by:

- mosquitoes;
- casual contact such as shaking hands, or lavatory seats; or
- through food, water or the respiratory route.

Control programmes. The main method of control is health promotion, and this should involve community leaders, religious organizations and non-governmental organizations (NGOs). Promotion can be to the general public to supply them with the correct information, or to specific groups. The most cost-effective health education will be to high-risk groups such as commercial sex workers, homosexuals and workers who are single or unaccompanied by their families. Promotion of condom use and making condoms available at both commercial and government outlets should be instigated. (See Section 4.6.2.) Thailand has had much success with its brothel-based 100% condom use, a model being tried in other countries.

As already noted, criminalization of sex workers and homosexuals only drives the practice underground and efforts should be made to rehabilitate these people into ordinary society by a change in law if necessary. Peer distribution of condoms was found to be very effective in Mumbai in reaching these disadvantaged groups. Men who have sex with men often have sex with women as well, making these women more vulnerable to infection too, so programmes to reach them may need to be developed. Needle and syringe exchange programmes in a number of countries have helped reduce the risk of infection in drug users. Prisons have been termed 'incubators of HIV', yet they are captive audiences and so much more could be done to reach this highly vulnerable group.

Girls should have the same opportunity for education as boys, with sex education an integral part of the school curriculum. Counselling and testing facilities need to be readily available, as well as programmes on mother-to-child transmission. Improved diagnosis and treatment facilities for STIs need to be made available, providing early and adequate treatment. Condoms can be dispensed at clinics, markets or at any suitable social marketing opportunity. (See Box 14.1.)

Treatment. Co-trimoxazole prophylaxis can be given to HIV-positive persons to prevent *P. jiroveci* pneumonia. The CD4 level and clinical staging decides when to start treatment. Treatment regimes must use a combination of drugs to prevent resistance from developing, generally two non-nucleoside reverse transcriptase inhibitors and a protease inhibitor, but each patient must be individually assessed. The following should be started on ART:

- patients with TB and hepatitis B (HBV) co-infection irrespective of CD4 count;
- symptomatic persons (including pregnant women) with clinical stage 3 or 4, irrespective of CD4 count; and
- asymptomatic or symptomatic persons (including pregnant women) with clinical stages 1 or 2 and with a CD4 count of less than 350.

The following first-line treatment regimes can be used (although efavirenz should not be used in the first trimester of the pregnant woman:

- zidovudine + lamivudine + efavirenz (or nevirapine); and
- tenovir disoproxil fumerate + lamivudine (emtricitabine) + efavirenz (or nevirapine). (This regime to be used for HIV/HBV co-infection.)

Second-line therapy will depend upon the regime used in first-line therapy. (The management of the HIV-positive pregnant woman and her newborn is covered in Section 18.1.7.)

People must be counselled before starting ART because missing as few as three doses in a month can result in a rise in viral load, the development of drug resistance and treatment failure. As with TB, a family member or friend should be chosen as a treatment supporter, ensuring that tablets are taken and that the person attends regularly for follow-up. The spouse or sexual partner is the ideal choice, as preventive methods, such as using a condom, must be maintained despite being on treatment. The supporter should come with the patient and be given information leaflets, treatment diaries and other aids to help in maintaining the patient's regular attendance. Mobile phone numbers can be used to recall late attendees and pill counts made to check adherence. ART cards and registers should be used in a similar way to that in TB programmes.

All HIV-positive persons should be tuberculin skin tested for TB, and information on any active symptoms asked for. If the TB test is positive and/or there are no symptoms related to TB, isoniazid prophylaxis should be given for 6 months. Any opportunistic infection must receive specific treatment for the condition. (See the WHO 'Integrated management of adolescent and adult illness' (IMAI) guidelines, Section 4.4.4 and under Further Reading at the end of the chapter.)

Surveillance. Voluntary testing of all persons should be made available at health facilities, but more active provider-initiated HIV testing should be encouraged when attending health facilities for other reasons. Numbers of newly diagnosed HIV-positive persons give an indication of the progress of the epidemic and are reported to WHO using the case definitions above. Population-based surveys have been conducted in a number of countries and give a more accurate picture of the prevalence.

Box 14.1. The control of sexually transmitted infections (STIs).

There has been a considerable increase in STIs, with new ones appearing or their relative importance changing. Some of the reasons for these changes are:

- increasing world population, especially of younger age groups;
- urbanization and migrant labour;
- increasing travel and mixing of populations.
- alteration of social values and increasing promiscuity;
- development of contraceptive practice;
- vulnerability of women biologically, culturally and socio-economically; and
- inadequate treatment, and the development of resistant organisms.

International travel has allowed a mixing of cultural groups that would otherwise have remained isolated, leading to the spread of different types and strains of STIs. The development of resistant strains has posed a problem to the developed world, but has left the developing world with an intolerable situation that they are economically unable to deal with.

STIs are more prevalent in young people, yet with an increasing world population it is predominantly these younger age groups that are expanding at a more rapid rate than others. This increase in the youth of the world has thrown a greater strain on the education services, so that health education, especially of STIs, is neglected.

Change has also occurred in social structure, whereby traditional values and the monogamous married couple are no longer regarded as the norm. In other cultures, where polygamy was accepted practice, the male freed from the bounds of society has the opportunity to seek multiple partners.

Married women are particularly vulnerable when they are abandoned or their husbands have to find work away from the confines of the family. STIs are often asymptomatic in women, so they do not seek treatment, putting their lives and those of any future children at greater risk. Inadequate treatment, often by private practitioners or the medically unqualified, encourages the development of resistant organisms.

Control and prevention is mainly by:

- health education;
- education of women and recognition of their equal place in society;
- family planning with readily available contraceptives;
- adequate diagnostic and treatment facilities and the development of standard treatment protocols;
- contact tracing; and
- routine testing of pregnant women.

Generally, the risk of developing an STI is more recognized than previously, rather than the shock that led to concealment or recourse to treatment from a medical quack. Also, contraceptive practice should not be discouraged, for it is the problem of the rapidly expanding young population that is a major contributory factor to STIs. The key is health education, with a combined approach of contraceptive advice and STI information. If this is to succeed there must be a considerable increase in treatment facilities, especially in urban areas. Standard regimes should be decided by specialists, and administered by primary health-care workers.

Improved treatment facilities, contact tracing, training of health workers and more effective drugs will not only reduce the prevalence and seriousness of STIs, but also of HIV infection.

14.11   Hepatitis B (HBV)

Organism. Hepatitis B virus (HBV).

Clinical features. After an insidious onset, with anorexia, nausea and abdominal discomfort, dark urine is produced and jaundice develops, from which the majority of patients recover. The symptoms are more severe than with hepatitis A (HAV; Section 8.9) and in a small proportion of cases a chronic active disease develops in which low-grade infection continues with periods of jaundice alternating with remissions. Illness can continue for many years/ invariably resulting in cirrhosis. (For differential diagnosis of jaundice see Table 8.2.)

In many parts of the developing world, HBV infection is common, but only about 30% of cases will show any symptoms, the severity of the disease being dose dependent. The disease is more serious in those over 40 years old, in pregnant women and newborn infants. Hepatocellular carcinoma is associated with chronic HBV infection.

Diagnosis can be made by finding the surface antigens (HBsAg). There are four subtypes, adr, adw, ayr and ayw, which vary in their geographical distribution and so provide useful epidemiological markers. Several simple test kits for HBsAg are available, and consist of a small strip with a well at one end for the blood sample and the result read as a positive band or dot. A further antigen e (HBeAg) is a marker of increased infectivity as well as indicating active viral replication in hepatocytes (which may result in liver damage).

Transmission can occur from blood, serum, saliva and seminal fluid. It is a hazard of blood transfusions, renal dialysis, injections and tattooing. It can be transmitted by sexual intercourse and during delivery. In the developing world, most infections arise from the infected mother to her child during delivery, or in the reuse or poor sterilization of syringes and needles. HBV is 50–100 times more infectious than HIV. The virus has been found in some bloodsucking insects (e.g. bedbugs) but transmission by this means has not been shown to occur.

Certain people with HBV are more infectious than others, resulting in a carrier state, the period of communicability being considerable. The risk of an infant becoming infected from a carrier mother can be 50–70% in some ethnic groups. There is a greater likelihood of the mother passing on the infection if she has acute HBV in the second or third trimester or up to 2 months after delivery. A high titre of the surface e antigen or a history of transmission to previous children increases the risk of a mother infecting her infant. The carrier state is more common in males and in those who acquired their infection in childhood.

Incubation period. 6 weeks to 6 months (usually 9–12 weeks), a larger inoculum of virus probably resulting in a shorter incubation period.

Period of communicability is from several weeks before the onset of symptoms until the end of clinical disease, unless the person becomes a carrier, in which case it is lifelong.

Occurrence and distribution. The carrier state has been estimated to be present in over 350 million people, with varying rates in different parts of the world: Western Europe 1%, South and Central America 2–7%, and Africa, Asia and the Western Pacific more than 8%. Infection occurs commonly in infancy or early childhood in the more endemic areas, with young children more likely to develop chronic infection. The disease kills about 600,000 persons annually, but once there is a good vaccination status in the general population this can be expected to rapidly decline.

HBV is an occupational hazard of health professionals so they should all be vaccinated, as well as taking precautions against contact with blood and body fluids, by the routine wearing of gloves.

Control and prevention. HBV vaccine should be given to all children as soon after birth as possible, then either a second dose with the first DTP (diphtheria, tetanus, pertussis vaccine) and a third with the third DTP or a dose with each DTP. Immunity is thought to last for at least 15 years in the fully vaccinated. There is convincing evidence that reduction of carriers will prevent the development of primary liver cell cancer.

Preventive methods are strict aseptic precautions in giving blood transfusions, injections and the handling of blood. All blood donors should be screened, with contributions to pooled blood being particularly scrutinized. The control of sexually transmitted infections has been covered above. Homosexual practice is particularly liable to lead to HBV infection. Persons at risk should be vaccinated.

Treatment. There is no specific treatment, but alpha-interferon and lamivudine have a limited effect in some people, particularly in the early stage of infection. Long-term treatment may also be of value. Its expense rules out its use in the majority of people.

Surveillance. Blood obtained in antenatal clinics, STI clinics or for other purposes can be anonymously tested for HBsAg. Surveys in developing countries have demonstrated high levels of carriers, so by implementing routine vaccination follow-up surveys the effectiveness of the vaccination programme can be monitored.

14.12   Hepatitis C (HCV)

Organism. Hepatitis C virus (HCV). There are many types of the virus, type 1 being the most serious.

Clinical features. Similar in many respects to HBV, HCV produces a milder disease, but as many as 10–20% will progress to cirrhosis and 1–5% to liver cancer over a period of 20–30 years. (See also Table 8.2.)

Diagnosis is by EIA to detect HCV-specific antibodies, with confirmation by HCV recombinant immunoblot (RIBA) assay and HCV RNA testing. PCR is now commonly used. Simple screening tests are available that are similar to those for HBV, many of them manufactured in developing countries. When a diagnosis is made, it should be confirmed by a more sensitive test.

Transmission is due to the use of poorly sterilized needles, giving sets and other methods of parental administration, so is common in developing countries and in those that abuse drugs in developed countries. Sexual or perinatal transmission probably occurs only rarely.

Incubation period. 2 weeks to 6 months (usually 6–9 weeks).

Period of communicability. Weeks before the start of clinical symptoms to lifelong.

Occurrence and distribution. Infection is found worldwide in the general population in developing countries, and mainly in drug users sharing equipment in the developed countries. However, there are probably many more cases than present figures suggest, and WHO estimates that there are 200 million infected, 3% of the world's population. This means that there are about 170 million chronic carriers who could go on to develop cirrhosis or liver cancer. Some 3 to 4 million persons are newly infected each year. The worst affected regions are Africa with 5.3% prevalence, Eastern Mediterranean with 4.6% and the Western Pacific with 3.9%. (See Fig. 14.2.)

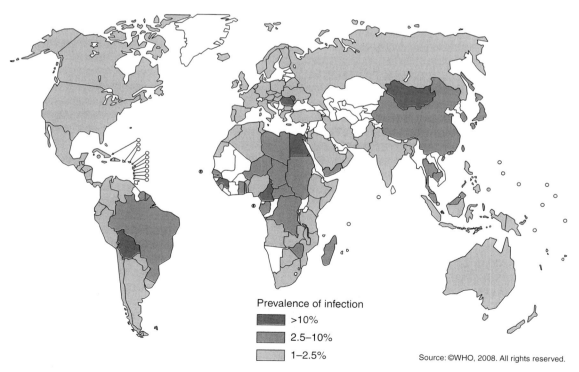

Prevalence of infection

■ >10%
■ 2.5–10%
■ 1–2.5%

Fig. 14.2. Hepatitis C prevalence, 2007. (Reproduced by permission of the World Health Organization, Geneva.)

Control and prevention. There is no vaccine for HCV so all precautions need to be taken to prevent further spread by rigorous adherence to the sterilization of needles and instruments, and the use of blood screened for HCV in transfusions. Needle and syringe exchange facilities should be made available for injecting drug users.

HBA and HBV vaccinations should be given to prevent co-infection, thereby protecting the liver from further damage.

Treatment. A combination of interferon plus ribavirin will prevent the virus from causing further liver damage but may not cure the disease completely. Much depends on the type of virus, with type 1 particularly hard to treat.

Surveillance. HBV is often diagnosed as a result of the person feeling lethargic and having symptoms of liver damage without jaundice. In certain communities, such as high prevalence areas in developing countries and among drug abusers, it may be worth conducting surveys.

14.13   Hepatitis Delta (HDV)

Organism. Hepatitis delta virus (HDV) infection is dependent on the person also being infected with HBV. Either both viruses can infect at the same time or HDV infects an HBV carrier.

Clinical features. With co-infection (both viruses infecting at the same time) there is normally a self-limiting infection with only about 5% continuing into the chronic form of HDV. However, superinfection (HDV infection of an already HBV-infected person) leads to a severe acute hepatitis with 80% continuing to chronic active hepatitis, often progressing to cirrhosis. Hepatocellular carcinoma due to HDV occurs with about the same frequency as with HBV. Mortality from HDV is between 2 and 20%, making it some ten times greater than from HBV alone. (See also Table 8.2.)

Diagnosis is made by detecting antibody to HDV using a serological assay.

Transmission is the same as for HBV, with the main route of transmission via infected blood and blood products percutaneously, or via the sexual route. Superinfection produces the greatest amount of virus and chance of HDV transmission.

Incubation period. 2–8 weeks.

Period of communicability. It is probably most infectious in the weeks prior to symptoms, becoming negligible once the disease is manifest.

Occurrence and distribution. Areas of high prevalence are Russia, Romania, Albania, southern Italy and the Mediterranean countries, West and Central Africa, Northern India and certain Pacific Islands (e.g. Okinawa). In the Amazon Basin, there is a particularly fulminant genotype (III), which carries a high mortality. In Western Europe and North America, infection is endemic in the injecting drug user community. Worldwide, WHO estimates that more than 10 million people are infected. Infection is disproportionately low in some countries with high HBV levels, such as China.

Control and prevention. As HDV is dependent on HBV infection, then the main strategy of control is to reduce HBV by vaccination. However, once a person is chronically infected with HBV, vaccination offers no protection so all the other methods for the control of HBV are relevant.

Treatment and surveillance. See HBV above.

14.14   Ebola Haemorrhagic Fever

Organism. Virus of the Filoviridae group of organisms, with four distinct subtypes; Zaire, Sudan, Côte d'Ivoire and Reston.

Clinical features. Illness presents with sudden onset of fever, headache, muscle pains, sore throat and profound weakness. This progresses to vomiting, diarrhoea and signs of internal and external bleeding, with (generally) liver and kidney damage. Mortality is 50–90%. The Ebola Reston subtype found in the Western Pacific causes asymptomatic illness.

Diagnosis is by ELISA for specific IgG and IgM antibodies, or by PCR, but should only be carried out in laboratories with maximum facilities for protecting staff. New tests on saliva and urine provide a safer method of making a diagnosis.

Transmission is by person-to-person contact via blood, secretions, semen or tissues of an infected person. Infected blood, especially via syringes, causes the most serious infections, while transmission has occurred via semen up to 7 weeks after clinical recovery.

Fruit bats have been found to carry the filovirus, and infection can occur from direct contact with bats, or possibly from their excreta. Several caves in sub-Saharan Africa have been found to harbour bats carrying the virus, so should be avoided. This suggests that Ebola may be a zoonosis, with indigenous people acquiring some immunity from contact with the virus at an early age, but the link has not been sufficiently established.

Infection has also occurred through handling ill or dead chimpanzees, gorillas and forest antelopes. The Ebola Reston strain has been contracted through handling cynomolgus monkeys (crab-eating macaques).

Incubation period is 2–21 days.

Period of communicability. From the start of symptoms, and for up to 10 weeks for seminal fluid. Health-care workers are particularly liable to become infected, especially during the phase of vomiting and diarrhoea. Contact with blood is invariably fatal.

Occurrence and distribution. The main focus of infection is the rainforest of Central Africa, outbreaks having occurred in Sudan, Democratic Republic of Congo (DRC), Gabon, Côte d'Ivoire and Uganda. Another focus of an Ebola-related virus has been found in monkeys in the Philippines exported for experimental purposes. This focal nature (again) suggests a zoonosis, but despite extensive search no reservoir has been found. Bats have been infected experimentally, but do not die from the disease, so might be responsible for maintaining the virus in the wild.

Control and prevention. The strictest level of barrier nursing is required, taking particular care to avoid contact with blood and all secretions. Soiled clothes and bed linen must be disposed of properly as they can also spread infection. Patients that die must be buried or cremated immediately using the same precautions, relatives being forbidden to touch or take the body away for burial. Patients that recover must be counselled about the dangers of sexual intercourse and the infective nature of semen.

All contacts of a case and accidental contacts by health-care workers must be quarantined and the temperature checked twice a day. Surveillance should continue for 3 weeks from the date of contact.

Caves known to be inhabited by fruit bats in sub-Saharan Africa should be avoided.

Treatment. There is no specific therapy and hyperimmune serum does not offer any long-term protection.

Surveillance. Outbreaks should be reported to WHO, neighbouring countries and those with air connections, so that surveillance can be mounted on travellers.

14.15 Marburg Disease/Haemorrhagic Fever

A closely related virus (the Marburg virus) causing an infection first identified from laboratory monkeys in Marburg, Germany, produces a similar illness to Ebola haemorrhagic fever but with a mortality of about 25%. Cases have occurred in Uganda, Kenya, Zimbabwe and the DRC. In all other respects, Marburg disease is similar to Ebola haemorrhagic fever, to which reference should be made above.

14.16 Lassa and Crimean–Congo Haemorrhagic Fevers

Lassa and Crimean–Congo haemorrhagic fevers have similar presentations to Ebola and Marburg disease and are highly infectious through blood, urine and other body fluids, but as they are both primarily zoonoses they are covered in Sections 17.9 and 16.10.2, respectively.

Summary

- A number of important infections are transmitted by the body fluids of blood, serum, semen, saliva and various other discharges, and include the sexually transmitted diseases, HIV, hepatitis viruses and haemorrhagic fevers.
- Sexual transmission is increased by contact with commercial sex workers and having multiple partners, and then generally transferred to the spouse, also often affecting the children.

- Health education of both sexes, the use of condoms, provision of detection and treatment facilities, screening of blood and the use of disposable needles and syringes are methods of prevention.
- HBV vaccination should be started following birth, while an effective vaccination for HIV infection is still hoped for.

Further Reading

Clutterbuck, D. (2004) *Sexually Transmitted Infections and HIV*. Mosby-Wolfe, London.

Family Planning New South Wales (2011) *Reproductive and Sexual Health: An Australian Clinical Practice Handbook*, 2nd edn. Family Planning New South Wales, Sydney.

Reithinger, R., Kamya, R.M., Whitty, J.M., Dorsey, G. and Vermund, S.H. (2009) Interaction of malaria and HIV. *British Medical Journal* 338, elocator b2141, 1400–1401.

Rogstad, K. (ed.) (2011) *ABC of Sexually Transmitted Infections*, 6th edn. Wiley-Blackwell, Oxford and Chichester, UK/Hoboken, New Jersey.

World Health Organization (2007) *Tuberculosis Care with TB-HIV Co-management: IMAI*. WHO, Geneva. Also available at: http://www.who.int/hiv/pub/imai/TB_HIVModule23.05.07.pdf (accessed 6 March 2012).

World Health Organization (2010) *Antiretroviral Therapy for HIV Infection in Adults and Adolescents: Recommendations for a Public Health Approach, 2010 Revision*. WHO, Geneva. Also available at: http://whqlibdoc.who.int/publications/2010/9789241599764_eng.pdf (accessed 6 March 2012).

15 Insect-borne Diseases

By adopting a more specific means of transmission, some parasitic organisms have become dependent on vectors for carriage to a new host. Several vectors may be used, but often the parasite is restricted to only one kind of vector. This would at first appear to reduce the chance of infection, but instead of the haphazard scattering of large numbers of organisms into the environment, in the hope that one of them will find a new victim, using a vector will have a more certain chance of success. The vector carries the parasite right to the new host and, in many cases, introduces it directly into them. Often a development stage takes place in the vector and the infective stage continues to be produced for the rest of the vector's life. However, transmission depends on the vector being able to find a new host, often within a limited period of time, a vulnerable step in the life cycle and one where control methods are most likely to succeed.

Vector transmission is one of the commonest methods of spreading disease and many of the infections transmitted this way are of major importance, so large sections of the book are devoted to them. Such is their importance that they are best divided into two: this chapter, which includes all the vectors that use flight, such as mosquitoes and biting flies; and the next chapter on ectoparasites that attach to the host, such as fleas and lice.

15.1 Mosquito-borne Diseases

The mosquito is the most important vector of disease, because it is abundant, lives in close proximity to man and needs to feed on blood (the female must have a blood meal for the development of her eggs). Incredibly, it is a very delicate insect, being easily blown by the wind, a weak and slow flier and susceptible to climatic change. Its success lies in its opportunism and rapid developmental cycle, allowing large numbers to be produced in a short period of time. Once a suitable breeding place appears, be it a few puddles after a rain storm or a man-made water storage tank, a mosquito will quickly lay its eggs. These develop within a short period of time into a large number of adults. Each may become a vector, and although many will die, there will be sufficient to seek out suitable blood meals and transmit infection.

Some parasites are specific to certain types of mosquitoes, e.g. malaria and the anophelines, while others, like the arboviruses, are less selective and utilize many different species. Different kinds of mosquitoes may be required in a complex transmission cycle such as yellow fever.

Development of the parasite within the mosquito may be morphological without multiplication (as with filaria), or may involve asexual (arbovirus) or sexual (malaria) reproduction. Each of these methods confers advantages, such as the huge number of organisms produced by asexual reproduction, or the opportunity to develop strains of varying type with sexual reproduction, but if the mosquito does not live long enough for these developmental stages to take place then all is lost.

There are two main groups of mosquitoes, the anophelines (which include *Anopheles*) and the culicines (which include *Aedes*), which are distinguished by characteristics found in all of the development stages (Fig. 15.1). The adult *Anopheles* mosquito raises its hind legs away from the surface, easily remembered by its stance being like one side of a letter 'A', while the larva lies horizontal to the surface. The eggs are laid singly and have little floats on each side. In contrast, culicine mosquitoes rest horizontal to the surface, their larvae hang down from a single siphon and their eggs have no floats, often being laid in rafts. It is better to try to differentiate an adult male from a female, with its bushy antennae, before subsequently separating anophelines from culicines by the length of the palps. More precise species identification is required to identify

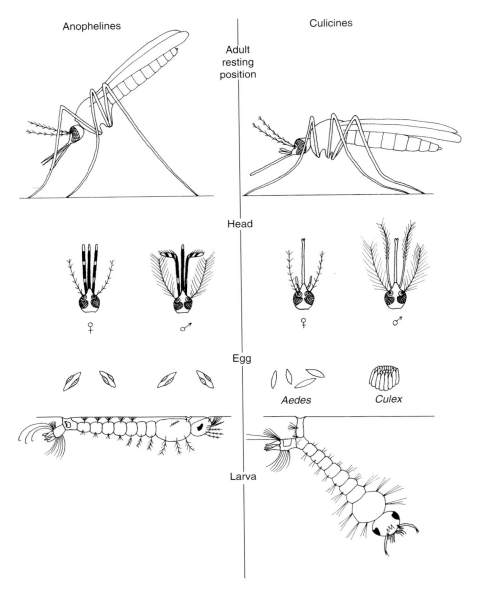

Fig. 15.1. The main differences between anopheline and culicine mosquitoes.

which mosquitoes are the principal vectors, but this needs entomological help.

Mosquitoes differ in their habits, some preferring to take blood meals on humans (*anthropophilic*) and others on animals (*zoophilic*), while some are non-specific, depending on which type of meal is most readily available. They also have particular biting times, either only indoors, only outdoors or a mixture of the two. The biting period can be mainly during the night or predominantly in the daytime. All these different parameters need to be measured in determining the importance of each type of mosquito as a vector.

15.2 Arboviruses

Arthropod-borne-virus (arbovirus) infections occur in epidemic form in a number of different parts of the world. Many viruses have been identified (see

Table 15.1 and Chapter 20), but they are best grouped into three symptom complexes.

15.2.1 Those producing mainly fever or arthritis

Chikungunya, O'nyong-nyong, West Nile, Orungo, Oropouche and Ross River fevers

This group of infections is summarized in Table 15.1. They present as a dengue-like disease (see below) with headache, fever, malaise, arthralgia or myalgia, lasting for a week or less. Rashes are common in Chikungunya, O'nyong-nyong and West Nile fevers. The arthralgia of Chikungunya fever can be debilitating, hence its name 'to become contorted' (from Tanzania) and may present as a haemorrhagic fever in India and South-east Asia. West Nile and Oropouche fevers can present as encephalitides, especially in the elderly. Ross River fever predominantly presents as a polyarthritis and rash. There are many other arbovirus infections that also present as fever listed in Chapter 20.

Table 15.1. The important arbovirus infections of humans.

Virus	Distribution	Vectors	Reservoir
Mainly fever or arthritis			
Chikungunya	Africa, South and South-east Asia	*Aedes (Ae.) aegypti, Ae. africanus, Ae. albopictus*	Baboons, bats, rodents, monkeys
O'nyong-nyong	East Africa, Senegal	*Anopheles (A.) gambiae, A. funestus*	Mosquitoes?
West Nile	Africa, Asia, Europe, USA	*Culex pipens molestus, C. modestus, C. univittatus*	Birds
Oropuche	Trinidad, South America	Mosquitoes, possibly *Culicoides*	Monkeys, sloths, birds
Orungo	West Africa, Uganda	*Ae. dentatus, Anopheles* spp.	Humans?
Ross River	Australia, New Zealand, Pacific Islands	*C. annulirostris, Ae. vigilax, Ae. polynesiensis*	Mosquitoes
Fever and encephalitis			
Western equine	Americas	*C. tarsalis, Culiseta (Cs.) melanura*	Birds
Eastern equine	Americas, Caribbean	*Cs. melanura, Aedes* and *Coquillettidia* spp.	Birds, rodents
St Louis	Americas, Caribbean	*C. tarsalis, C. nigripalpus, C. quinquefasciatus*	Birds
Venezuelan equine	Central/South America, Caribbean, parts of USA	*C. tarsalis* and other *Culex, Aedes, Mansonia, Sabethes, Psorophora, Anopheles, Haemagogus* spp.	Rodents
Japanese	East, South and Southeast Asia	*C. tritaeniorhynchus, C. gelidus, C. fuscocephala*	Birds, pigs
Murray Valley	New Guinea, Australia	*C. annulirostris*	Birds
Rocio	Brazil	Probably mosquitoes	Birds? Rodents
Haemorrhagic fevers			
Yellow fever	South America and Africa	*Ae. aegypti, Ae. africanus, Ae. simpsoni, Ae. furcifer/taylori, Ae. luteocephalus, Haemagogus* spp.	Monkeys, mosquitoes
Dengue 1, 2, 3 and 4	Asia, Pacific, Caribbean, Africa, Americas	*Ae. aegypti, Ae. albopictus, Ae. scutellaris* group, *Ae. niveus, Ochlerotatus*	Human/Mosquito, (monkeys in jungle cycle)
Rift Valley	Africa, South-west Asia	*Ae. caballus, C. theileri, C. quinquefasciatus* and other *Culex* and *Aedes* spp.	Sheep, cattle, etc., mosquitoes
Kyasanur Forest	South India	*Haemaphysalis* (hard ticks)	Rodents, monkeys
Crimean–Congo	Europe, Africa, Asia	*Hyalomma* spp. (hard ticks)	Domestic animals

Diagnosis of all the arbovirus infections is generally made on clinical grounds once the initial cases have been identified by virus isolation in a specialist laboratory. Specific ELISA and reverse transcriptase-polymerase chain reaction (RT-PCR) can be used. A rise in specific IgM in serum or cerebrospinal fluid (CSF) is a useful diagnostic, if available.

Incubation period is from 3 to 15 days.

Period of communicability of all the arbovirus infections is as long as there are still infected mosquitoes remaining.

Susceptibility is general but infection leads to immunity, probably lifelong. In endemic areas, these are diseases of children, otherwise they are epidemic affecting all age groups and both sexes. In 2002, there were epidemics of West Nile virus in Israel, Canada and the USA (resulting in 3231 cases and 176 deaths in the latter), countries where this infection has not occurred before. While most people suffered minor illness, individuals with weakened immune systems, such as people with chronic diseases, those on chemotherapy or the elderly suffered more serious effects, including meningitis and encephalitis. Infection has now spread to many countries in Central America, the Caribbean Islands and Colombia in South America. In August 2011, West Nile virus infection reached Europe, with most cases in Greece and Russia.

Outbreaks of Chikungunya fever in the Indian Ocean Islands of Comores, Madagascar, Mayotte, Mauritius, La Réunion, and the Seychelles occurred in 2006–2008, with one third of the population of La Réunion affected and resulting in several cases being imported to Europe. A much larger outbreak developed in India in 2006–2007, with 1.43 million cases (see also Section 19.4).

15.2.2 Those presenting as fever and encephalitis

Western equine, Eastern equine, St Louis, Venezuelan, Japanese, Murray Valley and Rocio encephalitis

This group of diseases presents with a high fever of acute onset, headache, meningeal irritation, stupor, disorientation, coma, spasticity and tremors. Fatality rates are variable, with up to 30% in Japanese, Eastern equine and Murray Valley encephalitis. The distribution, vectors and reservoirs of these viruses are summarized in Table 15.1. Japanese encephalitis (JE) is covered in more detail below.

From the reservoir bird or animal, the organism is often first transmitted to another host, such as horses in the equine arbovirus infections. Humans are then mainly infected from mosquitoes feeding on the horses (but see also Section 16.10.3).

Incubation period is from 5 to 15 days. Susceptibility is highest in the very young and old, with inapparent infection occurring in other age groups.

15.2.3 Haemorrhagic fevers

Yellow fever, Dengue, Rift Valley fever, Kyasanur Forest disease and Crimean–Congo haemorrhagic fever

As well as dengue and yellow fevers, which will be covered in more detail below, a group of generally mild viral fevers including Rift Valley fever, Crimean–Congo haemorrhagic fever and Kyasanur Forest disease, at certain places and on certain occasions take on a severe form resulting in vascular permeability, hypovolaemia and abnormal blood clotting. Infection commences as an acute fever, malaise, headache, nausea or vomiting, with petechial rashes, severe bruising and bleeding taking place from various sites. Blood can be vomited, passed in the faeces, come from the nose or gums and bleed into the skin. After a few days, sudden circulatory failure and shock may occur, producing a mortality of up to 50%. In Rift Valley fever there are also less fatal forms, ocular (blurring and decreased vision with 50% experiencing permanent loss of sight) and meningoencephalitic (disorientation, convulsions and coma, with low death rate, but often permanent neurological deficit).

Rift Valley fever is normally a disease of cattle, sheep, camels and goats, in which high mortality can cause considerable economic loss, but spread to humans also occurs. A large number of unexplained abortions in livestock is often the first sign of an impending epidemic. The virus infects humans through wounds and broken skin, or can be inhaled from the aerosol produced when an animal is being slaughtered; infection can occur via mosquitoes as well. There is a suggestion that drinking the raw milk of an infected animal can also infect the person. The disease was normally restricted to Africa, but in 2000 it spread to Saudi Arabia and Yemen, raising the fear that it could infect other parts of Asia and Europe.

Incubation period. 3–12 days.

Period of communicability. This lasts as long as there are infected animals and live mosquitoes that have fed on them, but the virus can also be spread transovarially in the mosquito, with the eggs remaining viable for many years. Permanent foci of Rift Valley fever can therefore become established.

Some arbovirus infections can also be spread by non-mosquito arthropods, such as Kyasanur Forest disease and Crimean–Congo haemorrhagic fever. (See Sections 16.10.1 and 16.10.2.)

15.2.4 Control and prevention of arbovirus infections

The main method of control is the destruction of vector mosquitoes and breeding places. The most important vector mosquitoes are *Culex* and *Aedes*, which live in collections of water close to the home. Search is made for larvae and all breeding places destroyed. Water tanks, blocked drains, discarded tin cans or old tyres are favourite breeding places. A simple method is to use schoolchildren, making a game or giving a reward for the number of breeding places found. Large breeding areas (such as water tanks) can be covered, screened, treated with insecticides, or natural predators introduced (e.g. fish or dragonfly larvae). An improvement on just covering water pots and containers is to use an insecticide-treated cover rather than place the insecticide in the container.

Where there is an epidemic in a compact area, such as a town, then the quickest and simplest (although expensive) method of bringing the epidemic to an end is to use fogging or ultra-low volume (ULV) aerial spraying (see Section 3.4.1). Compared to lost working hours this can be a cost-effective procedure.

Personal prevention with repellents (Section 3.4.1) can protect the individual. The infected case should be nursed under a mosquito net so as not to infect mosquitoes. A vaccine is available for Venezuelan, Eastern and Western equine encephalitis, which can be used both for humans and horses.

Where an animal reservoir is involved, then restriction of animal movement or the reduction of rodents can be of value. In Rift Valley fever, special precautions should be taken in handling domestic animals and their products, including the wearing of gloves and protective clothing. The milk of infected animals should not be drunk, neither must they be slaughtered and their meat consumed. Blood and other body fluids of patients are also infectious so barrier nursing should be instituted. All animals should be vaccinated prior to the outbreak. During an outbreak, newly infected animals maybe viraemic but not display any symptoms, and there is a danger that reuse of needles and syringes may actually increase spread. An inactivated cell culture vaccine for use in humans is available, but has not been fully evaluated.

Treatment. There is no specific treatment, supportive therapy being given. (Ribavirin may be of value.)

Surveillance. Regular checks should be made on mosquito breeding places and control methods instituted where mosquitoes are found. People can be taught to regularly search their home areas for mosquito breeding. (See further under dengue Section 15.4 and yellow fever Section 15.5.) Outbreaks are often associated with heavy rainfall (which provides conditions for mosquito breeding) so can often be forecast.

15.3 Japanese Encephalitis (JE)

Organism. The Japanese encephalitis virus (JEV) is a member of the flavivirus family, the same group of viruses as the West Nile, St Louis, dengue and yellow fever viruses.

Clinical features. Japanese encephalitis (JE) presents as a sudden onset of fever, headache, body aches and pains. Mild cases recover completely but a high proportion develop encephalitis and progressive coma. Children under 10 years of age may present with gastrointestinal symptoms and convulsions, rapidly leading to death. Those that survive the severe disease may have residual neurological or psychiatric disabilities.

Diagnosis is by finding the specific IgM in CSF or serum. The virus can be cultured in specialist laboratories.

Transmission. The main vectors are *Culex tritaeniorhynchus*, *C. gelidus* and *C. fuscocephala*, mosquitoes that predominantly breed in rice fields. The reservoir of infection is probably in wading birds, but domestic pigs also harbour the virus, from which it is transferred to humans. The mosquito breeds when the rice fields are flooded and the first green shoots appear, dying off when the rice grows and shades the water, which produces a marked seasonality, with a peak period in Thailand in July and August, in China in August, and in India/Nepal in September and November. In irrigated areas, mosquito breeding can occur throughout the year, while outbreaks have occurred in urban areas where suitable standing water permits the breeding of vector mosquitoes.

Incubation period. 4–14 days.

Period of communicability. This lasts as long as there are infected mosquitoes continuing to bite people. Mosquitoes can also become infected by feeding on a clinical case at any time during the illness.

Occurrence and distribution. Serological surveys indicate that most people living in endemic areas contract subclinical infection before the age of 15 years. However, young children and adults who have not been infected as children (including visitors) may get clinical disease, and possibly severe disease, with 20–30% mortality. There are about 50,000 cases reported annually and 10,000 deaths.

The endemic area is South and South-east Asia, particularly Cambodia, Laos, Vietnam, Thailand, Malaysia, Myanmar, Indonesia, Philippines, the Indian subcontinent and Russia, with a decreasing incidence in China, Japan and Korea. Risk within any of these countries is greatest during the rice-growing season and when an epidemic is ongoing. JE has recently spread to New Guinea and northern Australia.

Control and prevention. Agricultural methods such as drying out rice fields when no crop is growing or decreasing the number of crops can reduce the period of risk. Personal protection with long-sleeved clothing, the wearing of trousers and use of repellents can reduce mosquito biting. The mosquito bites during the daytime, so babies and young children should be made to sleep under insecticide-treated mosquito nets (Box 3.1). The main method of prevention though is to vaccinate all children in endemic areas, but after the age of 1 year so as not to interfere with remaining maternal antibodies. A booster dose should be given a year later for all types of vaccines and then every 3 years up to 10–15 years of age for the mouse-brain derived vaccine. An alternative strategy is vaccination of the pig reservoir.

Treatment. There is no treatment.

Surveillance. Notification of cases should be reported to WHO so that neighbouring countries and visitors can take precautions.

15.4 Dengue

Organism. Dengue virus has four serotypes (1, 2, 3 and 4).

Clinical features. Dengue presents as a sudden onset of fever, retro-orbital headache, joint and muscle pains, and facial signs of flushing, puffy eyelids and red eyes. A maculopapular or scarlatina-form rash usually appears after 3–4 days. Depression and prolonged fatigue often occur following the acute manifestations. Dengue haemorrhagic fever (DHF; recently designated severe dengue), in which there is profound bleeding into skin and tissues, is now a serious feature of many epidemics. After the initial symptoms, the condition suddenly worsens with facial pallor, abdominal pain and cyanosis. The liver may become enlarged and then signs of bleeding occur, such as into the gastrointestinal tract, with concurrent shock.

DHF is probably due to a sensitization with a previous dengue serotype, either acquired at birth or from a previous infection, type 2 being the most potent and types 3, 4 and 1 being responsible in decreasing importance. Differential effects on racial groups suggest that host factors may also have a role, as does the geographical origin of the dengue strain.

Diagnosis. Virus can be isolated from the blood in acute cases. IgM-capture ELISA on a single specimen indicates recent infection, which is confirmed by a rising titre in paired sera.

Transmission. Mosquitoes of the *Aedes* group, especially *Ae. aegypti*, *Ae. albopictus* or a member of the *Ae. scutellaris* group are responsible for transmission. These mosquitoes are more easily identifiable than most by their black colour, with distinctive white markings (Fig. 15.2). They like to breed close to humans, taking advantage of any water containers, old tyres, empty tins or other small collections of water in which they can breed. They are daytime biters and can be found in large numbers in urban and peri-urban areas. *Ae. albopictus* has comparatively recently become established in the USA, Central America and the Caribbean owing to the trade in used tyres.

Virus is maintained in a human/mosquito cycle in many parts of the world, but in Africa and Southeast Asia a monkey/mosquito cycle is involved.

Incubation period is 3–15 days (commonly 4–6).

Period of communicability. The mosquito is able to transmit infection 8–12 days after taking an infective blood meal and remains infective for the rest of its life. Humans and monkeys are infectious during and just before the febrile period.

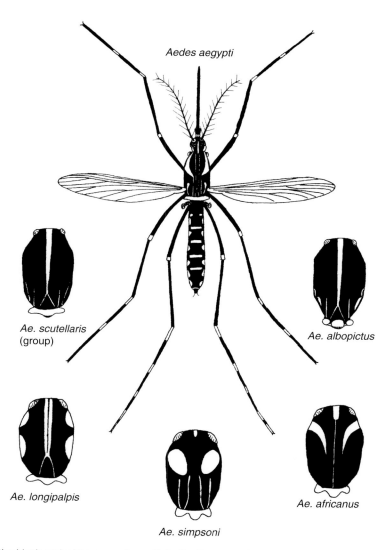

Fig. 15.2. *Aedes*, the black and white mosquitoes. Note the thorax markings of the different species.

Occurrence and distribution. Dengue is now endemic in South and Central America, sub-Saharan Africa and South and South-east Asia (Fig. 15.3). In more isolated communities, large epidemics have occurred, especially in island countries of the Caribbean and Pacific, with devastating effect. The epidemic can be so massive as to immobilize large segments of the population, disrupt the workforce and cause a breakdown in organization. The development of DHF has been variable, producing a number of deaths. It is estimated that there are about 50 million cases of dengue and 0.5 million of DHF, with 12,000 deaths due to dengue every year. Children are the main sufferers of both dengue and DHF.

Control and prevention. The main method of control is to reduce mosquito breeding, especially of the *Aedes* mosquito, by depriving it of collections of water or covering them so that mosquitoes cannot enter. All water tanks, pots or other containers must be covered at all times, treating the covers with insecticides if there is not a perfect fit. Guttering around the roof can also allow pools of water to collect, so should be of sufficient slope for good drainage and be cleaned out regularly. Old tyres should have holes cut in them or be removed altogether (one answer to the disposal problem is to weight them and bury them at sea to form artificial reefs).

People should check round their gardens and the immediate vicinity at regular intervals to remove any cans, coconut shells or other temporary collections of water. Children are very effective at doing this and can be encouraged with a marks or reward scheme.

Screening of houses and mosquito nets are of little use because people are often outside their houses when the mosquito bites, but these measures are of value for young children. ULV spraying, either by fogging or by aircraft, is of value in the presence of an epidemic, but only adult mosquitoes are killed, which are soon replaced by young adults, unless simultaneous larval control is also in operation.

Treatment. There is no specific treatment, but hypovolaemic shock must be treated with rapid fluid replacement and oxygen therapy.

Surveillance. Regular checks should be made on mosquito breeding, especially of *Ae. aegypti*.

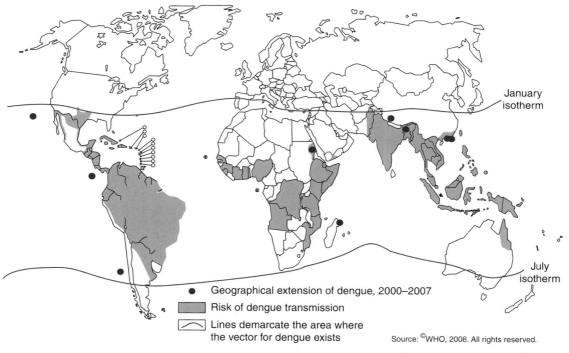

January isotherm

July isotherm

- ● Geographical extension of dengue, 2000–2007
- Risk of dengue transmission
- Lines demarcate the area where the vector for dengue exists

Fig. 15.3. Dengue transmission in 2007. (Reproduced by permission of the World Health Organization, Geneva.)

Samples are taken and the number of larvae breeding is counted to give an indication of the risk of transmission. Further details will be found under yellow fever (Section 15.5).

15.5 Yellow Fever

Organism. The yellow fever virus is a flavivirus.

Clinical features. One of the haemorrhagic group of arbovirus infections, yellow fever presents with a sudden onset of fever, headache, backache, prostration and vomiting. Jaundice commences mildly at first and intensifies as the disease progresses. Albuminuria and leucopenia are found on examination, while the haemorrhagic symptoms of epistaxis, haematemesis, melaena and bleeding from the gums can all occur. In endemic areas, the fatality rate is low except in the non-indigenous. The death rate may reach 50% in epidemics.

Diagnosis is made on clinical grounds after initial identification of an outbreak. Virus can be isolated from blood in specialist laboratories, such as the Pasteur Institute in Dakar, and IgM tested by ELISA techniques. Viral isolation and typical liver histology from fatal human cases and in monkeys thought to have died from the disease can assist in the evaluation of epidemics. A revised case definition developed by the World Health Organization (WHO) is:

- **Suspected,** acute onset of fever, with jaundice appearing within 14 days. (See Table 8.2 for differential diagnosis of jaundice.)
- **Probable,** presence of yellow fever IgM in the absence of yellow fever immunization within 30 days. Epidemiological link to a confirmed case or an outbreak.
- **Confirmed,** detection of yellow fever-specific IgM or fourfold increase of yellow-fever IgM or IgG antibody titres or detection of yellow fever-specific neutralizing antibodies in the absence of yellow fever immunization within 30 days. If no yellow fever immunization within 14 days, then either the detection of yellow fever virus genome in blood or other organs by PCR or of antigen in blood or other organs by immunoassay or the isolation of yellow fever virus.

Transmission. Yellow fever is a disease of the forest, maintained in the monkey population by the sylvatic transmission cycle, which involves *Haemagogus, Sabethes* and *Aedes* mosquitoes in America, and *Aedes* in Africa (Fig. 15.4). The monkeys are generally not affected by the disease but occasionally start dying, indicating that spread to the human population may soon begin. In South America, it may be a reduction in the monkey population that will make the canopy mosquito look for another blood meal and perhaps feed on humans. More commonly, it is the person who goes into the forest to cut wood or hunt that becomes bitten incidentally. When they return to their village or town they are fed on by *Ae. aegypti*, and an urban yellow fever transmission cycle is set up (see Fig. 15.4). In Africa, three different kinds of mosquitoes are involved. *Ae. africanus* remains in the jungle canopy rarely feeding on humans, but should the monkey descend to the forest floor or even enter areas of human habitation it is fed on by *Ae. simpsoni, Ae. furcifer-taylori* or *Ae. luteocephalus*. The mosquito then bites a person on the edge of the forest (the rural cycle) who returns to the village soon to suffer from yellow fever. Fed upon by the peri-domestic mosquito *Ae. aegypti*, an urban cycle is started (Fig. 15.4). The extrinsic (within-mosquito) cycle of infection takes 5–30 days, depending on the temperature and type of mosquito. Transovarian (transovarial) infection can also occur.

Incubation period is 3–6 days.

Period of communicability is from before the fever commences to 5 days after, so the patient should be nursed under a mosquito net to prevent new mosquitoes from becoming infected.

Occurrence and distribution. Yellow fever nearly always presents as an epidemic in humans, affecting all ages and both sexes, although adults (particularly males) who go into the forest are likely to be the first to contract the disease. Yellow fever is restricted to the areas of Africa and South America shown in Fig 5.1. WHO has established a special initiative to assist Benin, Burkina Faso, Cameroon, Côte d'Ivoire, Ghana, Guinea, Liberia, Mali, Nigeria, Senegal, Sierra Leone and Togo, the 12 highest risk countries (see further below).

Control and prevention. The most important part of the complex mosquito transmission cycle is *Ae. aegypti*. With its proximity to man, it is capable of infecting a large number of people as well as being

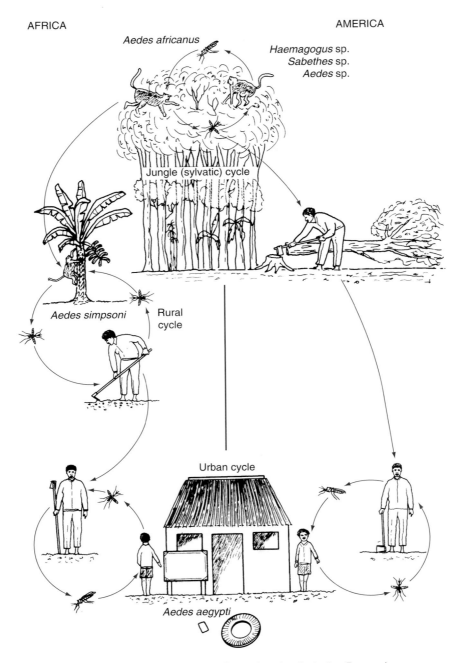

AFRICA

AMERICA

Aedes africanus

Haemagogus sp.
Sabethes sp.
Aedes sp.

Jungle (sylvatic) cycle

Aedes simpsoni

Rural cycle

Urban cycle

Aedes aegypti

Fig. 15.4. Yellow fever transmission cycles in Africa and South America (including Panama).

the easiest mosquito species to control. It breeds in small collections of water near to people's houses so a careful search for larvae and the destruction of breeding places can do much to reduce the dan-

ger. Simple clearance is the most effective method of reducing the mosquito population (see under dengue above), but insecticides such as temephos (Abate) can be used where collections of water cannot be destroyed or covered. In the event of an epidemic, then emergency reduction by fogging or ULV spray from aircraft will rapidly destroy the adult population (but not the larvae).

One attack of yellow fever confers immunity for life if the person survives the disease. Inapparent infections can also occur. A very effective vaccine has been developed, which provides immunity for at least 10 years and probably longer, so all those at risk in the known endemic areas should be vaccinated (Fig. 5.1). This has been attempted by offering vaccination at markets and meetings, or systematically offering it to schoolchildren. WHO now recommend that yellow fever vaccination be included in the childhood vaccination programme in the 33 countries of Africa in the yellow fever zone; the vaccine is to be given at the same time as the measles vaccine. The countries of South America have already implemented childhood vaccination programmes. In the event of an epidemic, then ring vaccination can be performed; the epidemic is surrounded by a circle of vaccinated persons, progressively closing in on the centre of the outbreak. Areas of Africa and South America have been designated as yellow fever areas (Fig. 5.1) and all visitors to this zone require vaccination. If a person has visited a country where there is a risk of transmission and they are not vaccinated and then enter another country where the vector of yellow fever is present, then the authorities can quarantine that person for 6 days.

In view of the rapid urbanization of African cities and the increase in migration, WHO is concerned that major outbreaks could occur, exhausting vaccine supplies, so is proposing to pre-emptively vaccinate some 48 million people (17% of the population) in the 12 high-risk countries. The priority groups for vaccination will be determined from the past history of yellow fever outbreaks in the particular district or its proximity to an outbreak, and the proportion of vaccinated persons in the district (the lower the proportion the higher the priority). In order to do this, WHO has established a stockpile of vaccine that can be drawn upon for preventive mass vaccination and emergency use.

In these days of rapid air transport, it has always been surprising that yellow fever has not been transported to Asia where there are the vectors and conditions for transmission. A suggested reason is that there is some cross immunity with other Group B arboviruses (flaviviruses), and that the level of such induced immunity may be sufficient to prevent epidemic spread. A precaution is to spray all aircraft coming from a yellow fever area.

Treatment. There is no specific treatment, but supportive therapy is given to combat shock and renal failure.

Surveillance. All cases of suspected or confirmed yellow fever should be reported to WHO as an event of international public health importance. The prevalence of the urban vector can be measured by the *Ae. aegypti* index. This is the number of houses found with *Ae. aegypti* breeding within a specified area of 100 houses. Alternatively, the Breteau index can be used, which is the number of containers in which larvae are found out of 100 samples. If this is kept below 5%, or preferably 1%, then the danger of an epidemic is minimized.

15.6   Malaria

Organism. There are four human malaria parasites, *Plasmodium falciparum*, *P. vivax*, *P. malariae* and *P. ovale*. *P. falciparum* causes the most serious disease and is the commonest parasite in tropical regions, but differs from *P. vivax* and *P. ovale* in having no persistent stage (the hypnozoite) from which repeat blood-stage parasites are produced. *P. vivax* has the widest geographical range, being found in temperate and subtropical zones as well as in the tropics. *P. vivax* infection will lead to relapses if a schizontocidal drug only is used for treatment, and some strains, e.g. the Chesson strain in New Guinea and Solomon Islands, requires a more prolonged radical treatment. *P. malariae* produces a milder infection but is distinguished from the fever caused by the other three species by having paroxysms of fever every fourth day. *P. malariae* can persist as an asymptomatic low-grade parasitaemia for many years, to multiply at a future date as a clinical infection. *P. ovale* is the rarest of the parasites and is suppressed by infections with the other species.

The malaria parasite *Plasmodium* may be the cause of one of the oldest parasitic infections of humans, dating from at least 60 million years ago when it inhabited the guts of reptiles. The parasite was transferred to bird and mammalian predators where forms evolved that entered the bloodstream. At some time, it adapted to the mosquito, with separate species evolving to parasitize different kinds of birds and mammals, including humans.

The malaria parasite reproduces asexually in the human and sexually in the mosquito (Fig. 15.5). A merozoite attacks a red blood cell (RBC), divides asexually rupturing the cell, and each newly formed merozoite attacks another RBC. Toxins are liberated when the cell ruptures, producing the clinical paroxysms. After several asexual cycles, male and female gametes (gametocytes) are produced which are ingested when a mosquito takes a blood meal. These go through a complex developmental cycle in the stomach wall of the mosquito, culminating in the production of sporozoites, which migrate to the salivary glands ready to enter another person when the mosquito next takes a blood meal.

The sporozoite enters a human liver cell, in which development to a schizont takes place. This ruptures, liberating merozoites, which attack RBCs, so starting an erythrocytic cycle all over again. In *P. vivax* and *P. ovale*, a persistent liver stage, the hypnozoite, is formed, meaning that if parasites are cleared from the blood, relapses can occur, often continuing for many years unless radical treatment is given.

Clinical features. Infection commences with fever and headache, soon developing into an alternating pattern of peaks of fever followed by sweating and profound chills. Classically, these take on a pattern of either 3 days (tertiary malaria) or 4 days (quaternary malaria). However, falciparum malaria can present in many different forms, including cerebral malaria (encephalopathy and coma), and acute shock, haematuria (blackwater fever) and jaundice. The higher the parasitaemia the more severe the morbidity and the higher the mortality. Cerebral malaria in children presents as febrile seizures, making it difficult to differentiate it from other causes, but malaria should be considered the most likely diagnosis and treatment started without delay.

Partial treatment leads to recrudescences of fever, whereas relapses can occur many years after initial infection with *P. vivax* and *P. ovale*.

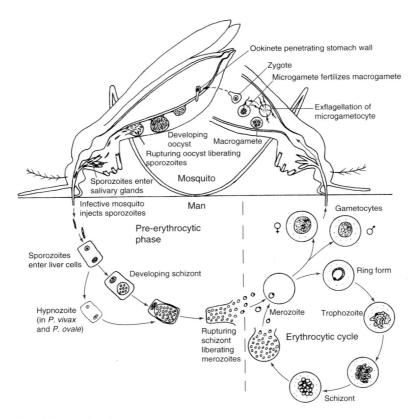

Fig. 15.5. The malaria (*Plasmodium* spp.) life cycle.

Interaction between malaria and HIV infection has now been shown to produce more severe clinical disease in persons already infected with human immunodeficiency virus (HIV), as well as an excess of cases.

Diagnosis is from a thick blood smear (to detect parasites) and a thin smear (to determine species) (Fig. 15.6). Rapid diagnostic test (RDT) dipstick methods have made the diagnosis of malaria simpler, but need to be evaluated for each country in which they are to be used. They are particularly useful for surveys.

Transmission is by *Anopheles* mosquitoes (Table 15.2). The efficiency of the vector will depend upon the species of *Anopheles*, its feeding habits and the environmental conditions. This varies widely, from *A. gambiae*, the most efficient of all malaria vectors, to a species such as *A. culicifacies*, which is comparatively inefficient. Vector efficiency is determined by a number of factors, such as the preferred food source (man or animal), the time of biting (easier in the middle of the night when people are sleeping) and whether the mosquito lives inside the house or outside; but the most important factor is the mosquito's length of life. Only a few *A. culicifacies* will survive longer than 12 days and so become infective (i.e. most die before completion of the extrinsic cycle), whereas 50% of a population of *A. gambiae* will live longer than 12 days. Longer living mosquitoes are better vectors.

A female mosquito must have a blood meal before it can complete its gonotrophic cycle and lay a batch of eggs. The gonotrophic cycle is normally about 2–3 days but varies with temperature, species and locality. Long-living mosquitoes will be able to lay several batches of eggs, and this characteristic is used to estimate longevity of a mosquito species.

Another factor is mosquito density. A large number of mosquitoes have a greater transmission potential than a few. Some mosquitoes are produced in large numbers at certain favourable times of the year while others maintain more constant populations. The environment largely determines mosquito density.

The most important environmental factors are temperature and humidity, with wind, phases of the moon and human activity having lesser effects. Temperature determines the length of the development cycle of the parasite and the survival of the mosquito vector. This means that in temperate climates malaria can only be transmitted in brief periods of warm weather when the right conditions are available. In tropical regions, altitude alters the temperature, and highland areas will have less (although possibly epidemic) malaria.

Water is essential for the mosquito to breed. In arid desert countries, the mosquito cannot survive, but wells and irrigation have allowed mosquitoes to breed and malaria to appear. Rainfall generally increases the number of breeding places for mosquitoes, so there is more malaria in the wet season. However, the rain may be so great as to wash out breeding places, thereby instead producing a decrease in the population.

The mosquito, being a fragile flyer, is easily blown by the wind, sometimes to its advantage, but generally to its disadvantage. On windy evenings, mosquito biting may decrease considerably.

Nocturnal mosquitoes are sensitive to light so on a moonlit night there is a reduction in numbers. Measurements of mosquito density must be made on several nights, or ideally over a period of months.

Where the mosquito species is mainly zoophilic (feeds on animals), keeping domestic animals in proximity to the household will encourage mosquitoes to feed on them instead of on the human occupants. It is these environmental factors that determine whether malaria is *endemic* or *epidemic*. Where conditions of temperature and moisture permit all-year-round breeding of mosquitoes then endemic malaria occurs, but if there is a marked dry season or reduction in temperature, then conditions for transmission may only be suitable during part of the year, resulting in seasonal malaria. If conditions are marginal and only favourable every few years, then epidemic malaria can result. Epidemic malaria is devastating as large numbers of people who have no immunity are attacked. Endemic and epidemic malaria call for quite different strategies of control.

Malaria can also be transmitted by blood transfusion, from needles and syringes and rarely congenitally.

Incubation period depends upon the species and strain of the parasite:

- *P. falciparum*   9–14 days
- *P. vivax*   12–17 days, but in temperate climates it can be 6–9 months
- *P. malariae*   18–40 days
- *P. ovale*   16–18 days

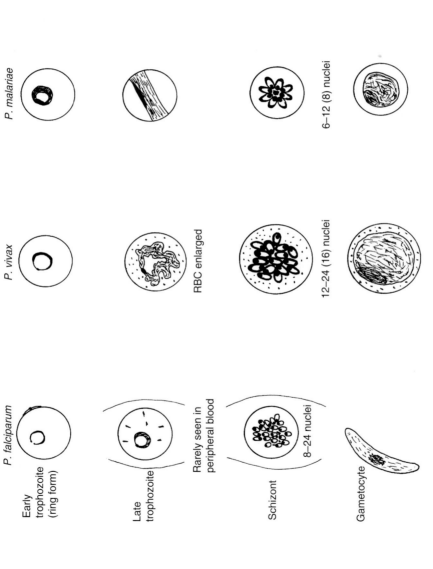

Fig. 15.6. Differential diagnosis of *Plasmodium* spp. RBC, red blood cell.

Table 15.2. The main malaria vectors and their behaviour in relation to control.

Geographical area	*Anopheles* species	Behaviour in relation to control
More arid areas of sub-Saharan Africa and Western Arabia	*A. arabiensis*	Feeds on animals and humans depending on availability. Some exit after feeding.
More humid parts of sub-Saharan Africa	*A. gambiae s.s.*	Bites humans in the middle of the night. Rests indoors after feeding. Breeds in temporary puddles, increasing considerably in wet season and declining in dry.
Sub-Saharan Africa, including highlands	*A. funestus*	Bites humans in middle of the night. Rests indoors after feeding. Breeds in more permanent water bodies, remaining a constant vector all year.
Turkey, Central Asia, Afghanistan	*A. sacharovi, A. superpictus*	Bites humans indoors.
Rural areas of Indian subcontinent and South-west Asia	*A. culicifacies*, species A, C, D and E	Feeds predominantly on animals but bites humans sufficiently to be the main rural vector in India and Sri Lanka. Tends to bite early in the night. Breeds in water tanks and pools, but not rice fields.
Urban areas of Indian subcontinent and South-west Asia	*A. stephensi*	Feeds on humans and animals throughout night except in cold weather when biting is early. Breeds in wells and water tanks.
Indian subcontinent	*A. fluviatilis* species S	Bites humans and rests indoors. Associated with hill streams.
South and South-east Asia	*A. sundaicus*	Mainly bites cattle, but also humans sufficiently to be a vector. Breeds in salt-water lagoons.
South-east Asia (including North-east India and South-west China)	*A. minimus*	Feeds on humans and rests indoors, but due to prolonged insecticide spraying has changed to outdoor resting and animal biting in some areas.
South-east Asia	*A. dirus*	Bites humans indoors, but then exits. Associated with forests.
	A. aconitus	Lives indoors. Breeds in rice fields.
Nepal, Malaysia, Indonesia	*A. maculatus*	Bites humans indoors. Breeds in rice fields.
Indonesia	*A. leucosphyrus*	Bites humans and rests indoors.
Philippines	*A. flavirostris*	Bites humans and rests indoors.
China	*A. sinensis*	Mainly bites animals, inefficient vector.
	A. anthropophagus	Bites humans, efficient vector. Both *A. sinensis* and *A. anthropophagus* breed in rice fields.
Melanesia	*A. farauti, A. punctulatus, A. koliensis*	Bites humans indoors and rests indoors. Breeds in temporary rainwater pools.
Central America, western South America and Haiti	*A. albimanus*	Bites outside and early in the night. More abundant during rainy season.
Central and northern South America	*A. pseudopunctipennis*	Bites humans indoors.
North urban South America	*A. darlingi*	Bites humans and rests indoors. Biting time variable in different parts of its range. More abundant during rainy season.
Northern South America	*A. nuñeztovari*	Bites humans indoors but exits during night.
	A. aquasalis	Bites outside early in the night. Breeds in brackish water.
South America	*A. albitarsis* complex (*A. marajoara*)	Bites humans outdoors. Associated with gold mining.

Period of communicability is as long as there are infective mosquitoes. For a mosquito to become infective it must live long enough for the parasite to complete the developmental cycle (the extrinsic cycle), which depends upon the temperature and species. *P. vivax* completes this more quickly than *P. falciparum*.

	Development time (days) at mean ambient temperature		
Species of parasite	30°C	24°C	20°C
P. vivax	7	9	16
P. falciparum	9	11	20
P. malariae	15	21	30

At 19°C, *P. falciparum* takes in excess of 30 days (beyond the life expectancy of the average mosquito), whereas *P. vivax* can still complete its cycle in less than 20 days; 17°C is the absolute minimum temperature for *P. vivax*, but the extrinsic cycle is longer than the lifetime of the mosquito.

Occurrence and distribution. In a non-immune population, children and adults of both sexes are affected equally. In areas of continuous infection with *P. falciparum*, malaria is predominantly an infection of children, in whom mortality can be considerable. The survivors acquire immunity, which is only preserved by the maintenance of parasites in the body, due to reinfection. Should the individual leave an area of continuous malaria, immunity may be reduced. The other time when immunity is reduced is during pregnancy, and severe malaria can occur in the pregnant woman, even one that has lived in an endemic area. This is worse in the first pregnancy than subsequently. (See also Section 18.2.9.)

The body responds to malaria by an enlargement of the spleen. The degree of enlargement and the proportion of the population with palpable spleens has been used as a measure of malarial endemicity:

- *Hypoendemic.* Spleen rate in children (2–9 years) not exceeding 10%.
- *Mesoendemic.* Spleen rate in children between 11 and 50%.
- *Hyperendemic.* Spleen rate in children constantly over 50%. Spleen rate in adults also high (over 25%).
- *Holoendemic.* Spleen rate in children constantly over 75%, but spleen rate in adults low.

In endemic areas, the gametocyte rate is highest in the very young, but in epidemic malaria or areas where transmission has been considerably reduced, gametocytes occur at all ages.

Malaria is found in the tropics and subtropics of the world (Fig. 15.7 and Table 15.2), mostly *P. falciparum*, but *P. vivax* is the predominant species in the Indian subcontinent. The disease used to be more extensive, with seasonal malaria in temperate regions, but extensive control programmes have confined it to its present limits. However, increase in population and the development of resistance, both by the parasite and the mosquito, means that malaria is still the most important parasitic disease in the world. Each year there are some 300 million cases, and over a million people die.

It has long been suspected that there is an interaction between malaria and HIV infection, and recent findings suggest that between the start of the HIV epidemic in the 1980s and 2006 there were almost 1 million excess malaria cases and 8500 excess HIV cases in one of the districts of Kenya alone.

Global climatic change has resulted in an increase in epidemic malaria (infecting new or infrequently involved areas), and in the development of endemic malaria in highland areas which were normally protected by their lower temperatures (see also Section 1.5.3).

Control and prevention. Mathematical models were introduced in Section 2.4, malaria being one of the best examples in which they can be used to work out the strategy for control. The parasite life cycle was described above and is illustrated in Fig. 15.5, while each of these stages can be represented mathematically on a diagram as shown in Fig 15.8. The stages and values for each of the places where the life cycle can be interrupted are:

1. In *humans*:

- Reduction of the duration of infection ($1/r$) by chemotherapy.
- Prevention of infections with gametocytes (b) by chemoprophylaxis and vaccination.

2. In *mosquitoes*:

- Prevention of human biting ($a \times a = a^2$) by personal protection and mosquito nets.
- Decreasing mosquito density (m) with larviciding and biological control.

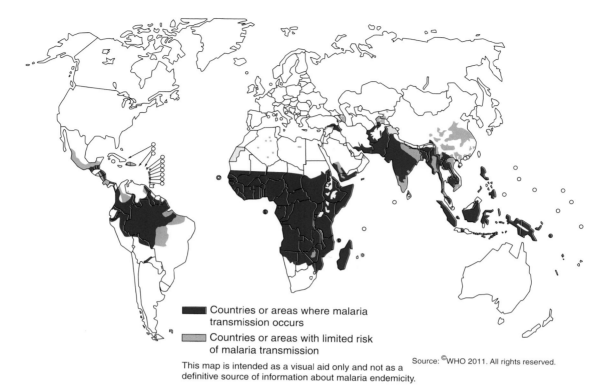

Countries or areas where malaria
transmission occurs

Countries or areas with limited risk
of malaria transmission

This map is intended as a visual aid only and not as a
definitive source of information about malaria endemicity.

Fig. 15.7. Malaria, countries or areas at risk of transmission, 2010. (Reproduced by permission of the World Health Organization, Geneva.)

- Reduction of the proportion surviving to infectivity (p^n) by residual insecticides and treated mosquito nets.
- Reduction of the mosquito expectation of life ($1/-\ln p$) by knock-down and residual insecticides, where p is the probability of a mosquito surviving through one day, n the time taken to complete the extrinsic cycle, and ln the natural logarithm).

The complete formula becomes

$$z_0 = \frac{ma^2bp^n}{-r(\ln p)}$$

where z_0 is the basic reproductive rate (see Section 2.2.3). Each of the parameters can be given values that have been measured in the field so that the level of control required to interrupt transmission can be calculated (reduce the basic reproductive rate below 1).

Some useful modifications of the formula are for the vectorial capacity:

$$\frac{ma^2p^n}{-r(\ln p)}$$

and for the critical density of mosquitoes below which the infection will die out:

$$\frac{-r(\ln p)}{a^2bp^n}$$

More complex models have been developed to overcome some of the shortcomings of this model, such as the development of immunity, but even in this limited form it is very valuable.

The effectiveness of any potential strategy can be estimated from the algebraic expression given to each part of the formula without making any calculations:

- $1/r$, the duration of infection reduced by chemotherapy, which demonstrates the small effect of just treating malaria cases, and that control efforts such as mass drug administration used in malaria eradication programmes, needs to be

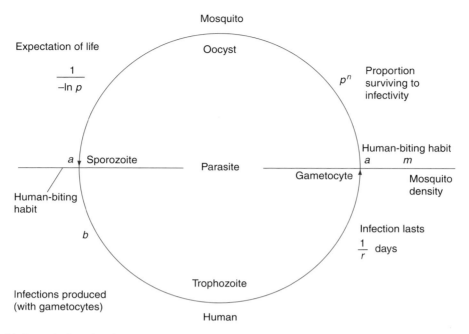

Mosquito

Expectation of life

Oocyst

$$\frac{1}{-\ln p}$$

p^n Proportion surviving to infectivity

Human-biting habit

a Sporozoite

a m

Parasite

Gametocyte

Mosquito density

Human-biting habit

b

Infection lasts $\frac{1}{r}$ days

Trophozoite

Infections produced (with gametocytes)

Human

Fig. 15.8. Mathematical model of malaria based on the schematic life cycle of the parasite. See text for explanation of variables.

total, covering every single person – virtually impossible to achieve.

- *b*, actually a notation normally applied to mosquitoes, being the proportion that ingest gametocytes so that the parasite sexual cycle can take place, but can be applied to the human part of the cycle as any method which prevents the production of gametocytes. This can either be by preventing infection in the first place with vaccination or chemoprophylaxis, the use of gametocidal drugs, or preventing the mosquito feeding on a malaria case by keeping the case under a mosquito net. However, *b* is only a unitary factor, so all of these methods will need to be nearly perfect to work.

- *a*, the number of bites that need to be made by the mosquito. One bite is needed to introduce infection and another to take up gametocytes, so the interruption of mosquito biting could be quite an effective strategy. Therefore, personal protection with clothing, repellents and mosquito nets is a valuable method of control.

- *m*, the density of mosquitoes, is only a unitary factor demonstrating the poor results of larviciding and biological methods in malaria control.

- *p*, mosquito survival, consists of two factors, the mosquito's expectation of life (short-lived vectors are poor transmitters) and the number of mosquitoes living long enough to complete the extrinsic cycle. In this, *p* is raised to the *n*th power, showing that reducing the length of life of the mosquito (mainly by the use of insecticides) is the best control strategy.

Personal protection. Methods of personal protection have been covered in Section 3.4.1. They include clothing, mosquito nets and repellents. Items of clothing such as socks and shawls can be treated with repellents, which retain activity for some time, or repellents can be applied directly to the skin. Some naturally occurring plants have repellent properties, such as *Tegetes minuta* in East Africa.

Mosquito nets are most effective if used properly. Providing subsidized mosquito nets can be used as a method of malaria control, especially for mothers and children who are liable to go to bed early (before mosquito biting starts). This can be improved by treating the nets with synthetic pyrethroid insecticides (such as permethrin, deltamethrin, alpha-cypermethrin or lambda-cyhalothrin). This repels mosquitoes and kills those that come into contact with the net. When used on a community scale, the concentration of insecticide-treated mosquito nets (ITNs) can produce a mass effect, reducing the mosquito population and the sporozoite rate. An improved technology is the manufacture of mosquito nets with the insecticide already in the net, known as long-lasting insecticidal nets (LLIN). These retain activity for at least 4 years, which avoids the regular retreating of nets, and holds considerable potential as the main method of malaria control. The method of treating mosquito nets and more on their use will be found in Box 3.1.

Mosquito bed nets are more effective and cheaper to maintain than screening the whole house, which is only recommended for people with a high standard of living. A small hole in the netting can render the rest ineffective. A knock-down spray can be used to kill mosquitoes that have entered a screened house.

The use of smoke from mosquito coils or vaporizing mats can be surprisingly effective and has the advantage that it is a cheap personal protection. Coils are easily manufactured locally and naturally occurring substances, such as incorporated pyrethrum. People often sit around fires in the evening and by the addition of certain plants a repellent smoke can be produced.

Mosquitoes can be encouraged to bite other animals if they are the preferred blood meal; however, if the animals are taken away, such as to market, then the mosquitoes may be forced to take their blood meals on humans. The habits of the malaria vectors will need to be known before encouraging this practice.

Residual insecticides. Use of residual insecticides has been covered in Section 3.4.1. These are applied to the inside surface of houses so that the resting mosquito (after it has taken its blood meal), absorbs a lethal dose of insecticide and dies before the parasites it has taken up in the blood can complete development. This was the main method of the malaria eradication programmes used in many countries of the world. Unfortunately, insecticidal resistance, organizational breakdown and reluctance by people to have their houses sprayed, resulted in an abandonment of the goal of eradication. This has been replaced by a policy of malaria control in which house spraying may be a component.

Larviciding and biological control. The number of larvae determines the density of mosquitoes,

so any method which reduces the larval numbers inadvertently reduces the potential number of adults. The larvae can be attacked by several different methods:

- using insecticides and larvicidal substances;
- modification of the environment; and
- biological control.

Larvicidal substances can be oils that spread over the water surface and asphyxiate the larvae or have insecticidal properties. The size and flow of the body of water will determine which is the preferred method to use. Modification of the environment by drainage or filling in is the most permanent and effective, but is an expensive undertaking. It is worth spending money on engineering methods in areas of dense population such as towns, while in rural areas much can be achieved by using self-help schemes. The considerable advantage of this method is that once done, it lasts for a long period of time, if not permanently, and in these days of resistant mosquitoes it is seen as an economic proposition in some circumstances (see also Section 3.4.1).

Biological control using fish or bacilli (*Bacillus thuringiensis* or *B. sphaericus*) will reduce mosquito larvae to a certain extent, but a balance, as with much of nature, often results. Biological control can also be used directly against adults with the sterile male technique. This has not been successful with mosquitoes because of the very large numbers involved and their short period of life. Another method that is being considered is species competition, whereby a non-malarial mosquito from another part of the world is introduced to compete with the resident vector. This has not met with any great success.

In epidemic malaria, using a fogging machine or ULV spray from aircraft can rapidly reduce adult mosquito density. This will cut short the epidemic by killing off flying adults, but needs to be repeated regularly as new adults will continually be produced from larvae that are not affected by the knock-down sprays.

Chemoprophylaxis. Attempts to use chemoprophylaxis on a large scale for pregnant women and young children have not met with much success, except in areas of seasonal malaria chemoprophylaxis (SMC, see Section 18.2.9), but could be given to persons at particular risk such as non-immune immigrants or migrant workers. Chloroquine 300 mg (two tablets) weekly can be used where chloroquine resistance is not a major problem, but local advice should be sought. It is preferable to give pregnant women and young children priority in the distribution of ITNs or LLINs, or to use chemoprophylaxis in combination with these.

Reducing the number of gametocytes. Quinine, chloroquine and amodiaquine are active against the gametocytes of *P. vivax* and *P. malariae*, but not against the more important *P. falciparum*. Proguanil and pyrimethamine act on the development of gametocytes within the mosquito on all four *Plasmodium* parasites. Primaquine has a highly active and rapid action on gametocytes of all species, whether in the blood or mosquito, and is used in combination with treatment in the individual. It has also been proposed as a method of reducing the level of gametocytes within the population, but would require an almost perfect mass treatment, as well as consideration of the danger of toxicity (especially with glucose-6-phosphate dehydrogenase deficient individuals) so is not considered a suitable method of malaria control.

Any person found to have malaria should, where possible, be protected by a mosquito net so as not to infect new mosquitoes. This is a particularly important measure during eradication and control campaigns, especially when endemicity is brought to a low level.

Vaccines. Attempts to produce a vaccine against malaria have been in progress since 1910. A vaccine made from killed sporozoites by irradiating mosquitoes is reasonably effective, but cannot be produced on a large scale. Easier to produce are vaccines made by isolating the DNA fragments of the circumsporozoite antigen and cloning them through bacteria or yeasts. This has allowed large quantities of pure antigen to be produced, and trials of candidate vaccines. A prototype vaccine, RTS,S, has recently been shown to reduce the chance of children contracting malaria in the trial areas of Kenya and Tanzania by 50%. However, even if a vaccine is developed, there will still be all the problems of vaccination programmes, such as coverage, administrative difficulties and response of the public (see Section 3.2).

Prospects for malaria control. Malaria attracts the wonder cure; first it was the eradication programme, now all hope is pinned on the vaccine, but the disease is more likely to be controlled by simple, non-dramatic methods, where care to detail is applied. It is the encouragement of simple protective methods that everybody can follow, like using ITNs (or LLINs), or community action to modify the environment to make it unsuitable for mosquitoes to breed (see Table 15.2 for the main vectors). A multiplicity of simple methods, carried out by many responsible people, is likely to be more successful in the long term than more complex methods.

Treatment of the uncomplicated case of *P. vivax*, *P. malariae* and *P. ovale* malaria is with chloroquine:

- 600 mg of chloroquine base as an initial dose,
- 6 h later, 300 mg chloroquine base,
- followed by 300 mg chloroquine base for 3 or more days.

However, chloroquine-resistant *P. vivax* has been reported from Western Pacific islands, including the island of New Guinea, as well as from Guyana in South America.

P. falciparum is resistant to chloroquine and many other antimalarials, largely as a result of their indiscriminate use. The artemisinin group of compounds, especially artesunate, artemether and dihydroartemisinin are mostly effective, and WHO recommends that they be used in combination with other antimalarials as an artemisinin combination therapy (ACT) to reduce the development of resistance. Unfortunately, the first cases of artimisinin-resistant malaria have appeared in Cambodia and Thailand, while reports suggest that resistance is also developing in Africa and South America. Intense efforts are being made to contain and eliminate these pockets of resistance before they spread more widely. ACT still remains effective in most places and one of the following regimes can be used:

- artemether/lumefantrine;
- artesunate plus amodiaquine (in areas where the cure rate of amodiaquine monotherapy is greater than 80%);
- artesunate plus sulfadoxine/pyrimethamine (in areas where the cure rate of sulfadoxine/ pyrimethamine is greater than 80%);
- artesunate plus mefloquine (insufficient safety data to recommend use in Africa); and
- dihydroartemisin plus piperaquine.

The addition of a single dose of primaquine (0.75 mg/kg body weight) will accelerate the removal of gametocytes, but care must be used in glucose-6-phosphate dehydrogenase deficiency areas.

While the microscope slide is being read (in many situations it may need to be sent to a centre for confirmatory microscopy) and the health worker has excluded other possible causes of fever, then presumptive treatment can be given. This is with a full course of therapy, which can be discontinued if the slide result is negative. Where cheaper treatment regimes, such as with chloroquine, are still effective, this is a reasonable strategy, but where ACT is required, then the increased cost of using an RDT is justified. (The cost of an RDT is about the same as a course of ACT.) Careful training is required.

In *P. vivax*, chloroquine will only clear parasites from the blood, and to effect radical cure, primaquine is administered in a dose of 15 mg base daily for 14 days (except in the island of New Guinea and other Western Pacific Islands where more prolonged treatment is required).

Case finding and treatment is an effective control strategy where there is a low level of malaria, but it needs to be used in combination with other methods.

Surveillance. In all areas where malaria is found, a blood slide should be taken from anyone with a fever. Where attempts are being made to eradicate or reduce the level of malaria then an active system of surveillance may be instituted as described in Section 4.5.2.

Where a control method is in operation, then regular checks should be made, such as the proportion of houses with ITNs and the number of people sleeping under them. More will be found on malaria programmes in Sections 4.1, 4.2, 4.3, 4.5 and 4.6.

15.7 Lymphatic Filariasis

Organism. *Wuchereria bancrofti*, *Brugia malayi* and *B. timori*, nematode worms. The life cycle is illustrated in Fig. 15.9. Microfilariae, the larval nematode form present in the peripheral blood, are taken into a mosquito's stomach when it feeds on humans (or an animal reservoir in *B. malayi*). The larva loses its sheath inside the mosquito, migrates through the stomach wall and burrows into the muscles of the thorax. It becomes shorter and fatter, commonly described as sausage shaped.

Developmental changes take place and it elongates to a third-stage, infective larva. Leaving the thoracic muscles it migrates to the proboscis where it waits for the mosquito to feed. Forcing its way out of the proboscis, it falls onto the human (or animal) skin, finding a way into the tissues, generally through the wound made by the mosquito. (This differs from malaria, in that the infective larva is *not* injected when the mosquito takes a blood meal.) This developmental stage in the mosquito, from the time of the blood meal until reinfection, takes 11–21 days (average 15) at an optimum temperature of 26–27°C (extremes are 17 to 32°C), a very similar length of time to the development of *Plasmodium*.

When the larva brakes out of the mosquito to enter the skin this is a very precarious time for the parasite and only 20–40% are successful. No multiplication has taken place in the mosquito, so one larva that was taken up in the blood meal becomes one adult in the human. However, many larvae are lost, with only about 1 in 700 succeeding. Because there are male and female worms, it is necessary for the two sexes to meet if the female is to be fertilized. Many are unsuccessful in finding a mate of the opposite sex and it is only when there is a heavy infection that the probability of them doing so is increased. So intensity of infection will determine the outcome. Once the worms mate the female produces huge numbers of microfilariae into the lymphatic system, and these reach blood vessels via the thoracic duct.

The parasite has timed its production of microfilariae to coincide with the biting time of the vector mosquito, a phenomenon called periodicity. Mostly this is a nocturnal cycle, with a peak around midnight, but it can also be diurnal, or in the Central and Eastern Pacific Islands it is aperiodic, with similar levels of microfilariae being found throughout the 24 h period.

Microfilariae live for about 6 months and adult worms 7–12 years, although they probably only produce microfilariae for 2–3 years.

Clinical features. In the human body, the larva reaches the lymphatics and settles down in a lymphatic node to develop into an adult. It is the obstruction of the lymphatic drainage system by the adult worms, especially the fibrotic reaction when they die, that causes the series of disease manifestations. A range of conditions result including fever, lymphangitis, lymphoedema, hydrocele, elephantiasis and chyluria. Night sweats are a common

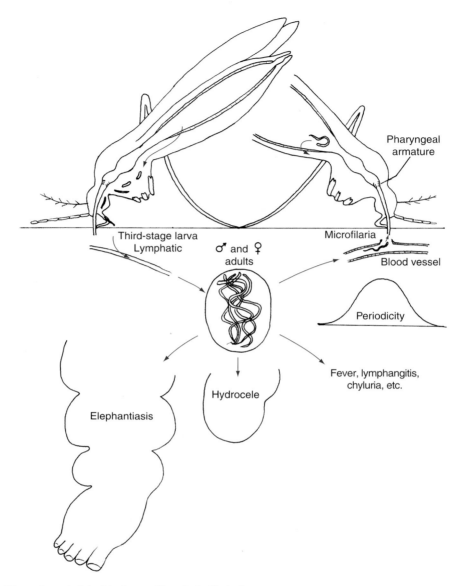

Fig. 15.9. Life cycle and clinical features of lymphatic filariasis.

early indication of infection, with high eosinophilia counts. An allergic reaction, tropical pulmonary eosinophilia syndrome, can also result. Although the signs and symptoms are diverse and variable, in an endemic area they are often known, and a blood sample will soon confirm the diagnosis.

Diagnosis used to be by finding microfilariae in a measured sample of blood using a thick blood smear, counting chamber or filtration technique, taken during the peak microfilarial output, which generally means collecting samples at night time. These laborious methods have now largely been replaced by circulating filarial antigen (CFA) detection either based on ELISA or on an immunochromatographic card. However, the card test only diagnoses positive or negative, while the ELISA is semi-quantitative, so where full quantitative measures are required, the measured blood sample methods will still need to be used. This will be the case in assessing control programmes, as a decrease in the number of microfilariae occurs before conversion to negativity. CFA detection is also not available for *B. malayi* or *B. timori*. Different microfilariae need to be differentiated, as seen in Fig. 15.10, as several filarial infections may be present in the same locality.

Transmission is by both culicine and anopheline mosquitoes (Table 15.3), producing quite different patterns of infection and, as a result, different strategies for control. If *Anopheles* mosquitoes are the vectors they are nearly always the same vectors as transmit malaria, so the mosquito might well have a double infection or its expectation of life be affected by being parasitized by filariasis and malaria.

As the microfilaria is quite large, it causes damage to the mosquito when it bores into the thoracic muscles, so the more microfilariae the mosquito ingests the more likely it is to be killed by a heavy infection. (In *Culex* and *Aedes* mosquitoes this occurs when the microfilarial density exceeds $50/20\,mm^3$ of blood.) This is seen in Fig. 15.11 at point E for both culicine mosquitoes (upper figure) and anopheline mosquitoes (lower figure). The line P represents the equilibrium level (basic reproductive level of 1), whereby above the line transmissions will increase and below it infection will die out, so when infection is excessively heavy mosquito mortality occurs and the infection dies out. In reality, the number of microfilariae will decrease below the point E, mosquitoes will survive sufficiently to transmit again and the level will approach E, or the level of equilibrium, again. This is always the case with culicine transmission, but in the bottom figure it will be noticed that there is also a lower point I, below which transmission is not sustained for anopheline mosquitoes. In other words, at low levels of microfilariae, the anopheline mosquito seems to be able to prevent itself from becoming infected. This is probably due to the pharyngeal armature in anopheline mosquitoes, which damages microfilariae. When there are many microfilariae ingested by the mosquito sufficient will remain undamaged to produce infection, but at low levels of microfilariae, every microfilaria will be damaged. This applies to both *W. bancrofti* and *B. malayi*, so for control purposes, the type of mosquito is more important than the species of parasite.

Filarial infection is determined by the number of infected bites, which can either be the result of a high intensity over a short period of time or of constant bites over a long period of time. Mosquito mortality occurs when density of microfilariae is excessive, so the chronic, long-term pattern is more common.

Incubation period. From infection to the development of adult worms is about 1 year, but the first symptoms may not occur until microfilariae are produced (fever) or worms die to produce lymphatic obstruction some years later.

Period of communicability. Because many infective bites are required to produce infection in humans, there will need to be a continuous supply of infected mosquitoes. The development cycle in the mosquito is 11–21 days (mean 15 days). The infected person can continue to produce microfilariae for in excess of 10 years, although maximum output is in the first 3 years.

Occurrence and distribution. Humans only are infected by *W. bancrofti*, but an animal reservoir exists for *B. malayi* in monkeys, cats and several other animals. All races, both sexes and all ages of persons are equally susceptible to infection. (There are marked differences between individuals developing elephantiasis, but these are immunological rather than ethnic.)

Three types of filariasis are seen: *rural* filariasis transmitted by nocturnal *Anopheles* mosquitoes with a generalized distribution similar to that of malaria; *urban* filariasis transmitted by *Culex*, with a tendency to invade new areas; and the Pacific Island variety, which has a homogenous (rural) distribution but is transmitted by day- and night-biting *Aedes* mosquitoes.

W. bancrofti is found in the tropical regions of the world, but with only a few foci in South America and the Caribbean. *B. malayi* is restricted to East and South-east Asia, overlapping with *W. bancrofti* in part of its range. *B. timori* is only found in the islands of Timor, Flores, Alor and Roti (Fig. 15.12). In 2010, there were estimated to be 1.39 billion people at risk of filarial infection in 72 countries and territories, approximately 18% of the world population. Some 120 million people in the world are infected and 40 million with disabling disease.

Control and prevention. A similar process to that used for malaria for identifying the best strategies

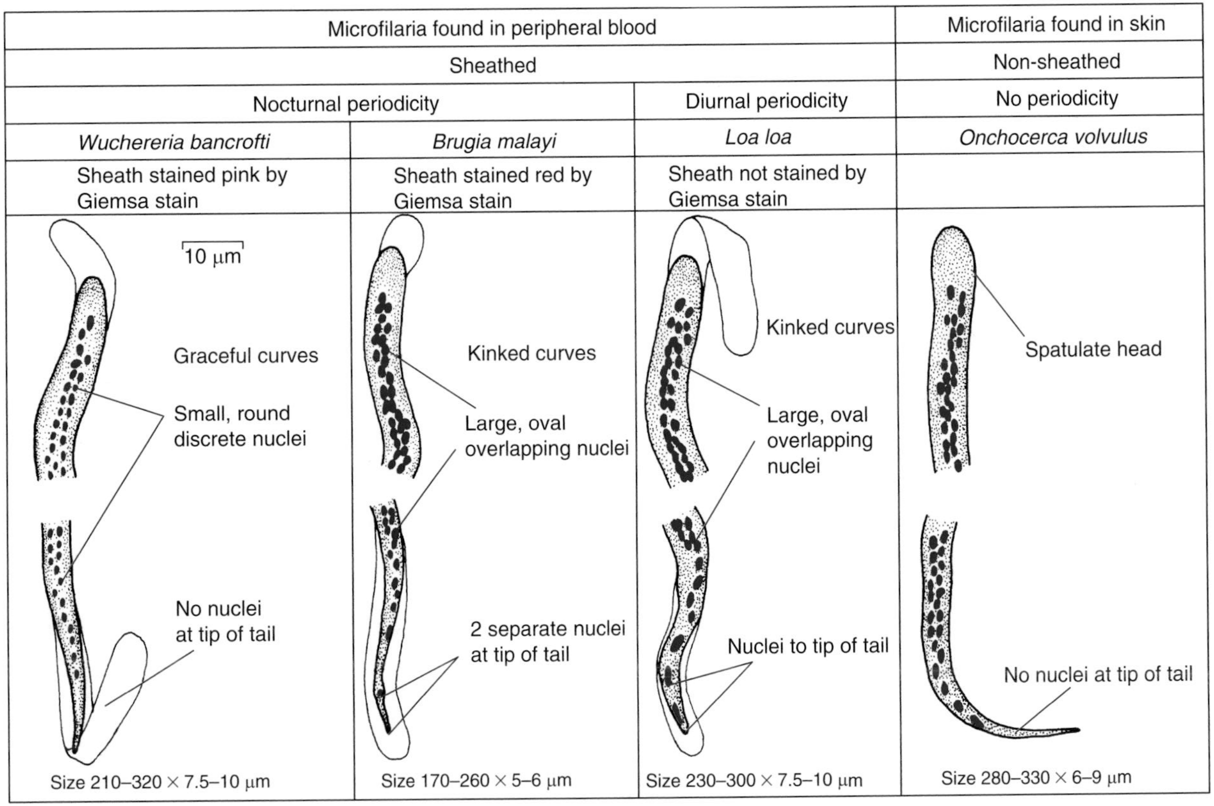

Fig. 15.10. Differential features of microfilariae of medical importance. (Courtesy Department of Medical Parasitology, London School of Hygiene and Tropical Medicine.)

Table. 15.3. The vectors of lymphatic filariasis (*A., Anopheles*; *Ae., Aedes*; *C., Culex*; *M., Mansonia*; *O., Ochlerotatus*).

Geographical area	Species transmitting *Wuchereria bancrofti*	Species transmitting *Brugia malayi*
West Africa, rural East Africa, Madagascar	*A. gambiae, A. funestus, A. arabiensis, A. melas, A. merus*	
Urban East Africa	*C. quinquefasciatus*	
Egypt	*C. pipiens molestus*	
India, Sri Lanka and Maldive Islands	*C. quinquefasciatus, A. minimus, Ae. niveus, O. harinasutai*	*M. amulifera, M. indiana, M. uniformis, M. annulata, M. bonneae, M. dives*
China	*Ae. togoi, A. sinensis, A. anthrapophagus*	*Ae. togoi, A. lesteri, A. sinensis, A. anthrapophagus*
Vietnam	*A. jeyporiensis*	
Rural Thailand	*O. hariniasutai*	*M. annulata, M. bonnae, M. uniformis, M. indiana*
Malaysia	*A. letifer, A. whartoni, A. maculatus, A. dirus, A. donaldi, A. letifer*	*M. annulata, M. annulifera, M. bonnae, M. dives, M. uniformis, A. campestris, A. donaldi*
Indonesia	*A. balabacensis, A. leucosphyrus, A. maculatus*	*M. annulata, M. bonnae, M. dives, A. barbirostris (B. timori)*
Philippines		*M. dives*
New Guinea (Papua New Guinea and Irian Jaya)	*A. farauti, A. punctulatus, A. koliensis, C. annulinostris, C. bitaneniorhynchus, M. uniformis*	
New Caledonia	*Ae. vigilax*	
Fiji	*Ae. polynesiensis, Ae. fijiensis, Ae. pseudoscutellaris, Ae. oceanicus*	
Polynesian Islands	*Ae. polynesiensis, Ae. samoanus, Ae. upolensis, Ae. kesseli, Ae. tutuilae, Ae. tabu, Ae. cooki*	
North-east Brazil	*C. quinquefasciatus*	

for control can also be applied to filariasis. The various places at which control can be implemented are:

- reduction of the number of infective bites by mosquitoes;
- decreasing the number of microfilariae in the human host;
- reduction of the mosquito's expectation of life;
- decreasing the mosquito density;
- alteration of the mosquito biting time; and
- reduction of the number of adult worms.

Reducing the number of infective bites. Multiplication does not take place when the larva enters the host so the disease process and its severity depends upon repeated entry of parasites to the body, many of which will be unsuccessful. The transmission process is surprisingly inefficient, requiring some 15,500 infected bites to produce a reproducing adult. This means that for *Anopheles* mosquitoes,

approximately eight bites per person per day can take place without the disease being transmitted.

The number of bites can be reduced by taking simple precautions of personal protection: mosquito nets, repellents, protective clothing, etc. ITNs or LLINs are effective in nocturnally periodic filariasis transmitted by anopheline mosquitoes (Box 3.1). This would be an additional benefit of a malaria control programme.

Decreasing the number of microfilariae (mass chemotherapy). Mass drug administration (MDA) is the main method used in the filariasis elimination programme. This is given as an annual single dose treatment to all the population for at least 5 years, preferably 7 years. Two regimes are used:

- albendazole 400 mg + ivermectin 150–200 mcg/kg, or
- albendazole 400 mg + diethylcarbamazine (DEC) 6 mg/kg.

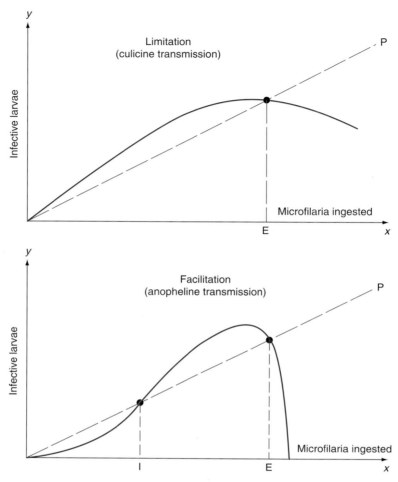

Fig. 15.11. The dynamics of culicine and anopheline transmitted filariasis. (Reproduced, by permission, from Pichon, G., Perrault, G. and Laigret, J. (1975) *Rendement parasitaire chez les vecteurs de filarioses*. (WHO/FIL/75.132), World Health Organization, Geneva.) See text for explanation of variables.

An alternative is to use DEC-fortified salt (or fortified Soy sauce in China) for 6–12 months, if total compliance can be assured. DEC cannot be used in an area that also has onchocerciasis.

This strategy is likely to work in areas in which filariasis is transmitted by *Anopheles* mosquitoes if the number of microfilariae can be maintained below the critical threshold (I in Fig. 15.11). One estimate suggests that this level is about 12 microfilariae/60 mm³. However, as *Anopheles* is also a vector for malaria, reducing the number of parasitizing microfilariae, which cause damage to the mosquito, will increase the mosquito's expectation of life and improve its chance of transmitting

malaria. Precautions should therefore be taken at the same time to prevent this from happening by the use of ITNs or LLINs (Box 3.1).

In areas in which culicine mosquitoes are the vectors, it is unlikely that MDA alone will succeed in eliminating filariasis, as can be seen from Fig. 15.11, and from past experience in control programmes in Samoa and Tahiti. Control of the mosquito also needs to take place, a simple strategy being the use of expanded polystyrene beads, as was used in latrines in Zanzibar and soakage pits in south India (see also below).

Before mounting a mass drug treatment control programme, a complete survey is needed. Follow-up

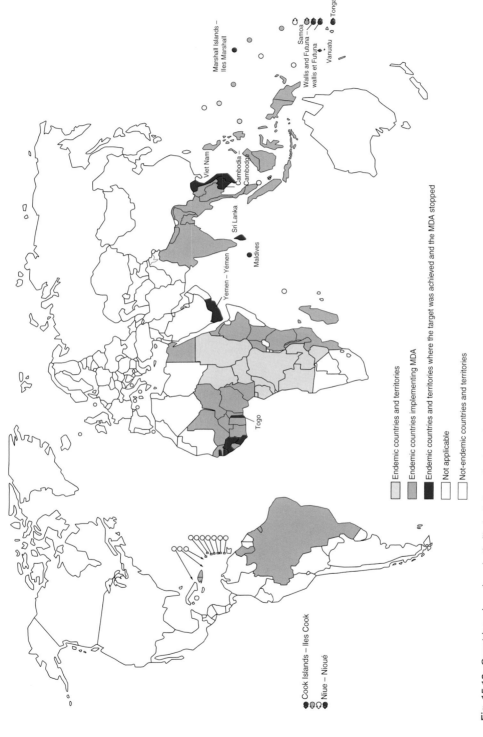

Fig. 15.12. Countries where lymphatic filariasis is endemic and status of mass drug administration (MDA) in those countries, 2010. (Reproduced by permission of the World Health Organization, Geneva.)

- Endemic countries and territories
- Endemic countries implementing MDA
- Endemic countries and territories where the target was achieved and the MDA stopped
- Not applicable
- Not-endemic countries and territories

surveys of samples of the population are made at annual intervals; 30% of the treated population should be sampled. Children less than 1 year old, pregnant and nursing mothers, the sick and the very old should be excluded from mass treatment. Side effects, especially itching, can be most unpleasant, and a pilot control study should precede the main campaign. Considerable care should be taken in areas where both filariasis and onchocerciasis co-exist. *Loa loa* infection in parts of West Africa may make it impossible to use the standard MDA regimes; instead a 4–8 week course of doxycycline can be used.

Reduction of the mosquito's lifespan (vector control). By reducing the lifespan of the mosquito to below that of the developmental period of the parasite within the mosquito (range 10–15 days), transmission of infective larvae will be halted. This can be done by spraying residual insecticides inside houses or treating mosquito nets.

Where the same vectors transmit both malaria and filariasis, then a joint control programme is cost-effective. ITNs or LLINs are particularly suitable for filariasis control where there is an anopheline vector and could be used as the only strategy or combined with MDA (see above). The degree of mosquito reduction required is much less for filariasis than it is for malaria; however, mosquito control needs to be for a prolonged period, at least 7 years and preferably 10 years.

Decrease mosquito density (larviciding). The number of mosquitoes able to bite man is dependent upon the number of larvae that develop into adults, so by reducing the number of larvae, mosquito density is also diminished. This is a supplementary method of malaria control and has also been covered in Section 3.4.1 on vector control. Various methods can be used, larvicides, genetic modification, and environmental or biological control. These methods are particularly appropriate to culicine-transmitted urban filariasis, although the degree of larval reduction required is often difficult to achieve. In enclosed areas of water such as latrines and septic tanks, expanded polystyrene beads are very effective.

B. malayi is transmitted mainly by *Mansonia* and *Anopheles* mosquitoes, *Mansonia* being particularly difficult to control because the larvae attach themselves to the underside of water plants (especially *Pistia*), where they are immune to surface oils and larvicides. Removal of these water plants by hand or with herbicides has produced some effect.

Alteration of mosquito biting pattern. The parasite has developed a periodicity of its microfilariae which coincides with the biting pattern of the vector mosquitoes. If it is possible to alter the time mosquitoes bite then the chance of them taking up microfilariae will also be reduced. This has happened in some places owing to the prolonged use of residual insecticides, and although it is probably not possible to utilize this as a main control method, it could be of subsidiary value.

Reduction of the number of adult worms. Unfortunately, there is no specific drug that kills adult worms, although DEC causes substantial mortality, a valuable secondary action to killing microfilariae. The worms lie embedded in the lymphatics so cannot be removed surgically, as practised in onchocerciasis control.

Adult worms live for approximately 10 years (range 7–12 years), so if reinfection can be prevented for this period they will die off and there will be no reservoir of infection. It is maintaining control methods for this period of time that is crucial with filariasis.

Treatment for established elephantiasis is unsatisfactory, with mutilating surgical procedures. If discovered in its early stages of intermittent swelling, before tissue damage has occurred, then pressure bandages can prevent gross elephantiasis from developing. In *B. timori*, repeat doses of DEC reduce lymphoedema and, to a certain extent, elephantiasis. In other areas, a single dose of DEC plus albendazole or a multi-week course of doxycycline (by its action on the endosymbiotic *Wolbachia* organisms and also as a macrofilariacide) may be tried. Moxidectin, which is used in veterinary practice, is being tried in humans against adult worms in onchocerciasis and could, theoretically, also kill adult *W. bancrofti*.

Surveillance. Hydrocele or lymph-node surveys can be of value in rapidly defining the area of filariasis. Detailed blood surveys are then made.

The year 2020 has been designated as the target for elimination of lymphatic filariasis worldwide. Surveillance and search for new cases will need to continue for a considerable period of time and for several years after a country has been found to be free of infection.

15.8 Onchocerciasis

Organism. Onchocerca volvulus, a nematode worm that has a predilection for the skin and eye, is transmitted by *Simulium* flies. Microfilariae are taken up by the fly when it bites the human, and undergo larval changes within the thoracic muscles, migrating to the head of the fly as infective larvae. When the fly bites again, microfilariae break out on to the skin to enter via any abrasion, especially the bite wound.

Clinical features. The microfilariae, as they migrate through the skin, cause itching and damage resulting in skin changes, loss of elasticity and discoloration, the so-called 'leopard skin'. As well as migrating through the skin, they also enter the eye, where the reaction caused by their death leads to eye damage, the person in time going blind, giving onchocerciasis its other name of 'river blindness'. Adult worms settle in subcutaneous nodules, making this a ready method of diagnosis. Lymphadenopathy is also a feature, sometimes being gross, e.g. 'hanging groin'.

Diagnosis is made by taking skin snips, which are placed in saline, and the liberated microfilariae identified (Fig. 15.10). Taking a measured area of skin with a special punch allows density measurements to be made. Slit-lamp examination of the eye may observe microfilariae in the anterior chamber or reveal characteristic eye damage. The adult worms live in palpable nodules in the skin so their presence and characteristic skin changes can suggest a clinical diagnosis.

Transmission. The vector *Simulium*, also called the blackfly, breeds in fast-flowing streams where it is found in huge numbers. The female fly attaches its eggs to the leaves of water plants in fast-flowing water, where they have the high oxygen levels they require for their development (Fig. 15.13). The fly has a painful bite and is persistent, making it a considerable nuisance, but is also a powerful flier, and assisted by the wind can travel up to 100 km in search of a blood meal.

The *Simulium* vectors and their usual breeding places are listed in Table 15.4. The African flies prefer to bite the lower body, whereas the South American flies attack the upper body. Although they can fly great distances, maximum density is at the breeding place, resulting in focal infection.

They are outdoor, daytime biters, but each species prefer different times of day to seek their blood meal. South American *Simulium* species have pharyngeal armatures, whereas African species do not, but mortality due to superinfection by *Onchocerca* is not important. The adult flies live for 2–3 weeks (with a maximum of 3 months) but prefer to feed on animals rather than humans. However, people need to collect water, so it is when they come to the river, to wash or collect drinking water, that they stand the greatest chance of being infected.

O. volvulus only infects humans (and epidemiologically insignificant chimpanzees and gorillas). Eye and skin pathology is related to the proximity of the nodules, so more nodules on the upper part of the body produces a higher prevalence of blindness. In Africa, the savannah infection produces more blindness than that acquired in forests.

Microfilariae are found only in the skin, a high density leading to the more severe clinical manifestations, as well as producing greater opportunity to infect flies. They survive for up to 2.5 years and have a periodic cycle with peak at 16.00–18.00 h, but this is relatively unimportant.

Incubation period is prolonged, normally taking about 1 year for symptoms to start following infection.

Period of communicability is some 16–17 years, adult worms producing microfilariae into old age. *Simulium* becomes infective after 6–13 days, depending on temperature.

Occurrence and distribution. Onchocerciasis is found only in tropical Africa, Yemen and South/Central America, with well-marked foci in much of this area (Fig. 15.14). In West and much of Central Africa the infection is more widespread with the most westerly part of the region covered by the Onchocerciasis Control Programme (OCP, see below).

Repeat infection and progressive damage from dying microfilariae means that blindness is more common in adults, children then having to lead them around until their turn comes to go blind. Because of these severe consequences, abandonment of good village sites close to rivers has frequently resulted, although control programmes have largely reversed this trend.

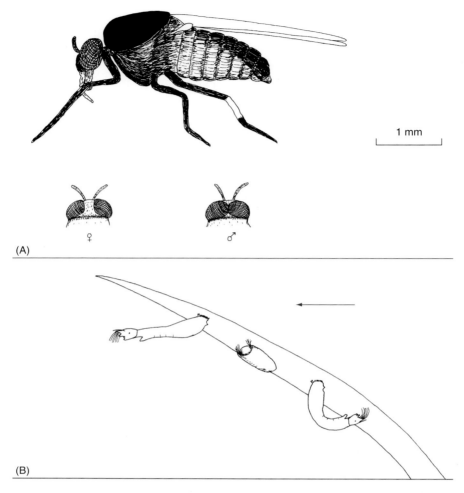

(A)

(B)

Fig. 15.13. *Simulium*, the vector of onchocerciasis. (A) Adult. (B) Larvae and a pupa attached to a water plant, the stream flowing in the direction of the arrow.

Control and prevention. Various approaches to control can be tried, as with lymphatic filariasis. These are:

- reducing the fly density;
- avoidance of fly breeding places;
- reducing the microfilarial density;
- reduction of the number of adult worms; and
- reduction in the number of *Simulium* bites.

Reducing the fly density (larviciding). The larvae breed in water, so insecticide is sprayed on streams and rivers. They are relatively sensitive to insecticides, so low-dose applications, 0.05 to 0.1 mg/l are effective.

Temephos (Abate) is suitable as it is effective in a very low dose, is relatively non-toxic to fish and retains some residual action. It exerts its effect for some 20–40 km downstream in the wet season. The main difficulty with larviciding is to ensure that every watercourse is treated. Owing to the flies' ability to cover large distances, recolonization soon takes place when insecticidal applications are discontinued. Although expensive, the extra cost of using aircraft and helicopters can be justified if many watercourses, spread over large areas of countryside, have to be covered.

Unfortunately, insecticidal resistance has occurred in a number of areas, so biological control with

Table 15.4. *Simulium* vectors of onchocerciasis.

Geographical area	*Simulium* species	Breeding place	Habitat
West Africa, Central African Republic (CAR), Sudan, Uganda, Ethiopia (Yemen?)	*S. damnosum* species complex	Large rivers	Savannah, sometimes forest
West Africa, CAR, Sudan	*S. sirbanum*	Large rivers	Savannah
West Africa, CAR, Congo	*S. squamosum*	Small-to-medium sized rivers in hilly areas	Forest, savannah, mosaic
West Africa	*S. soubrense*	Large rivers	Forest, savannah
West Africa	*S. sanctipauli*	Large rivers	Forest
West Africa	*S. yahense*	Small watercourses	Forest
Cameroon, CAR, Tanzania	*S. mengense*	Large rivers	Forest
Congo, Burundi, Uganda, Tanzania, Malawi	*S. kilibanum*	Large rivers	Forest
Congo, Burundi, Rwanda, Uganda, Sudan	*S. naevi* species complex	Heavily shaded small permanent rivers in forest	Forest
Ethiopia	*S. ethiopiense*	Heavily shaded small permanent rivers in forest	Forest
Tanzania	*S. woodi*	Heavily shaded small permanent rivers in forest	Forest
Guatemala, Mexico	*S. ochraceum*	Small mountain streams	Highlands
Guatemala, Mexico, Venezuela	*S. metallicum*	Small streams	Highlands
Colombia, Ecuador, Venezuela	*S. exiguum*	Large rivers	Lowlands
Brazil, Venezuela	*S. guianense*	Large, fast-flowing rivers	Highlands
Brazil, Venezuela	*S. oyapockense*	Large rivers	Lowlands

B. thuringiensis is an alternative. This does not have the spreading power of insecticides, so greater concentrations need to be used (in the order of 0.9 mg/l), and it has to be mixed with water before it can be applied.

Avoidance of fly breeding places. Maximum contact between humans and flies occurs near rivers where *Simulium* breeds, but these can be avoided by providing alternative water sources, such as wells or a piped water supply.

Reducing the microfilarial density. Ivermectin immobilizes microfilariae, which are flushed out of the skin and eye and killed in the lymph nodes. As microfilarial death occurs away from the skin and eye, irritation is minimized and ocular reaction reduced. Ivermectin can be given as a single dose of 200 µg/kg with retreatment at 6 and 18 month intervals. This means that MDA for onchocerciasis can be used as an adjunct to vector control. MDA given twice a year has been found to eliminate infection if continued for 15–17 years.

However, it cannot be used in areas where *Loa loa* infection is also found, in which case doxycycline can be used for 4–8 weeks.

Reducing the number of adult worms. Because the adult worms live for a considerable period of time, during all of which they are producing microfilariae, specific attack on the adult parasites can reduce both the symptoms and the potential for transmitting infection. Nodulectomy or the surgical removal of adult worms from skin nodules, can be a relatively effective procedure, practised particularly in the onchocercal areas of Guatemala, where nodules are more common in the upper parts of the body. Doxycycline continued for 6 weeks kills endosymbiotic Wolbachia on which the *O. volvulus* obtains nutrition, so that it also dies; it should be used on a selective basis and not given to pregnant women or children.

Reducing the number of *Simulium* bites. Personal protection is less effective against *Simulium* than with mosquitoes, with nets being inappropriate,

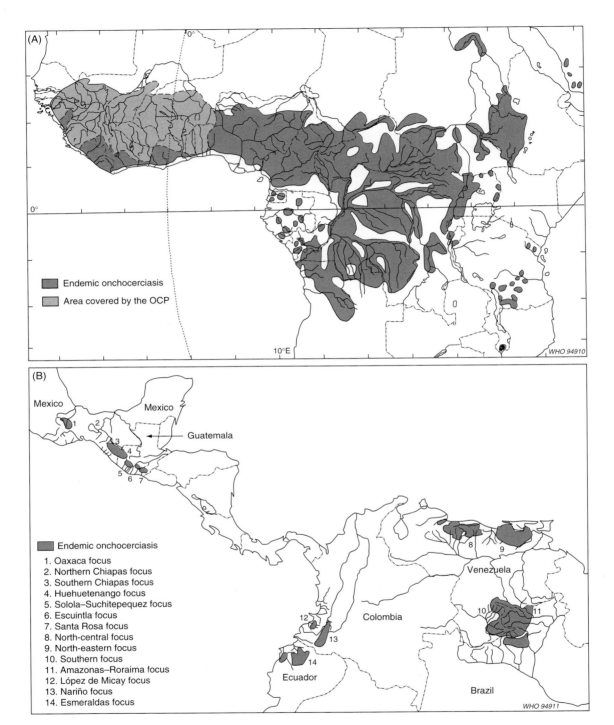

Fig. 15.14. Distribution of onchocerciasis. (A) Africa and Yemen. (B) the Americas. OCP, former Onchocerciasis Control Programme area. NB some of these foci have since been eliminated. (From World Health Organization (1995) *Onchocerciasis and its Control*. Technical Report Series No. 852. Reproduced, by permission of the World Health Organization, Geneva.)

although repellents have some effect. The wearing of long-sleeved shirts and long trousers with hat and net can be used by individuals investigating the disease, but are not methods that can be developed for mass use. Avoiding passage through breeding sites will reduce fly biting.

Onchocerciasis control programmes. As adult *O. volvulus* can live for 15–17 years, any control programme would need to be maintained for this length of time before eradication could take place. However, most programmes seek to reduce the intensity of infection to a level where symptoms are absent. The criteria used in the OCP in West Africa were:

- less than 100 infective larvae/person a year; and
- annual biting rates of less than 1000.

After many years of operation, the OCP finished in 2002, with delegation to individual countries to detect and treat all new cases.

The main method of control was larviciding, which can be extremely effective if carried out thoroughly. Species eradication of *S. naevi* was achieved in Kenya by methodically treating every watercourse with DDT. Where the disease covers a limited area, then such an intense programme could be considered. In a more diffuse focus, the borders of control need to be extended sufficiently to prevent reinvasion by *Simulium* flying in from outside. While resistance is a serious problem, resistant *Simulium* is less important in transmission.

Mass drug therapy, or selective therapy to persons with heavy infections, can be given right from the start of the programme. This will rapidly reduce the level of microfilariae and the potential for infecting flies. Preventing blindness (with ivermectin) has been particularly valuable in obtaining the cooperation of people. As lymphatic filariasis and onchocerciasis occur in the same areas in a number of countries (mainly in West Africa), and ivermectin is used to treat both diseases, then joint programmes (with the addition of albendazole) are cost-effective.

The mass drug therapy approach has been particularly valuable in the areas formerly covered by the OCP in Africa. Ivermectin therapy, which had been used for 15–17 years in Mali and Senegal, was stopped and no further infections were detected after 2 years, showing that the disease can be eliminated.

Mass drug administration with ivermectin is also used in the South/Central America Onchocerciasis Elimination Programme, with good progress being made in reducing foci in all countries. If no further transmission takes place, certificates of elimination are due for Colombia in 2011, Ecuador in 2013, Mexico and Guatemala in 2014 and Venezuela and Brazil in 2016.

Treatment. Ivermectin has been very effective, especially in the reduction of blindness. A 6 week course of doxycycline is effective in killing adult worms.

Surveillance. Skin and nodule surveys can be used to indicate areas that need more intense skin-snip examination. (See also the OCP programme above.)

15.9 Loiasis

Organism. *Loa loa*, a nematode worm. The life cycle of the parasite is essentially the same as that of *W. bancrofti*, except that the vectors are tabanid flies.

Clinical features. The disease is characterized by Calabar swellings (named after a town in eastern Nigeria) which are transient, itchy and found anywhere on the body. Fever and eosinophilia suggest that they have an allergic aetiology. *L. loa* is often confusingly called the eye worm (to be differentiated from *O. volvulus*), as the worm is sometimes seen migrating across the conjunctiva, but it produces no pathology in the eye.

Diagnosis. *L. loa* is diurnally periodic and diagnosis is made by examining daytime blood in which the microfilaria (Fig. 15.10) will be found. *Mansonella ozzardi*, *M. perstans* and *M. streptocerca* are also commonly found in blood and skin smears in the same area and need to be differentiated from *L. loa* as well as from *W. bancrofti* and *O. volvulus*.

Transmission. The vector is *Chrysops*, a large, powerful fly which inflicts a painful bite, attacking either within the forest or at the forest fringe.

Incubation period. Although microfilariae may appear in the blood after about 6 months, the first symptoms may take years.

Period of communicability. Like *O. volvulus*, the adult can live for up to 17 years, producing microfilariae all this time. *L. loa* takes 10–12 days to produce infective larvae in the fly.

Occurrence and distribution. Loiasis is found in west and central African rainforests, and especially in the Congo River basin.

Treatment. Both adult worms and microfilariae are killed by diethylcarbamazine, but caution needs to be exercised as allergic reactions can be profound. Low dosages of 0.1 mg/kg can be used to initiate treatment, gradually building up over 8 days to 6 mg/kg, which is continued for 3 weeks. Steroid cover may be required in those cases with more than 30 microfilaria/mm^3. Ivermectin will also reduce the microfilarial stage and produces less reaction, so is more suitable for mass control programmes. However, reactions do still occur, especially in those in whom the worm is seen crossing the eye, so a useful preliminary is to show people a picture of the worm in the lower eye and exclude those in which it has been seen.

Control and prevention. Extensive control measures are generally not warranted, the main preventive action being against the bites of *Chrysops* with protective clothing and repellents. Clearing the forest canopy, oiling of pools and mass treatment (with ivermectin) are methods that have been practised in areas of high transmission.

Surveillance. Surveys for Calabar swellings or a history of them will indicate the area in which to take a blood-smear survey.

15.10 African Trypanosomiasis (Sleeping Sickness)

Organism. There are two forms of human sleeping sickness in Africa, that due to *Trypanosoma brucei gambiense* and that due to *T. b. rhodesiense*. A third form (nagana), caused by *T. b. brucei*, is found in cattle, and causes considerable economic loss. (See Fig. 15.15.)

The trypanosome exists in several different forms during its life cycle. When seen in human blood, the trypomastigotes are long and slender, short and stumpy, or intermediate between the two, probably representing a cycle of antigenic variation (Fig. 15.19). They are introduced into the blood by the bite of the tsetse fly and multiply locally. After being

disseminated round the body they continue to multiply, rapidly in *T. b. rhodesiense*, less so in *T. b. gambiense*. They are infective to any tsetse fly when it bites, being taken up into the midgut. They multiply, migrate into the space between the peritrophic membrane and the gut wall, and pass forward to the salivary glands. The epimastigote developmental form changes into a trypomastigote, to infect the next person that is bitten.

Clinical features. The bite of a tsetse fly generally causes a local reaction, but 7–10 days after this initial reaction has subsided the site becomes red and inflamed, the first sign of infection having become established. Trypanosomes multiply at the bite site and aspirated fluid will contain the dividing forms. In *T. b. gambiense*; an enlargement of the lymph glands also takes place, especially those in the cervical region. This rarely occurs in *T. b. rhodesiense*, the disease progressing rapidly to involve the central nervous system (CNS), with invariably a fatal outcome, often from cardiac failure. The main clinical signs are fever and protracted headaches. In *T. b. gambiense*, the course is much more prolonged and personality changes may be the indication of infection, but inevitably the disease leads to progressive lethargy, emaciation, coma and death.

Diagnosis is by finding trypomastigotes in the blood, CSF or gland puncture. The blood smear should be repeated several times before a negative diagnosis is made. Parasite concentration techniques, such as capillary tube centrifugation or mini-anion exchange centrifugation are valuable. Antibodies may be detected by serological techniques, while a circulating antigen assay using the card agglutination test (CATT) in which a drop of finger-prick blood is mixed with a suspension of trypanosomes has revolutionized diagnosis for *T. b. gambiense*. This technique is particularly useful for surveys in the field.

Transmission is from the bite of the tsetse fly, in which the parasite goes through a developmental stage. However, as the infective form for the fly and the human is the same (the trypomastigote), mechanical transfer can occasionally happen if a contaminated fly bites another person within a short space of time. The trypanasome can cross the placental barrier so infection of the fetus can occur.

The tsetse fly (*Glossina*) is easily recognized by its characteristic stance and behaviour. A large and

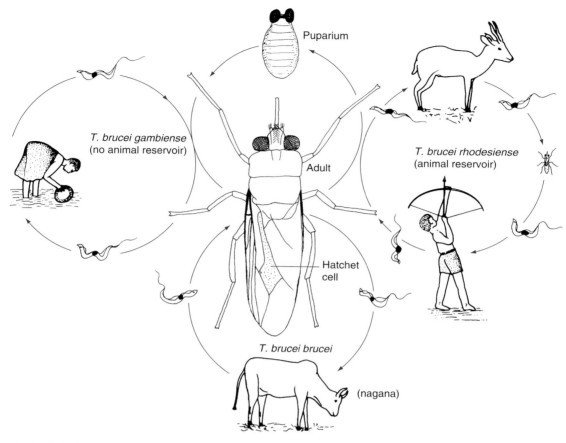

Fig. 15.15. African trypanosomiasis (caused by three subspecies of *Trypanosoma brucei*) life cycles and the tsetse fly.

powerful fly, it rests on a surface with wings folded like a pair of scissors. Within the venation of these wings a characteristic hatchet cell (Fig. 15.15) can be defined which helps in identification. However, when passing through 'fly' country, there is normally no doubt about its presence, as tsetse flies attack any moving object in large numbers, rendering the most painful bite. They are attracted by movement and will cling to the side of a vehicle travelling at 30–40 kph without being dislodged. They prefer dark colours and if there is a large object they will fly to that in preference. They are more abundant near their preferred breeding place in the sandy soil beside rivers.

The distribution of tsetse flies is shown in Fig. 15.16, in which it will be noticed that distinct species are often related to particular sleeping sickness areas (compare with Fig. 15.17). Table 15.5 is

a simplified guide to assist in identifying the species of *Glossina*, but professional confirmation should always be obtained.

Incubation period. 3 days to 3 weeks in *T. b. rhodesiense*, months to years for *T. b. gambiense*.

Period of communicability. The trypanosome takes 12–30 days to complete its developmental stage in the tsetse fly, depending on temperature, the fly then remaining infected for life. Humans can be infected for many years with *T. b. gambiense*, but due to the shorter life history with *T. b. rhodesiense*, the animal reservoir is probably more important.

Occurrence and distribution. Around half a million people live in sleeping sickness areas with

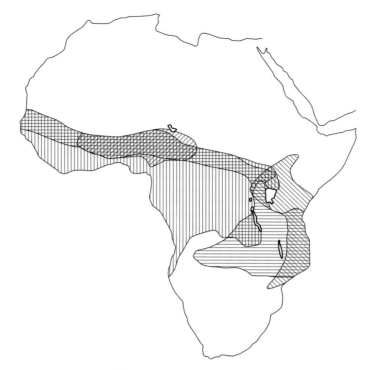

Fig. 15.16. Tsetse fly distribution in Africa. ▤, *Glossina morsitans*; ▧, *G. pallidipes*; ▥, *G. palpalis* and *G. fuscipes*; ▨, *G. tachinoides*.

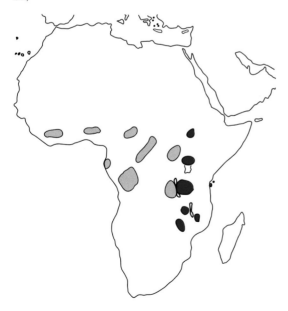

Fig 15.17. Sleeping sickness foci in Africa. Light blue, *Trypanosoma brucei gambiense*; dark blue, *T. b. rhodesiense*.

an estimated 100,000 new cases each year. *T. b. gambiense* mostly occurs to the west of the Central Rift Valley of Africa, containing the lakes of Tanganyika, Kivu, Edward and Albert, while *T. b. rhodesiense* is found mainly to the east (Fig. 15.17). *T. b. gambiense* infection is particularly prevalent in the Democratic Republic of the Congo (DRC), with over 70% of cases and *T. b. rhodesiense* in Tanzania and Uganda (where there might be overlap of the two types). These two diseases differ markedly in their epidemiology and control.

Gambian sleeping sickness. Sleeping sickness, as with other vector-borne diseases, is determined by the habits of the vector. In the gambiense type, the tsetse fly breeds in the tunnel of forest along the course of rivers (Fig 15.18). Although powerful flyers, they do not range far from this shaded protection, but travel extensively through this tunnel of forest in search of blood meals. Any mammals, including humans that come to the river to drink or cross it, are attacked and fed upon.

Humans are the main reservoir of *T. b. gambiense* infection (although the domestic pig may be

Table 15.5. A simplified key to *Glossina* of medical importance and their favoured habitats.

Hind tarsi	All segments dark above	*G. palpalis* group (1)
	Only 2 distal segments dark above	*G. morsitans* group (2)
	1. Abdomen obviously banded dorsally	*G. tachinoides*
	Abdomen dark, unbanded dorsally	*G. palpalis* (W. Africa)
		G. fuscipes (E. Africa)
	2. Distal 2 segments of front and middle tarsi *without* dark tips	*G. pallidipes*
	Last 2 segments of front and middle tarsi *with* dark tips	(3)
	3. Bands of abdomen very distinct and sharply rectangular	*G. swynnertoni*
	Bands on abdomen rounded medially and less distinct	*G. morsitans*
In summary, the vectors of *Trypanosoma brucei gambiense* are:		*G. palpalis*
		G. tachinoides
		G. morsitans
and those of *T. b. rhodesiense* are:		*G. morsitans*
		G. pallidipes
		G. fuscipes
		G. swynnertoni
		G. tachinoides (SW Ethiopia)
Favoured habitats are:	a. Lake and riverside fringing forest	*G. palpalis*
		G. tachinoides
		G. fuscipes (near Lake Victoria)
	b. Fringing forest without permanent water	*G. pallidipes*
	c. Miombo woodland, thickets and 'game' savannah woodland	*G. morsitans*
	d. Restricted to Northern Tanzania 'game' savannah woodland	*G. swynnertoni*

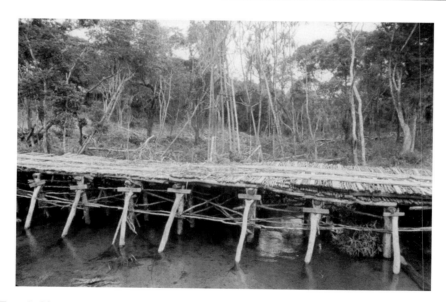

Fig. 15.18. Tunnel of forest along the banks of a river with selective clearance (leaving the big trees).

involved) and people whose jobs bring them into contact with the infected fly are more likely to succumb to infection. As women are involved in the collection of water, the preparation of food and the washing of clothes, they are more commonly infected in Gambian sleeping sickness.

The disease can occur in endemic and epidemic form. There are well-known foci from which people become infected at a constant rate (Fig 15.17), but movements of infected flies or, more commonly, people into new areas can initiate epidemics. Generally, infected flies are comparatively few in number, so that a large number of bites are required before a person becomes infected. Where the community that is fed upon is small and stable (less than 10 persons/km^2) then a few cases will only occur. When the community is much larger (above 10 persons/km^2), as when an infected person travels to a more densely populated area, then the infection can be transmitted to other people who, in turn, form a reservoir to infect more flies, and an increasing number of cases occurs. Epidemic sleeping sickness is more likely in *T. b. gambiense* infection as it is a more chronic disease and cases provide a reservoir (to infect flies) before symptoms cause them to seek medical attention. While endemic foci are difficult to eradicate, control measures should prevent epidemics from occurring.

In 1998, almost 40,000 cases of *T. b. gambiense* infection were reported although there were probably more like 300,000 cases. By 2005, after coordinated effort, the estimated number of cases had declined to 60,000 and by 2009 to 30,000.

Rhodesian sleeping sickness. The principal vector of *T. b. rhodesiense* is *G. morsitans*, which breeds along watercourses, but then travels widely throughout the extensive shade cover provided by the forest belt. This open type of forest, commonly called 'miombo' (mainly *Brachystegia* and *Julbernardia* spp.) is found in large areas of East Africa. Smaller wild animals inhabit it, especially the bushbuck, which forms a reservoir of infection. Towards the margins of this forest belt, the cover breaks up into thickets separated by savannah grassland in which large numbers of wild animals are found. The tsetse fly ranges widely over these areas, feeding mainly on animals and using the thickets for cover and shade. It is, therefore, humans that travel through the forest and fringing savannah in their occupational pursuits – the hunter and honey collector – that become infected. Adult males are then the main victims in Rhodesian sleeping sickness.

T. b. rhodesiense infection is not a focal disease, and because of its short clinical course, epidemics are uncommon. However, movements of people, such as the development of new settlements in forest areas, will expose a large number of people to infected flies all at the same time, so allowing an epidemic to start. The first signs that this is happening is where women, and especially children, become infected.

Although these are the main patterns for the two diseases, sometimes a riverine tsetse fly becomes the vector of Rhodesian sleeping sickness.

Sleeping sickness was far more widespread in former times, and in early history is thought to have extended as far as the Nile Valley. A major epidemic in Uganda between 1900 and 1920 claimed at least a quarter of a million lives and resulted in major resettlement and movement of the population. While there were probably many causes for this epidemic, it was preceded by several years of drought, followed by heavy rains, so that climate change might well have an impact on this disease in the future.

Control and prevention

Vector control. Knowledge of the habits and behaviour of the local vector is necessary before embarking on methods of vector control. The principal is to modify the environment so that it is unsuitable for the fly, but not to make so much damage that the water table is affected or soil erosion results. With the riverine type of habitat, areas of the forest tunnel are cleared, removing all the dense undergrowth but leaving the big trees with their extensive root systems to prevent erosion of the riverbank (Fig. 15.18). Clearance should be continued for half a kilometre on either side of a river crossing, water collection place or inhabited area.

In East Africa, where extensive forest provides a habitat for the fly, the forest margin is pushed back from any place of habitation. A band of at least 1 km, preferably 2 km, should be left between the area of habitation and the forest. This must also include any cultivated area, and regulations are required to prevent people from moving into the cleared part to start new cultivation. Ring barking is a more economical method of forest clearance than cutting down every tree.

Where forest clearance is impractical then insecticides can be used. This is easiest along the course of substantial rivers using a boat, spraying the forest on either side. In the savannah-type habitat, isolated thickets can be treated. Extensive insecticidal application to miombo forest is inappropriate. Insecticide applications have to be repeated, whereas forest clearance is permanent and the relative costs of these two techniques needs to be considered.

Trapping can also control the vector. A well-designed trap will collect enough flies to considerably reduce the biting risk. An effective trap has a fine metal mesh treated with insecticides, which is shaded to attract tsetse flies. These are rapidly killed when they touch the screen, but this must be cleaned regularly to work efficiently.

The fly can bite through thin clothing, so taking preventive action from being bitten in a tropical climate is difficult.

Alteration of the human habitat. Sleeping sickness has been responsible for large movements of people from their traditional homelands either by self-choice or by government action to avoid an epidemic. Moving people away from the sleeping sickness areas is the ultimate method of control, but one to be taken only when all else fails.

The preferable alternative to moving populations is to modify the habitat so that it is unsuitable for disease transmission. Methods of forest clearance have already been described, while providing water supplies will remove the reliance on obtaining water from rivers.

The density of population largely determines the endemicity, as mentioned above. Two different approaches can be taken:

- Keep the population close together and clear an area of forest around them.
- Encourage the people to spread out very widely so that they partially clear a large area of forest.

In the first method, the people are safe as long as they remain within the village, but once they pass through the forest they are subjected to a considerable number of bites. In the second alternative, people will become infected in the initial stages of forest clearance, but once this has been done then protection will be much greater and more use can be made of the land. In the initial period of forest clearance, a surveillance service will be required to find the pioneer cases. The most unsatisfactory solution is a moderately large population spread evenly over the area, as this is the potential situation for an epidemic.

Parasite reduction. A surveillance service should be set up and all cases treated (see below). Finding cases in the early stages of the disease not only increases the chance of successful treatment, but also removes a potential source of infection to tsetse flies.

Another approach to reducing the parasite reservoir in *T. b. rhodesiense* is to destroy the animal population. This used to be practised on a wide scale, but animal conservation has now questioned the wanton slaughter of animals. In most cases, it will be found that the human reservoir is more important than the animal reservoir, but where there is evidence that flies are becoming infected from this alternative source then game can be killed or driven off.

Treatment of cases requires hospitalization as the drugs used are highly toxic.

- First-line treatment (when the trypanasome has not crossed the blood–brain barrier) is with pentamidine for *T. b. gambiense* and suramin for *T. b. rhodesiense*.
- When the CNS is involved, then melarsoprol can be used for both, but is toxic, while eflornithine is very effective against all stages of *T. b. gambiense*.
- A combination of nifurtimox and eflornithine can also be used against *T. b. gambiense* but not against *T. b. rhodesiense*.

Pentamidine has been used as a prophylactic against *T. b. gambiense* infection in people at special risk. There is no prophylactic against *T. b. rhodesiense* infection.

Surveillance. A surveillance service should be set up in a sleeping sickness area. Sleeping sickness workers are recruited more on their knowledge of the local community than on their medical skills, as the simple techniques of gland puncture or making a blood slide can easily be taught. The workers cover a set area and take slides from people with symptoms of persistent fever and headache, or those who pursue a particular occupation, such as hunters, honey collectors or woodcutters. In *T. b. gambiense* infection, palpation of the neck glands can provide a useful estimate of prevalence. In an epidemic of *T. b. rhodesiense*, a mass blood slide examination can be performed in the worst affected areas to detect asymptomatic cases.

The illness in animals is more extensive than in the human population and veterinary services often set up extensive surveillance and control programmes, so combining efforts with them can be of value.

15.11 American Trypanosomiasis (Chagas' Disease)

Organism. *Trypanosoma cruzi.* The trypanosome in American trypanosomiasis undergoes a development cycle both in the vector bug and the vertebrate host, with trypomastigotes, the infective form, and pseudocysts forming in the muscle. The pseudocysts contain amastigotes, which grow a flagellum and become promastigotes and epimastigotes (Fig. 15.19) when the pseudocyst ruptures, finally developing into infective trypomastigotes (Fig. 15.20). The trypomastigote of the American disease has a larger kinetoplast and is more curved than that of the African one. The infection differs in that repeat cycles take place in the host's muscles, producing a chronic disease state.

Clinical features. American trypanosomiasis presents as an acute infection, generally in children, with fever, local swelling at the site of inoculation and enlargement of the regional lymph nodes. Muscular tissues are attacked, so that in adult life chronic conditions

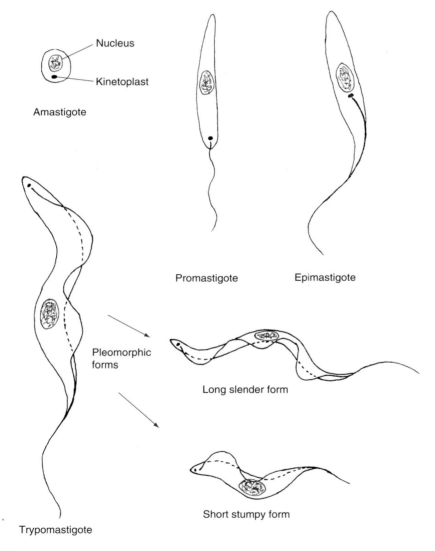

Fig. 15.19. Different forms of trypanosomes.

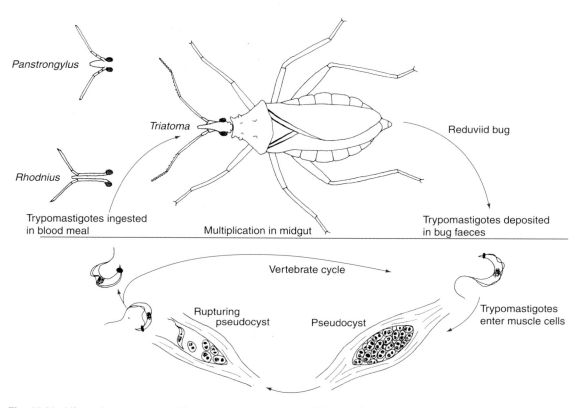

Fig. 15.20. Life cycle and vectors of American trypanosomiasis (Chagas' disease).

such as enlargement of the heart, oesophagus or colon develop. Heart failure and cardiac irregularities are common manifestations that lead in time to disability and an early death. The HIV-infected person can also develop acute myocarditis or meningoencephalitis. Oesophageal cancer can occur in a small proportion of patients with megaoesophagus. Congenital Chagas' disease results in small-sized infants with CNS and cardiac involvement.

Diagnosis is by finding the organism in the blood in the acute stage. Methods of concentrating the erythrocytes or xenodiagnosis (feeding of laboratory-reared clean bugs on the patient) are often required. In the chronic case, serological tests may be positive.

Transmission is by Reduviidae bugs, differing from area to area according to the species of reduviid and the reservoirs of infection. The main genera of bugs are *Triatoma*, *Rodnius* and *Panstrongylus*, which can be differentiated from each other by their antennae and mouthparts (Fig. 15.20). Essentially

there are two cycles, a wild and a domestic, which are illustrated in Fig. 15.21.

In the wild cycle, armadillos, opossums, raccoons and a number of other animals have been found to be infected, living in close proximity to the burrow-inhabiting bugs. This infection remains as a zoonosis until disturbed by a domestic animal, commonly a dog ferreting around the burrows of these wild animals. They are attacked by the bugs and acquire the infection. On returning to the house, the dog becomes a reservoir for the domestic bugs, which transmit the infection to any humans living or staying in the house.

In Central America, the cycle is semi-domestic with the reservoir maintained in the domestic rat (*Rattus rattus*) from which house-haunting bugs pass on the infection to people in the house. Although the bugs feed on people, it is the passage of trypanosomes in the bug faeces, which are rubbed into the wound or conjunctiva that produces the infection.

The bugs live in cracks in the walls and floors and within thatch in the roof. The mud and wattle type of structure is particularly suited to the conditions

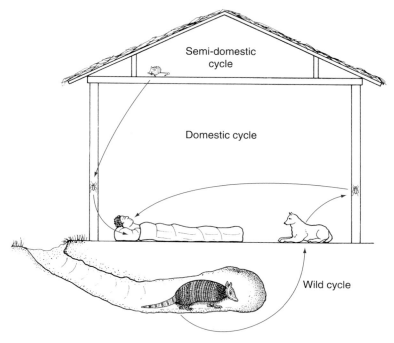

Fig. 15.21. Transmission cycles of American trypanosomiasis.

required. The number of bugs hiding within the cracks and crevices can be several hundreds.

Infection can also be transmitted by blood transfusion, and small epidemics in a group of people sharing the same food suggests that contamination of food by bug faeces could lead to transmission by the oral route.

The infected mother can pass infection on to her newborn either during pregnancy or childbirth. Organ transplants and laboratory accidents are rarer methods of transmission.

Incubation period. 5–14 days.

Period of communicability. Bugs become infected after 8–10 days and remain so for life, which lasts about 2 years. Infected persons have circulating trypanosomes in the acute and early chronic stages of the disease, but these may persist in small numbers for the life of the individual.

Occurrence and distribution. Chagas' disease is found throughout Central America and most countries of South America, with a prevalence of 13 million, annual incidence of 200,000 and deaths 13,000. Due to population movements, cases are now found in the USA, Canada, Europe and Western Pacific countries. Considerable progress has been made in controlling the disease, with Uruguay, Chile, Brazil and Argentina being declared free of infection and good progress being made in Bolivia and Paraguay.

Control and prevention. The methods of control are to reduce the number of bugs that come into close proximity with humans and remove the reservoirs of disease. These requirements are both satisfied by improvements to housing. Unfortunately, trypanosomiasis is a disease of poverty and building new and better houses is rather impractical in this segment of the population. If assistance can be given, then proper foundations and cement walls will not only deny a place for the bugs to live, but also prevent rats and armadillos from making their burrows underneath them. Even with existing houses, much can be done by applying a layer of mud plaster to the walls and erecting a simple ceiling. Where cost prohibits any of these methods, then residual insecticides can be sprayed on to the walls and ceilings. This can effectively be carried out as a control programme, using a similar methodology to that for malaria.

First, a pyrethrum spray is administered which draws the bugs out of their hiding places and marks the infected houses. In the attack phase, a residual insecticide is sprayed on all houses in an infected locality (not just applied to infested houses). A second spraying is made 90 days after the first to houses where bugs have been found either in the preliminary or attack phases. Spraying continues at this time interval until the number of infested houses falls below 5%. Maintenance is achieved by regular house searches and by instituting focal spraying when reinfestation is discovered.

The use of pyrethroid fumigant cans which release insecticide when lit, and of insecticidal paints, are simpler methods than residual spraying. An alternative is to protect the individual from being bitten by the use of insecticide-treated mosquito nets (see Box 3.1).

The dog is probably the most important domestic reservoir of the disease and householders should question the value of maintaining such animals if they are proving a threat to the health of the family. Good hygiene, trapping and poison will keep down rats (see Box 16.1). Control of the wild reservoir is unlikely to be successful.

In areas of high endemicity, screening of blood donors is required and gentian violet (a trypanosomicidal agent) can be added to the blood. Pregnant women should be questioned about possible infection and tested where necessary.

Treatment. Nifurtimox and benznidazole are effective in the acute and early chronic phase of the disease.

Surveillance. Regular monitoring of houses for signs of infestation or reinfestation should be maintained (see above).

15.12. Leishmaniasis

Organism. There are seven species of *Leishmania* and a number of subspecies:

Visceral leishmaniasis	*L. donovani* (*donovani*)
	L. infantum (*infantum, chagasi*)
Mucocutaneous	*L. braziliensis* (*braziliensis, peruviana, guyanensis, panamensis*)
New World cutaneous	*L. mexicana* (*mexicana, amazonensis, pifanoi, garnhami, venezuelensis*)
Old World cutaneous	*L. major*
	L. tropica (*tropica, killicki*)
	L. aethiopica

The parasites are all transmitted by the bite of the sandfly and undergo the same simple life cycle. Promastigotes enter humans with the bite of the sandfly, change into amastigotes (Fig. 15.19), and are engulfed by macrophages. They multiply and finally rupture the cell, invading other macrophages. When the sandfly takes a blood meal, the amastigotes change into promastigotes. These multiply continuously so that the number produced can be so large as to block the foregut of the sandfly. When the insect next bites, it is forced to regurgitate promastigotes into the host before it can take a blood meal (Fig. 15.22).

In cutaneous leishmaniasis, the amastigotes remain at the site of introduction, contained by the macrophages of the skin. In visceral leishmaniasis, large mononuclear cells and polymorphonuclear leucocytes become invaded and subsequently carry the parasites to the viscera, especially the liver, spleen and bone marrow. The mucocutaneous form is intermediate, the parasite restricting its attack to the reticuloendothelial system of the mucus membranes of the mouth, nose and throat.

Clinical features. There are four main clinical forms of the disease, cutaneous, mucocutaneous, visceral (kala-azar) and post-kala-azar dermal leishmaniasis. The cutaneous infection starts with a papule and enlarges to become an indolent ulcer, which either heals or persists for many years. In the New World infections, a more aggressive form of mucocutaneous leishmaniasis (espundia, Chiclero ulcer) results in nasopharyngeal destruction and hideous deformities. The visceral form is a chronic infection with fever, progressive weakness, hepatosplenomegaly, lymphadenopathy and anaemia. There is progressive emaciation and weakness, with generally a fatal outcome if not treated. Post-kala-azar dermal leishmaniasis produces nodular lesions and can occur after apparent cure of the visceral case. It is due to host response rather than to the parasite.

As in leprosy, host response largely determines the outcome of the disease and in any condition in which this is minimized a more florid disease results. Cutaneous leishmaniasis is normally a self-limiting condition, but in some individuals diffuse cutaneous leishmaniasis, in which metastatic lesions are disseminated around the body, can occur. The resulting nodular lesions resemble those of lepromatous leprosy and respond poorly to treatment. So any condition that compromises the host

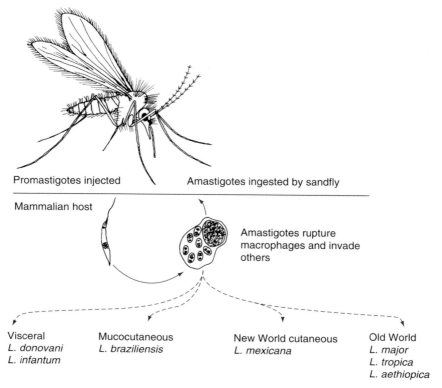

Promastigotes injected   Amastigotes ingested by sandfly

Mammalian host

Amastigotes rupture
macrophages and invade
others

Visceral	Mucocutaneous	New World cutaneous	Old World
L. donovani	*L. braziliensis*	*L. mexicana*	*L. major*
L. infantum			*L. tropica*
			L. aethiopica

Fig. 15.22. *Leishmania* vector, parasite and life cycle.

response, such as HIV infection, may lead to reactivation of latent disease or cutaneous disease progressing to visceral illness. Leishmaniasis, like tuberculosis (TB), is intertwined with HIV infection, so that in areas where leishmaniasis is found both conditions have a more serious outcome.

Diagnosis is by the detection of the intracellular Leishman–Donovan bodies in infected macrophages in the liver, spleen and bone marrow, or in cutaneous lesions, by stained smear or culture. PCR techniques can also be used. A dipstick method, K39, can be used for serological diagnosis and will be particularly valuable for field surveys.

Transmission is by the minute and fragile phlebotomine sandflies *Phlebotomus* and *Lutzomyia*. They are weak fliers, utilizing a hopping flight that only carries them a short distance from their habitat. This requires conditions of high humidity, as found in animal burrows and moist tropical forests. Typical habitats are tree holes, new or old animal burrows,

termite hills, rock crevices, foliage clumps and fissures that develop in the ground during the dry season.

The life cycle, from oviposition to emergence of the adult sandfly, can take 30–100 days depending on species and temperature, while the adult lives for approximately 2 weeks. Only the female sucks blood, and lizards, birds and mammals are satisfactory alternative food sources to humans.

Most species of sandfly feed out of doors during the evening and night, but will do so in the day when there is shade, or the weather is overcast. If it is windy they are unable to fly. They are not able to bite through clothing and mainly attack the lower parts of the body. The main vectors are summarized in Table 15.6.

A range of reservoirs are found in this complex of diseases. In Central Asia, cutaneous leishmaniasis is a zoonosis, the gerbil being the main reservoir. In India, there is a domestic reservoir, mainly of dogs, but direct human-to-human transmission also occurs. The vectors and reservoirs involved are summarized in Table 15.6.

Table 15.6. The vectors and reservoirs of leishmaniasis.

Type and parasite (*Leishmania* species)	Geographical area	Main vector (*Phlebotamus* or *Lutzomyia* species)	Reservoir
Visceral			
L. donovani	Mediterranean, SW Asia	P. peniciosus, P. ariasi, P. major syriacus, P. longicuspis	Dogs, foxes
	Central Asia	P. major syriacus, P. smirnovi, P. longiductus	Dogs, jackals, foxes
	China	P. chinensis	Dogs
	India, Bangladesh	P. argentipes, P. papatasi	Humans
	Sudan, Chad	P. orientalis, P. martini	Wild rodents and carnivores
	Kenya	P. martini	Dogs
	Central and South America	L. longipalpis	Dogs, foxes
L. infantum	Mediterranean	P. peniciosus	Dogs, foxes
Mucocutaneous			
L. braziliensis	Central and South America	L. wellcomi, L. umbratilis, L.trapidoi	Rodents and forest animals
Cutaneous (New World)			
L. mexicana	Mexico, Belize, Guatemala	L. olmeca	Forest rodents
	Amazon Basin	L. flaviscutellata	Forest rodents
	Peru	L. peruensis, L. verrucarum	Dogs
Cutaneous (Old World)			
L. major	Mediterranean	P. papatasi	Rodents, dogs, gerbils
	SW Asia	P. papatasi, P. sergenti	Dogs, rodents
L. tropica	Central Asia	P. papatasi	Rodents, gerbils
	India	P. sergenti	Dogs
	West Africa	P. duboscqi	Dogs, rodents
L. aethiopica	Ethiopia	P. longpipes	Hyraxes
	Kenya	P. pedifer	Rodents

Transmission can also take place directly through needles and other instruments contaminated with blood of an infected person. Sadly, this is also the method by which HIV is transmitted in many developing countries.

Incubation period. 2 weeks to 6 months, but can be years.

Period of communicability. The untreated case can remain infectious to sandflies for up to 2 years.

Occurrence and distribution. Leishmaniasis is found in Central/South America, Africa, the Mediterranean, South-west, Central and South Asia, and part of China, as shown in Fig. 15.23 and Table 15.6. Some 90% of all visceral cases are found in Bangladesh, Brazil, India, Nepal and Sudan; the majority of mucocutaneous cases are in Brazil, Bolivia and Peru; and 90% of cutaneous cases are in Afghanistan, Brazil, Iran, Peru, Saudi Arabia and Syria.

Population movements, both of persons from endemic rural areas into towns and during large man-made projects such as dams in endemic foci, have brought an increasing number of people into contact with leishmaniasis. Several large-scale development projects have been seriously hampered by epidemics of the diseases. Also, the spread of HIV infection has made what was largely a curable condition into a persistent source of parasites for the vector sandfly and a resulting more serious disease. It is estimated that 12 million people are infected worldwide, with 2 million new cases occurring annually.

Immunity develops following infection with the parasite, but there is little cross immunity. *L. tropica* has been used for a long time as an inoculum to induce a sore on a hidden part of the body so as to prevent a more disfiguring lesion developing on the face. *L. major* will protect against *L. tropica* as well as *L. major* lesions, and suspensions of living organisms have been prepared for this purpose. There is no cross immunity with kala-azar and the

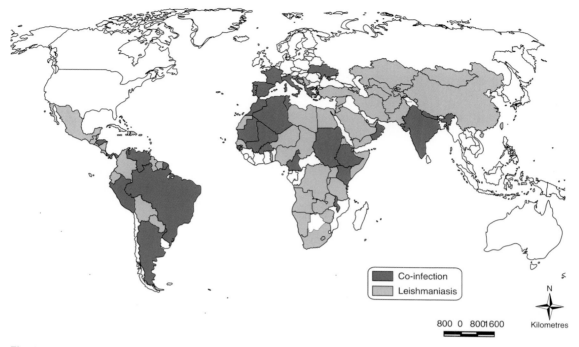

Fig. 15.23. The worldwide distribution of leishmaniasis and countries reporting *Leishmania*/HIV co-infection, 2000. (Reproduced by permission of the World Health Organization, Geneva.)

other species of *Leishmania*, but an attack of kala-azar will protect against developing kala-azar in any other part of the world.

Control and prevention. Cases of the disease are normally sporadic so should be treated to prevent flies from becoming infected. Early diagnosis via an adequate health infrastructure is an essential part of control, as well as reducing the morbidity and mortality of the disease.

Repellents and personal protection adequately protect the individual from being bitten. Sandfly nets can be used, but a more effective solution is ITNs or LLINs (see Box 3.1). Insecticide-treated sheeting in refugee shelters was found particularly useful in an epidemic in Afghanistan. The use of residual insecticides has been effective in areas where leishmaniasis overlaps with malaria, but owing to insecticide resistance and the replacement of this strategy by the use of insecticide-treated materials it is not justified to use this method except under epidemic conditions.

Because of the fragile nature of the vector, it is easily attacked with insecticides either as a residual house spray if the vector comes indoors, or by insecticide powder blown into mammal burrows,

ant hills and similar microhabitats. A longer term solution is to alter the micro-environment such as by the destruction of termite hills and killing of rodents. Proper control of domestic animals, especially dogs, can be effective where they are important reservoirs. The use of deltamethrin-treated collars has been found to be effective. A vaccine for use in dogs would be valuable.

Low-dose inocula and attenuated vaccines have been developed to minimize the severity of disease in some endemic areas. The concomitant problem of HIV infection has added to the seriousness of dual infection, so a simultaneous programme of sexually transmitted infection (STI) control is required with information produced on how to avoid both diseases.

Due to the lack of an animal reservoir in India, the availability of new diagnostic tests (the K39 dipstick) and effective treatment (with miltefosine) there is a real possibility of eliminating visceral leishmaniasis from the subcontinent based on the following strategy:

- early diagnosis and complete treatment of cases;
- integrated vector management;

- effective disease surveillance through passive and active case detection;
- social mobilization and partnership building at all levels; and
- clinical and operational research, as required.

Treatment has been with sodium stibogluconate or meglumine antimonate, but pentamidine or liposomal amphotericin B may be required in cases that do not respond, especially in mucocutaneous leishmaniasis. Because of the toxicity of the preparations treatment should be undertaken in hospital. Miltefosine has shown considerable promise in the treatment of visceral leishmaniasis, with high cure rates and in those cases resistant to antimony therapy. Its other advantage is that it can be administered orally, but it should not be given to pregnant women because of its teratogenicity. Miltefosine may be particularly valuable in the treatment of leishmania patients who also have HIV.

Paromomycin has been shown to be a safe and effective drug, possibly best given in combination with sodium stibogluconate, as the development of resistance to single-treatment regimes has a high probability. Other dual therapies are liposomal amphotericin B and miltefosine.

A unique way of treating cutaneous leishmaniasis is with methyl-aminolevulinic acid applied to the skin with phototherapy; this is under trial.

Surveillance. Outbreaks should be reported to neighbouring countries so that they can take control measures in border areas. Patients with HIV infection should be examined for reactivated leishmaniasis.

Summary

- Vectors are a more specific way of carrying the infective organism direct to the host.
- The most important flying vector is the mosquito, but *Simulium*, tsetse flies, sandflies and the reduviid bugs transmit other serious infections.
- The dynamics of the vector need to be understood in defining the parameters of the infection and how to control it.
- Control is aimed at reducing the vector numbers, the biting rate and length of life to below a level where the parasite is unable to develop or is of a sufficiently small number to be unable to propagate the infection.

- Insecticide-treated nets are the main method of control, with residual spraying, larviciding, environmental modification and MDA also being used.

Further Reading

Duffy, P.E. and Fried, M. (2001) *Malaria in Pregnancy: Deadly Parasite, Susceptible Host.* Taylor & Francis, London/Informa Healthcare, New York.

Githeko, A.K., Lindsay, S.W., Confalonieri, U.E. and Patz, J.A. (2000) Climate change and vector-borne diseases: a regional analysis. *Bulletin of the World Health Organization* 78, 1136–1147. Available at: www.who.int/bulletin/archives/78(9)1136.pdf (accessed 22 February 2012).

Halstead, S. (2009) *Dengue* (Tropical Medicine: Science and Practice). World Scientific Publishing, Singapore/Hackensack, New Jersey/London.

Malaria Consortium (2007) *Malaria: A Handbook for Health Professionals.* Macmillan, Basingstoke, UK.

Maudlin, I., Holmes, P.H. and Miles, M.A. (eds) (2004) *The Trypanosomiases.* CAB International, Wallingford, UK.

Reithinger, R., Kamya, R.M., Whitty, J.M., Dorsey, G. and Vermund, S.H. (2009) Interaction of malaria and HIV. *British Medical Journal* 338, elocator b2141, 1400–1401.

Service, M.W. (ed.) (2001) *The Encyclopedia of Arthropod-transmitted Infections of Man and Domesticated Animals.* CAB International, Wallingford, UK.

Service, M.W. (2008) *Medical Entomology for Students,* 4th edn. Cambridge University Press, Cambridge, UK.

Warrell, D. and Gilles, H.M. (2002) *Essential Malariology,* 4th edn. Hodder Arnold, London.

World Health Organization (1992) *Lymphatic Filariasis: The Disease and its Control. Fifth Report of the WHO Expert Committee on Filariasis.* Technical Report Series, No. 821, WHO, Geneva.

World Health Organization (1995) *Onchocerciasis and its Control. Report of a WHO Expert Committee on Onchocerciasis Control.* Technical Report Series, No. 852. WHO, Geneva.

World Health Organization (2000) *Expert Committee on Malaria, 20th Report.* Technical Report Series, No. 892. WHO, Geneva.

World Health Organization (2000) *Management of Severe Malaria: A Practical Handbook,* 2nd edn. WHO, Geneva.

World Health Organization (2006) *Pesticides and Their Application: For the Control of Vectors and Pests of Public Health Importance,* 6th edn. Publication No. WHO/CDS/NTD/WHOPES/GCDPP/2006.1, Geneva.

World Health Organization (2007) *Long-lasting Insecticidal Nets for Malaria Prevention,* 3rd edn. WHO, Geneva.

World Health Organization (2010) *Guidelines for the Treatment of Malaria,* 2nd edn. WHO, Geneva.

16 Ectoparasite Zoonoses

Ectoparasites are non-flying vectors of disease, such as fleas, lice and ticks. They are responsible for an important group of zoonotic infections (those that are naturally transmitted between vertebrate animals and humans), which are often associated with animals in which the reservoir of infection is found. Because of the close interrelationship between the ectoparasite and the animals on which it feeds, focal zoonoses (synanthropic or exoanthropic zoonoses; see Section 1.3.5) result. Humans are often the accidental victims of these zoonotic infections, so knowledge of their biology and how to avoid these foci can often be all that is needed to prevent being infected. At other times, specific methods against the ectoparasite, the animal, or both, are required.

16.1 Plague

Organism. *Yersinia pestis*, the fragile organism that causes plague is a small oval-shaped bacillus (coccobacillus) that stains negative with Gram stain. With Giemsa or Wayson, the organism has a characteristic bipolar staining. It is sensitive to heat above 55°C, 0.5% phenol for 15 min and exposure to sunlight.

Clinical features. The disease in humans, which develops after the bite of an infected flea, is called bubonic plague, after the bubo or swelling that develops at the regional lymph nodes draining the site of inoculation. This is commonest in the groin and second most common in the axilla, but it can also occur in the cervical lymph nodes. This latter site is more likely in the case of sylvatic plague as infection can result from ingesting the organism when eating the reservoir rodent. (Some people eat rodents as a normal item in the diet, while in famine conditions others may be driven to eat whatever they can find, including rats.)

The bubo is painful and tender, becomes fluctuant and often breaks down to discharge pus. There is an associated high fever, confusion, irritability and signs of haemorrhage may develop. These may be subcutaneous, into the stomach or intestines, leading to prostration and shock, with death soon after.

In a few cases, with septicaemic plague, the disease may be overwhelming from the start. All the signs are more severe and develop so rapidly that a bubo is not formed and the patient is dead within a few days. In the generalized spread of the organism around the body it can invade the lungs and should a case of bubonic or septicaemic plague start coughing out bacteria, then transmission can occur via the respiratory route. This leads to pneumonic plague, where spread is from person to person and the flea is not involved; it is highly infectious and lethal, so stringent protective action must be taken. About 5% of bubonic patients develop terminal pneumonia and transmit infection via the respiratory route. The onset of pneumonic plague is very quick, with shallow, rapid breathing, watery blood stained sputum, high temperature, pulmonary oedema and shock. Death occurs between the third and fifth day.

Meningeal plague can also occur, generally owing to inadequate antibiotic treatment, and this is associated with axillary buboes. A mild form of the disease with swollen glands and slight rise in temperature can occur as pestis minor, but many of these cases go undiagnosed and tend to occur towards the latter part of an epidemic. During an epidemic, routine throat swabs may detect *Y. pestis*, but there is no good evidence that transmission can occur from these cases.

Diagnosis and case definition. Fresh aspirate from a bubo, blood or sputum will contain organisms that stain negative with Gram but show bipolar staining with Giemsa or Wayson. Culture on to blood agar or desoxycholate can be made from blood, throat swabs, sputa and material aspirated from buboes. Detection of the F1 antigen by fluorescence assay, ELISA, serological detection of anti-F1 antibody (also by ELISA) and agglutination testing or immunoblot are specific immunological tests. Conversion of the anti-F1 IgG titre in paired serum samples is the best confirmatory method. Asymptomatic cases of plague are common during epidemics and can be detected near foci by the passive haemagglutination test (PHA).

The (modified) World Health Organization (WHO) case definition for a confirmed case is:

- Meets the definition for a suspect case (clinical presentation and history of exposure to infected animals or humans or flea bite, or contact with a known focus within the last 10 days);

plus

- Microscopy of material from bubo, blood or sputum contains Gram-negative bipolar coccobacilli with Wayson or Giemsa staining *and* two of the following four tests must be positive: phage lysis of cultures at 20–25°C and 37°C; F1 antigen detection; PCR detection of *Y. pestis*; *Y. pestis* biochemical profile;

or

- A fourfold rise in anti-F1 antibody titre in paired serum samples;

or

- A positive rapid diagnostic test using immunochromatography to detect F1 antigen (in epidemic areas when no other confirmatory test can be performed).

Transmission. Figure 16.1 illustrates the different transmission cycles of plague, the trio of bacillus, rodent and flea, into which humans can be fatally drawn. In the established focus of wild rodent plague, infection is maintained in a comparatively resistant colony of animals, which suffer little from the disease. If a person strays into this focus as a hunter or trapper, then fleas from a wild rodent they have killed may bite them and cause plague. This is sylvatic plague, and is generally an isolated case with little epidemiological significance.

The more important event is when some change takes place in the wild rodent focus and domestic rodents become involved. Wars of nature are similar to wars of man and a replacement of one group of plague-resistant rodents by another of no resistance could cause a change in the ecological balance. Or from the opposite approach, an increase in the domestic rodent population may expand into the wild rodent one. Whichever of these alternative mechanisms takes place, the deprived flea seeks a new host and settles on a domestic rodent. The domestic rodent, being highly susceptible to plague, is rapidly killed, which makes the flea of the domestic rodent search for a new host, and because of his proximity, man is likely to become the next victim.

In Africa, the multimammate rat (*Mastomys natalensis*) acts as an intermediary between the feral rodent reservoir and the domestic rat, feeding on the remnants of the harvest. However, when the rains come it is driven to look for alternative stores of food and enters the home, bringing it into contact with the occupants. This brings a seasonal pattern of plague. If there is a drought, the situation is even more serious, because there is no food for the desperate multimammate rat, so it is forced early into conflict with the domestic rat and an epidemic occurs in the dry season as well.

A focus of plague is determined by three factors: the organism, the reservoir host and the flea vector. Many fleas have been incriminated as possible vectors, but species of *Xenopsylla* are the most important (*X. cheopis*, *X. brasiliensis* and *X. astia*). An identifying characteristic of fleas is that they can either have a comb on the top of the head, or they are combless. *Xenopsylla* is combless, differentiating it from *Ctenocephalides*, which is the common dog and cat flea. The common human flea, *Pulex*, is also a combless flea, but lacks the other distinguishing feature of *Xenopsylla* – the presence of a meral rod (these important features are illustrated in Fig. 16.1).

Fleas are able to survive for considerable periods (6 months) without taking a blood meal, and the larval and pupal stages are well adapted to changing fortune. If there is a limited food supply or a low temperature then the larva may prolong this stage from 2 weeks to more than 200 days and the pupae remain cocooned. When vibrations in the habitat, or the emission of carbon dioxide, or a rise in humidity, indicate that an inhabitant has returned, the larva rapidly develops and the emergent flea feeds on the new host. Fleas are not specific, but prefer their normal host species, and fertility may be reduced if they cannot feed on this host. They rapidly abandon a dead host and use

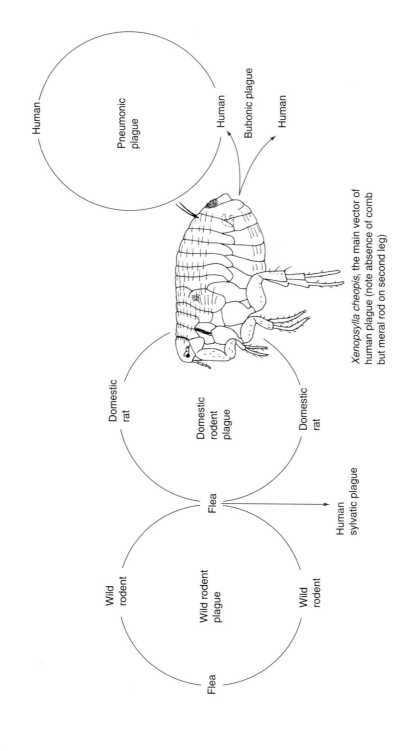

Human

Pneumonic plague

Human

Bubonic plague

Human

Xenopsylla cheopis, the main vector of human plague (note absence of comb but meral rod on second leg)

Domestic rat

Domestic rodent plague

Domestic rat

Flea

Human sylvatic plague

Wild rodent

Wild rodent plague

Wild rodent

Flea

Fig. 16.1. Plague vector and life cycles.

their powerful hind legs to help them hop on to a new one. Once re-established they tend to crawl around and settle to a regular feeding pattern. If fleas take in *Y. pestis* with their blood meal, these bacteria multiply in the proventriculus and lead to a blockage of the feeding apparatus. When the flea tries to feed again it regurgitates bacteria into the bloodstream while trying to take up blood. It is unsuccessful, so moves to a new host and tries again. Blocked fleas are therefore important in rapidly infecting many people.

Over 340 species of mammals have been found to be susceptible to plague, including rabbits, monkeys, dogs, cats and camels, but the main reservoir is in rodents, particularly rats. They differ in their susceptibility, so that a focus will die out where there is a highly susceptible colony, but persist where resistance is high. While it is the resistant rodents that maintain a focus, it is the movement of susceptible animals which is responsible for extending plague. Where the speed of mortality is high and the pool of susceptible animals limited, then the exacerbation will collapse and the focus return to its original boundary, but when a coincidence of susceptible rodents abuts on to domestic rodents,

then the stage is set for an epidemic in the human population. Foci of infection have been delineated (Fig. 16.2), some of which have given rise to plague outbreaks, while others have all the potential, but human disease has not occurred.

Pneumonic plague is transmitted by droplets of <5 μm so the organism is not aerosolized nor remains in the air. Face-to-face exposure is normally required when the patient coughs within 2 m of another person.

Incubation period. 2–6 days.

Period of communicability. An unblocked infected flea can remain alive for several months, able to transmit infection. Pneumonic plague is highly infectious and can spread rapidly within a concentration of people, although infected individuals will remain alive for only a few days.

Occurrence and distribution. Plague is a classic example of an ectoparasite zoonosis. The greatest of all epidemic diseases, it has ravaged the Orient, Asia and Europe, altering the course of history. The first recorded epidemic was in China in 224 BC.

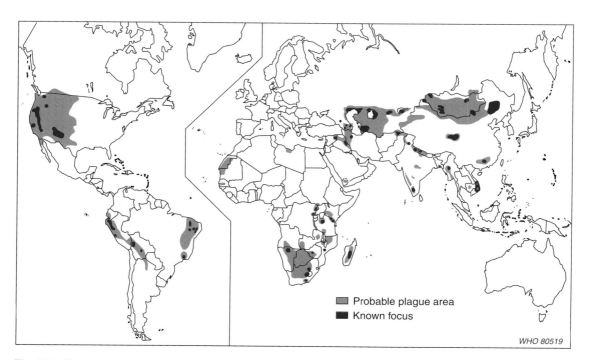

Probable plague area
Known focus

WHO 80519

Fig. 16.2. Known and probable foci of plague. (Reproduced by permission of the World Health Organization, Geneva.)

Today, the disease is confined to established foci (Fig. 16.2), from which it erupts from time to time but, fortunately, effective control now prevents the uncontrollable pandemics of the past.

Plague is a disease of civil disturbance and war. In recent history, the largest human outbreak has been in Vietnam. Most cases now come from Africa, with Madagascar and the Democratic Republic of Congo (DRC) accounting for 96% of the world cases since 1990. Other countries in Africa with persistent foci are Mozambique, Uganda and Tanzania. In 2003, there was a plague outbreak in two villages in Algeria. In the large focus in Central Asia sporadic cases are reported from Kazakhstan, Mongolia and north and west China, while the persistent focus in southern China has also produced an increase in cases. Outbreaks have occurred in the Andean focus in South America, particularly in Peru and Ecuador.

Control and prevention. The methods of control depend upon the transmission cycle involved (Fig. 16.1).

Wild rodent plague foci are often extensive and harmless, and to try and destroy them is a considerable task. If they are localized and close to habitation then it might be feasible to alter the environment by cultivation or in a way that discourages rodents, but precautions need to be taken so that a plague epidemic is not generated by such activity. Where hunters or soldiers have to pass through a plague focus then personal protection can be obtained from long trousers tucked into socks, treated with repellents or insecticides. Warnings should be given about the danger of touching or eating any animals killed.

Domestic rodent plague depends upon the two components of the rat and the flea, but the order in which they are attacked is crucial according to the stage of the disease. To kill rats during a plague epidemic only makes the infected fleas search for a human host and so increases spread. In the presence of plague, the fleas must be controlled first using insecticide powder (permethrin, bendiocarb or fenitrothione). Using a blower, burrows can be insufflated and rat runs liberally dusted. Rats pick up insecticide on their fur and take it into their nests with them. Fleas do not like cleanliness and people should be encouraged to wash with soap and warm water. Clothes can be searched and fleas picked off, but it is preferable to boil clothing to kill off larvae or missed adults. An even simpler method is to place clothing in a plastic bag and put it in the deep-freeze overnight. Once flea control has been carried out then efforts are made to reduce the rat population (see Box 16.1).

Plague vaccine will protect persons at risk from bubonic plague, but not from pneumonic plague. It is given as a course of three doses, with the second after 1–3 months and the third after 5–6 months, with boosters every 6 months in high-risk conditions. Chemoprophylaxis with tetracycline 250 mg four times a day or doxycycline 100 mg a day for a week should be given to close contacts of cases with pneumonic plague, or after exposure to *Y. pestis* or to a plague-infected flea, and also to medical workers at risk.

Quarantine of all close contacts, whether taking prophylaxis or not, is for 7 days. All persons should be dusted with insecticides to remove fleas and precautions taken to prevent aerosol spread from pneumonic cases. Any cases dying of plague should be buried or burnt with aseptic precautions.

Treatment. Effective treatment depends upon the speed of making a diagnosis and treating early. If plague has already been diagnosed in the area then a confirmatory test should not be awaited. The clinical presentation of fever and bubo in a severely ill patient is sufficient and treatment needs to be started immediately. This is with:

- streptomycin 1 g followed by 0.5 g every 4 h, up to a total of 20 g; or
- tetracycline 3 g immediately, followed by 1 g three times a day for 12 days; or
- doxycycline 100 mg every 12 h for 7 days; or
- chloramphenicol 500 mg every 6 h for 7–10 days.

Another drug, gentamicin, has the advantage of only requiring a single daily dose and was successfully used in treating a recent outbreak in DRC. Unfortunately multi-drug-resistant plague has developed in Madagascar.

Streptomycin is the treatment of choice, but can cause a Herxheimer reaction, so tetracycline is preferable in the critically ill. Resistant strains have occurred and the sensitivity of the organism should be monitored.

Isolation of cases is mandatory and the terminal bubonic case with pneumonia or pneumonic plague is highly infectious, so extreme precautions should be taken. Gowns and full face masks should be worn, as well as goggles to protect the eyes as *Y. pestis* can be absorbed through the conjunctiva.

Box 16.1. Rat control.

The control of rats can be by cats, traps or poisoning. A well-trained cat can be most efficient. Trapping is an effective means of rat control if carried out properly. Traps can be made out of scrap pieces of metal and are easily manufactured in developing countries. A knowledge of the rat runs is gained and the trap left baited, but unsprung. Once the bait has been taken, then the trap is set. Traps must be visited regularly, all dead rats disposed of (by burning) and the trap set again.

Prior to any rat control programme, a full survey should be carried out using holes, rat runs and droppings as indicators. Poisoning can be with either an acute or chronic poison. The number of poisons is considerable and, where available, it is preferable to solicit professional advice. Poisons strong enough to kill rats are also able to kill other animals that may eat them. They are also dangerous to humans, especially children, so proper safety precautions must be observed. A coloured dye should be incorporated to warn against their accidental use. Chronic poisons are preferable to acute poisons as rats die some time after taking the bait, so do not associate it with the meal. They also give a longer period for treatment (usually with vitamin K_1) should accidental poisoning have occurred. The most commonly used chronic poison is warfarin, which is mixed with bait in a ratio of 1:19. Others are diphacinone, a powder or water-soluble concentrate, and chlorophacinone, an oil-based concentrate, while a large number of chronic poisons are sold as prepared baits or wax blocks. The bait is first left without the poison and only if it is taken is it mixed with poison on subsequent applications. Zinc phosphide is a useful acute poison mixed in a proportion 1 part poison to 10 parts bait.

Broken maize or rice using cooking oil to dissolve the poison makes a good bait. Alternatively, the poison can be mixed with water and the bait left to soak. After drying out, it is then put in the traps. If the bait is to be used in damp conditions then it can be mixed with wax. If no bait has been taken for 2 weeks and there is no further sign of activity then poisoning can be discontinued. Rat protection with shields and guards should be used after rats have been eliminated and all sources of food and shelter removed.

There is a danger from the dust and gases produced when preparing baits, so a mask and gloves should be used. If poison is swallowed, copper sulfate can be administered in 0.25 g portions orally every 10 min until vomiting is induced.

Another method is to use poisonous gas (hydrogen cyanide) which is very effective as it kills both rats and fleas, but strict safety precautions, including the wearing of masks and protective clothing, must be observed. This method is especially useful for rodents that live in burrows. All exits are blocked before the gas is introduced.

Surveillance of foci should be maintained with regular trapping of rodents to examine them for infection and their flea populations. Notification of any confirmed or suspected case of plague must be made to WHO and neighbouring countries.

16.2 Typhus

There are many similarities between the epidemiology of typhus and plague, and it is convenient to approach the disease in the reverse order to which it is normally described in order to assist in its description. While plague is a composite disease of three different cycles utilizing the same organism and vector, there are three different forms of typhus (scrub, murine and epidemic) each with its own organism and vector (Fig 16.3).

Organism. The causative organism of typhus is a species of *Rickettsia* or *Orientia*, intracellular bacteria which require cellular tissue of the host or ectoparasite to develop and reproduce. The organisms can survive in the environment if suitable conditions prevail (e.g. in louse faeces); otherwise they are sensitive to heat (being killed by a temperature of 60°C for 30 min) and are easily killed by antiseptics.

The typhus-producing organisms and their ectoparasites are as follows:

Scrub typhus	*Orientia tsutsugamushi*	Trombiculid mites
Murine typhus	*Rickettsia typhi* (*R. mooseri*)	Flea, *Xenopsylla cheopis*
Epidemic typhus	*R. prowazekii*	Human louse

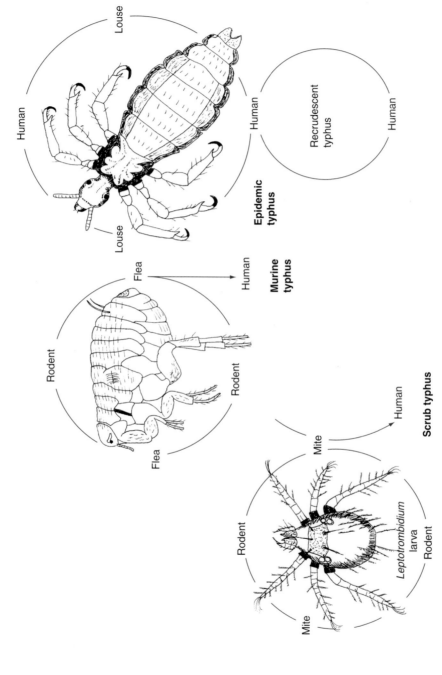

Epidemic typhus

Louse

Human

Human

Louse

Recrudescent typhus

Human

Human

Murine typhus

Flea

Human

Rodent

Rodent

Flea

Scrub typhus

Human

Mite

Rodent

Leptotrombidium larva

Rodent

Mite

Fig. 16.3. The transmission cycles and vectors of scrub, murine and epidemic typhus.

Clinical features. Typhus was confused with typhoid for a considerable period of time because they both produced fever, prostration and a rash. Indeed, typhoid obtained its name only when it was finally separated from typhus as being a less infectious disease, with markedly abdominal symptoms and a milder rash.

In the most severe form, epidemic typhus, there is a sudden onset with headache, pains, rigors and malaise as the temperature rapidly rises to 40°C or more. The temperature remains at this high level for the duration of the illness. The characteristic rash appears between the fourth and seventh days and consists of petechial haemorrhages on the trunk and limbs, but sparing the face, palms and soles. As the disease progresses, the patient becomes semi-stuporous, with confusion, anxiety and considerable dullness. Patients appear unable to hear, talk nonsense and have to be fed. By the third week, if treatment has not been given, the patient will progressively recover or else sink further into heart failure, bronchopneumonia and death.

In scrub typhus, the illness similarly commences with fever, progressive prostration and a macular rash, but after a few days the infective mite bite develops into an eschar. This is a red indurated area with a central vesicle that subsequently breaks down to leave a black scab. The severity of the disease varies markedly from area to area, being a severe and fatal illness, similar to epidemic typhus in some places, while in others, it is so mild and innocuous that it passes as 'flu'. I remember visiting a school near to a well-known mite island which expected all new students to have a minor illness for a day or two and then be immune for the rest of their academic stay.

In murine typhus, there is fever, followed by a rash, but the illness is milder than epidemic typhus, mortality is low and complications rare, so that most people fully recover in 7–10 days.

Diagnosis will probably be on clinical grounds, the eschar of scrub typhus being characteristic, but where available, the indirect fluorescence antibody test, labelled enzyme with ELISA or PCR can be used.

Transmission

Scrub typhus. Like wild rodent plague, scrub typhus is a zoonosis in which humans are not involved. Well-defined areas, called mite islands, harbour rodents, mites and the *Orientia* which is transmitted between them. A large number of rodents have been incriminated, including rats, and it is their system of burrows, runs and range of activity that determines the limit of the mite island. The rodents are fed upon by the larval stage of various leptotrombiculid mites (*Leptotrombidium*) that need to take blood so that they can develop into a nymph and subsequently an adult. The larva climbs on to grass or vegetation and awaits the passage of a rodent or any other mammal to which it attaches itself. Once it has fed, it drops off and continues its development in the soil. If during its feeding it sucks up *O. tsutsugamushi*, these develop in the nymph and adult and are passed on transovarially to infect the next generation of blood-sucking larvae. The mites appear unaffected by this infection, acting as a reservoir, hardly requiring the mammalian host except to provide a blood meal for their own continuity. Such is the balance of this arrangement that a mite island can persist undisturbed, causing harm to no one unless accidentally entered by humans. The larval mite will attack people just as it will attack birds and other mammals that come crashing through its hunting ground; transmitting the infection to its unusual host.

Scrub typhus is a disease of the wandering farmer, hunter or travelling army that is passing through, or accidentally camping in a mite island. The islands can be very small and localized or cover extensive areas, but generally they are associated with transitional vegetation or fringe habitats such as areas separating different vegetation zones (e.g. forest and grassland). Mite islands are nearly always the result of human activity, where forest is destroyed either for timber or in 'slash and burn' agriculture. The land regenerates as secondary growth, rats and other rodents move in and provide suitable conditions for the trombiculid mites.

Murine typhus. Scrub typhus has been given the alternative name of rural typhus, which adequately distinguishes it from urban typhus, the main characteristic of the flea-borne disease. Murine typhus is, then, a disease of towns and habitation, maintained there by domestic rodents, the rats *Rattus rattus* and *R. norvegicus*. In contrast to scrub typhus, the mammal in murine typhus is the reservoir of the disease and the common rat flea, *X. cheopis*, acts only as a transmitter. Many other mammals have been found infected – mice, cats, opossums, shrews and skunks – but the key in all these alternative sites is always the domestic rat.

The flea becomes infected by biting the host, the infection appearing not to have any effect on the flea and not shorten its lifespan. *R. typhi* is not transmitted by the bite of the flea but is passed in its faeces. If infected faeces are rubbed into an abrasion or inhaled as an aerosol, other rats become infected. The body of the flea is also highly contagious and if crushed, the organism is liberated. While *X. cheopis* is the main vector, the organism has also been isolated from *Pulex irritans*, the common human flea, and from lice, mites and ticks. These probably do not form an important means of transmission, but could explain epidemics in which *X. cheopis* is not found.

Humans are infected by their close association with domestic rodents. When a flea is squashed or scratched into an abrasion, its tissue juices or faeces contaminate the wound. The habit of some people when catching fleas of crushing them between their teeth is also a potential method of infection. However, it would seem that direct attack by the essentially healthy rat flea is uncommon and the more important method of transmission is from an aerosol of organisms in the flea faeces. These are carried on the rats' fur or sent into the air when disturbed. *R. typhi* can be inhaled, swallowed or enter through other mucus membranes, such as the conjunctiva. Murine typhus is common where rats live in constant contact with humans.

Epidemic typhus. While scrub typhus and murine typhus are zoonoses, epidemic typhus is an infection where only humans and the body louse, *Pediculus humanus corporis*, are involved. The louse can spend its entire life cycle on the same host, laying its eggs in the seams of clothing and finding all the food and shelter it requires. Female lice lay some 5–10 eggs a day, and these hatch in 6–9 days depending on the temperature. If the clothes are kept on the body then the temperature is maintained and hatching takes place rapidly, but if they are removed and cool down, development may take 2–3 weeks. One month is the maximum period the lice can survive under these conditions, so clothes that are not worn for this length of time will be free of lice.

The egg hatches into a nymph, which in all respects resembles a small adult, and sucks blood. Three nymphal stages are passed through before it becomes an adult louse. Lice, both males and females, can only survive by taking blood meals, and if deprived of these can last no longer than

10 days. They are sensitive to temperature and will abandon a dead person as well as one with a high fever. The lifespan of an adult louse is about 1 month and during this time a female may lay some 200–300 eggs.

R. prowazekii is ingested in the blood meal of the louse and can infect both males and females, and all nymphal stages. The rickettsiae develop in the epithelial lining cells of the stomach which they distend to such an extent that rupture takes place, liberating them back into the damaged gut lumen. These are then passed into the louse faeces in which they can survive for 100 days or more. The damage caused to the louse can be sufficiently severe to kill it within 10 days and this helps to explain why few lice are found on a person suffering from typhus.

Humans become infected by scratching the louse faeces into abrasions or the puncture wound left by the feeding parasite, or if the louse is crushed on the skin or in the mouth. Dried lice faeces can remain infectively viable for a considerable period of time and fine particles that are inhaled or enter the conjunctiva can be a potential hazard to those not infested with lice.

Lice thrive in conditions of deprivation and poverty, where clothing is worn without changing and people live in close proximity to each other. They cannot travel far, or survive for long without a blood meal, so it is the crowding together of people that allows lice to crawl across and infest a new host. Where clothing is changed or washed, or the ambient temperature is high, body lice do not occur and typhus is not found. But in times of human disruption brought about by war, famine or social upheaval, the crowding together of people, in conditions of poor sanitation, provides the stage for an outbreak of typhus. A similar situation can occur in the highland areas of tropical countries, where people live close to each other to keep warm.

Various claims have been made for non-human reservoirs of *R. prowazekii*, but humans appear to be an adequate reservoir and the louse an ideal vector. The difficulty is what happens to the organism when an epidemic has subsided? The probable answer is found in Brill–Zinsser disease, more suitably called recurrent typhus. In this condition, people are found to have *R. prowazekii* in their bodies long after they had the disease. The organism remains dormant until some event causes a breakdown in host resistance and overt disease reappears. Cases have been found 20 and 40 years after the person was in a typhus area and where lice have been absent for this length of time, but if lice are fed on these cases they become infected and can transmit epidemic typhus.

Incubation period. 1–2 weeks (up to 3 weeks in scrub typhus). The length of the incubation period is related to the infecting dose.

Period of communicability. Lice can become infected during the febrile illness, which may last for 2 weeks, but because lice will leave a febrile person, communicability is probably only during the earlier part of the illness. A chronic carrier (with Brill–Zinsser disease) can infect lice for up to 40 years. Lice excrete rickettsiae 2–6 days after an infected blood meal, but continue to be a source of infection for weeks after they have died. Fleas in murine typhus remain infected for life (about 1 year).

Occurrence and distribution. Like plague, typhus is a disease of history, particularly associated with the conflicts of man. When the anger of man causes war, disruption of civilizations, famine and refugees, then the disease of war, typhus, enters into the attack. At the present time it is a particular risk of refugee camps.

Epidemic typhus can occur in highland areas, particularly during the rainy season, with outbreaks occurring in Rwanda, Burundi, Ethiopia, Guatemala, Bolivia and Peru. The three countries in Africa have reported the most cases in recent times. In 1997, there were 24,000 cases of typhus in Burundi.

Murine typhus is endemic in Pakistan, India and Peninsular Malaysia, but may become epidemic in any part of the world where rats are found, such as in ports.

'Mite or typhus islands' are found in East, South and South-east Asia, including Siberia, China, Japan, Thailand, Pakistan, Australia and Pacific Islands. The disease is one of the few health problems in the Maldives.

Control and prevention of scrub typhus is by the wearing of clothing treated with repellents or insecticides to prevent the larval mite from attacking humans. Long trousers tucked into boots with high lace-up sides, or gaiters to cover the gap, should be treated with diethyltoluamide (DEET), dimethyl phthalate or a synthetic pyrethroid. Repellents should also be smeared on to arms and necks, because it is these sites that are attacked when working in the undergrowth. If an area of scrub typhus is known and it is desired to clear it permanently, then the undergrowth should be cut down and burnt, leaving the ground to thoroughly dry out before it is safe to use. A less permanent method is to spray the area with insecticides. Tetracycline can be taken as a prophylactic by those at particular risk, but such methods are never reliable.

Control of murine typhus is the same as for plague (Section 16.1), where the subject is covered in more detail. Essentially, it is the control of fleas and rats with the use of insecticide powders to kill the fleas first, followed by measures against rats. Buildings should be protected against reinfestation and new structures built with rat proofing (Box 16.1).

Control of epidemic typhus is control of the louse. In an epidemic, this is most effectively done by blowing an insecticide powder into people's clothing. This can be by a blower with a long nozzle that is pushed up the arms of clothing, down through necks and up trousers and skirts. The clothing should be thoroughly treated, remembering that the lice live between the underclothing and the body; 2% temephos, 1% propoxur, 0.5% permethrin or other synthetic pyrethroids can be used. Samples of lice should be tested for insecticidal resistance before and during mass treatments. As it is conditions of overcrowding that generate epidemics it is often not too difficult to disinfect large numbers of people in a comparatively short space of time. Dead bodies should be dusted with insecticides before burial. A longer term preventive method is to treat underclothing with insecticides in the same way as mosquito nets are treated, to give a target dose of $0.65–1 \text{g/m}^2$ permethrin. Clothes can be washed but treatment should be repeated every 6 weeks.

Prophylactic antibiotics, generally tetracycline, can be given to contacts to reduce the extent of the reservoir. Treatment centres should be set up to discover cases early, and antibiotics given.

Vaccines have been successful in controlling epidemics, but they suffer from various disadvantages. A killed vaccine (Cox) is painful when injected and does not give complete immunity, whereas a live attenuated vaccine appears to give solid immunity for over 5 years, but must be prepared carefully as virulence can increase. Vaccines can either be used for mass administration in the face of epidemics or be given to individuals at increased risk, such as medical personnel.

In the long term, typhus will only disappear when all lice are removed. People should be encouraged to wash themselves and their clothes. Clothes must be boiled or washed at over 70°C, which is a higher temperature than most washing machines achieve. Ironing clothes kills both adults and eggs. A simple means of killing lice is to place clothing in a plastic bag and put it in the deep-freeze overnight.

Treatment should be commenced as soon as possible, even before the diagnosis is confirmed, as speed is of the essence if treatment is to be effective. A single dose of 200 mg doxycycline, irrespective of age, is the treatment of choice. Alternatively, tetracycline at a dose of 500 mg four times a day and, where both of these are unavailable, chloramphenicol. Careful nursing is of the utmost importance.

Surveillance is the cornerstone of prevention by conducting louse surveys at clinics, prisons, institutions and collections of people. Cases of proven or suspect epidemic louse-borne typhus should be notified to WHO. All contacts of a case should be placed under surveillance for 14 days.

16.3   Louse-borne Relapsing Fever

Organism. *Borrelia recurrentis*, a Gram-negative spirochaete indistinguishable from *B. duttonii* (see Section 16.4) in stained preparations, and with some cross immunity between the two.

Clinical features. Louse-borne relapsing fever is an epidemic disease occurring in the same situations or even at the same time as epidemic typhus. The disease is very similar to tick-borne relapsing fever (see Section 16.4 below), with periods of fever lasting for a few days and then recurring after 2–4 days, ending in a crisis, but the number of relapses is generally less. The onset of fever is sudden with headache, myalgia and vertigo. A transitory petechial rash can occur and other symptoms such as bronchitis and hepatosplenomegaly may develop.

Diagnosis is by dark field illumination of fresh blood or smears of stained blood taken during a pyrexial episode, when spirochaetes will be seen.

Transmission. *P. h. corporis* is infected when it feed on humans during the pyrexial period. The spirochaete invades the haemocoel of the louse and is transmitted when the louse is crushed. The spirochaete is not transmitted when the louse feeds, but enters the bite wound or an abrasion when the louse is crushed. It can also enter through mucous membranes and possibly even unbroken skin. The greatest risk then is to the attentive parent or acquaintance delousing a member of the family or a friend. Crushing lice between the fingernails or teeth is a possible way of acquiring infection.

Infection of the louse is sufficient to kill it, as occurs in subclinical infection because the lice die even though the person does not show any symptoms. Humans are the only reservoir of the louse-borne infection.

Incubation period. 5–15 days, normally 8 days.

Period of communicability. Humans are most infectious during periods of pyrexia, but as reservoirs they can infect lice at any time. The louse becomes infectious 4–5 days after an infected blood meal.

Occurrence and distribution. The disease is associated with poor personal hygiene and overcrowding, in which lice flourish. Distribution is similar to that of epidemic typhus, being found in the highland areas of Africa, India and South America. There is an endemic focus in Ethiopia from which epidemics appear to originate, all the conditions being favourable about once every 20 years.

Control and prevention is the same as for epidemic typhus in Section 16.2 above, with delousing and improvement of hygiene.

Treatment is with a single dose of procaine penicillin (300,000 units) on the first day, followed by tetracycline 250 mg the next. Severe reactions to antibiotic therapy are commoner in louse-borne than tick-borne relapsing fever.

Surveillance. Cases of louse-borne relapsing fever must be notified to WHO and neighbouring countries. Routine inspections for lice should be carried out where facilities permit, such as in prisons, institutions and in new arrivals coming into refugee camps.

16.4 Tick-borne Relapsing Fever

Organism. *Borrelia duttonii*, which is indistinguishable from *B. recurrentis* (see Section 16.3) in stained blood films.

Clinical features. A fever develops with a recurring or relapsing pattern, as the name of the disease indicates. The period of fever lasts for a few days and then recurs after 2–5 days, with up to ten or more relapses occurring in the untreated case. The onset of fever is sudden with headache, myalgia and vertigo; a transient petechial rash can occur and a variety of other systems may be involved. There can be bronchitis, nerve palsies, hepatosplenomegaly and signs of renal damage. The disease is serious in young children.

Diagnosis. Spirochaetes are found in the blood during febrile periods when blood slides should be taken and either stained or viewed by dark ground illumination. An improvement on this technique is the direct centrifugal method.

Transmission, occurrence and distribution. Two different patterns of tick-borne relapsing fever occur; an endemic in Africa and epidemic in other parts of the world (Fig. 16.4).

In Africa, the vector tick *Ornithodorus moubata* is domestic in habit, living in and around the house, and transmitting the disease within the household. The reservoir is the tick, but humans act as a source of organisms. When a tick feeds on an infected person spirochaetes are ingested with the blood, multiply in the gut and enter the haemocoel, where they increase to enormous proportions. The spirochaetes pierce all organs of the tick's body, including the salivary gland, the coxal organ and the reproductive system, leading to transovarial infection. Nymphal stages may already be infected when they take blood meals, or can become so from their hosts. People are infected both by the bite of the tick and from the

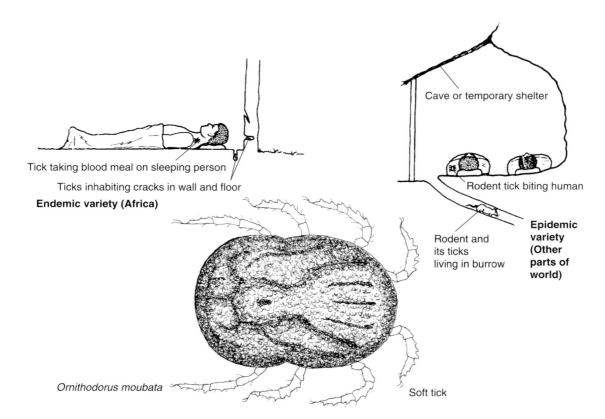

Tick taking blood meal on sleeping person
Ticks inhabiting cracks in wall and floor
Endemic variety (Africa)

Cave or temporary shelter
Rodent tick biting human
Rodent and its ticks living in burrow
Epidemic variety (Other parts of world)

Ornithodorus moubata
Soft tick

Fig. 16.4. The vector and epidemiology of tick-borne relapsing fever.

coxal fluid (see below), but not from the faeces. In *O. moubata* adults, the coxal fluid is the main source of spirochaetes, but in the nymphs and other species of *Ornithodorus* (see below), it is the salivary glands.

Babies and young children are particularly susceptible to infection in endemic areas, with adults exhibiting immunity. However, immunity is lost in pregnancy, and congenital infection can occur. Relapsing fever is a cause of abortion, stillbirth and premature delivery. This is particularly the pattern in Central and East Africa.

In other parts of the world, the infection is a zoonosis with a transmission cycle maintained between rodents and their parasitic ticks. People enter this cycle as intruders or by accident, in a similar way to sylvatic plague or scrub typhus. Rodent-inhabited caves, or campsites near rodent burrows, are areas where sporadic infection can occur. When temporary shelters or log cabins are erected near a zoonotic focus, then rats invade these buildings and their ticks begin to feed regularly on humans. An endemic pattern, similar to that in Africa, may then develop. Ticks responsible for transmitting relapsing fever in parts of the world other than Central and East Africa are *O. tholozani* in Asia, *O. erraticus* in North Africa and *O. rudis* and *O. talaje* in Central and South America.

The soft ticks (Argasidae), which include *Ornithodorus* spp., have a retracted head and no scutum, which differentiates them from the hard ticks (Ixodidae, see Section 16.5.1 below). As their name implies, soft ticks do not have a rigid structure, but a leathery body that looks like a collapsed bag. This hangs over the body structures, so viewed from above only the legs can be seen protruding from it (Fig. 16.4). When the tick takes a blood meal its collapsed body fills and becomes greatly distended. The tick digests the blood meal utilizing a structure called a coxal gland, which is like a filter to remove excess fluid.

After hatching, the soft ticks have several nymph stages (four in *O. moubata*), each needing to take a blood meal before passing on to the next. Finally, the fourth instar changes into an adult and egg laying commences after the female has become engorged with blood. The ticks can live for several years, so that many eggs can be laid in a lifetime, for in contrast to the hard ticks, the female soft tick does not die after egg laying but is able to continue taking blood meals, laying eggs after each.

Ticks rest in cracks and crevices of poorly built houses, emerging at night to feed on sleeping occupants. They can remain alive for up to 5 years after a single blood meal, and are able to attack again after the owner reoccupies a house following a prolonged absence. The eggs are coated with a waxy protective layer, allowing them to remain viable for several months; laid in walls, floors and furniture they will hatch in 1–4 weeks if conditions are suitable. Soft ticks, once established, are very persistent occupants.

Incubation period is 3–10 days.

Period of communicability. All stages of the tick are able to transmit infection and they remain infective for life.

Control and prevention. Ticks can be controlled with insecticides such as malathion, diazinon, permethrin or propoxur sprayed around houses. Special attention needs to be paid to any cracks and crevices where ticks may hide. In addition, insecticides can be mixed with the floor or wall plaster during construction or repair work. Benzene hexachloride applied as 140 mg base/m^2 is a suitable preparation. Infants (and adults) can be protected from house-invading ticks by sleeping under a mosquito net. Repellents such as diethyltoluamide or dimethyl phthalate smeared on skin or as a solution to impregnate clothing are effective in preventing ticks from biting. Items such as socks can be treated with insecticides in the same way as mosquito nets (see Sections 3.4.1 and 3.4.4). Ticks are also deterred from entering rooms in which a night light is glowing.

The rodent reservoir is of major importance in bringing ticks close to human habitation so all the methods mentioned in plague to control rodents should be used (Box 16.1). Improved house construction will prevent rodents from burrowing underneath.

Treatment is with a single dose of 300,000 units of procaine penicillin immediately, followed the next day by tetracycline 500 mg four times daily for 10 days. This regime provides adequate treatment while at the same time minimizes reactions.

Surveillance. Mass screening using fresh or stained blood slides can be used to delineate the infected population prior to a control programme.

16.5   Diseases Transmitted by Hard Ticks

16.5.1   Hard Ticks (Ixodidae)

Hard ticks are responsible for the transmission of several different kinds of organisms, including rickettsiae, *Borrelia* and arboviruses. The genera of medical importance are *Amblyomma*, *Dermacentor*, *Haemaphysalis*, *Hyalomma*, *Ixodes* and *Rhipicephalus* (Table 16.1). A female *Dermacentor* is illustrated in Fig. 16.5 to characterize the group of hard ticks. The feature that distinguishes hard from soft ticks is the presence of a scutum (shield) and protruding mouthparts. Care has to be taken in identifying the engorged specimen, for the body is so greatly distended as to obscure the head and mouthparts (Fig. 16.5). The female has a smaller scutum than the male, but as both males and females take blood meals, there is no need to distinguish between them.

Eggs are laid in a large mass on the ground, hatching after weeks or months into six-legged larvae. These larvae resemble mites, but are differentiated from them by prominent mouthparts and a scutum. The larvae climb on to grass or prominent vegetation to await a passing mammal on to which they then cling. Once attached, they crawl around to find an area of soft skin, such as in the ears, eyelids or below the belly of the animal. On humans, they may surreptitiously climb up the leg and attach themselves to the scrotum or between the buttocks. Once in a favourable site, they pierce the skin with their powerful mouthparts, inject saliva and feed on the host's blood. Larvae will remain attached for 3–7 days, after which they drop to the ground and seek a place to moult. After developing into an eight-legged nymph, the tick repeats the feeding pattern, being attached for 5–10 days and then falling to the ground once more for the final moult. From the nymph develops a male or female adult, which subsequently quests for a new host on which it remains for a considerable period of time (up to 1 month), becoming greatly engorged with blood. When it finally drops off, the female digests her blood meal and begins egg laying; after which she dies.

The life cycle of ticks is modified by temperature and humidity, so that if it becomes too cold the cycle of development will be delayed until more favourable conditions return. Larvae and nymphs tend to feed on small mammals and humans, whereas adults prefer larger animals such as cattle and game animals.

Control of ticks is mainly through the use of insecticides and repellents. Permethrin, malathion and propoxur are suitable insecticides, and are administered as dusting powders or solutions to infested animals. Cattle are commonly treated by making them swim through an insecticidal bath, or dip. This should be carried out on a regular basis, with monitoring of ticks for insecticidal resistance. Dogs are important carriers of ticks and should be similarly treated by insecticidal baths, making sure that they are totally immersed as the ears are a common site for ticks to attach. Dogs should wear tick-repellent collars to prevent them becoming infested in the first place.

Repellents such as diethyltoluamide or dimethyl phthalate smeared on skin or as a solution to impregnate clothing are effective in preventing ticks from becoming attached. Items such as socks can be treated with insecticides in the same way as mosquito nets (see Box 3.1 and Section 3.4.4).

Ticks take some 2h to attach themselves and start feeding, so a careful search of the body, paying particular attention to the upper legs, groin and buttocks, should be made after passing through tick-infested country. Larval and nymph stages can be very small, appearing to be just black dots, but they are often the main transmitters of infection so every endeavour should be made to find and remove them. Ticks should not be pulled off directly as the mouthparts may be left behind, which will continue to cause irritation; instead, they should be twisted out. Special tweezers can be used which are slid under the body of the tick to grab the mouthparts; then the tick is twisted out. Applying methylated spirit, ether, benzene or similar solutions will kill the tick and sterilize the wound.

16.6   Tick Typhus/Fever

Going under a host of names, Boutonneuse fever, Mediterranean spotted fever, African tick typhus, Indian tick typhus, Siberian tick typhus, Queensland tick typhus, to give but a few, this similar group of infections has been reported from a number of different parts of the world.

Organism. *Rickettsia conori*, *R. africae*, *R. siberica* and *R. australis*.

Table 16.1. Diseases transmitted by ticks. (**Bold** mentioned in the text.)

Disease	Clinical features	Vector	Distribution
Absettarov	Fever	*Ixodes* sp.	Europe, Russia
Babesiosis	Fever and haemolytic anaemia	*Ixodes* sp.	USA, Mexico, Europe, Russia
Bhanja	Fever, encephalitis	*Dermacentor*, *Haemaphysalis*	Africa, Asia, Europe
Colorado tick fever	Fever	*Dermacentor*	USA, Canada
Crimean–Congo haemorrhagic fever (Section 16.10.2)	Haemorrhagic fever	*Hyalomma* sp.	Africa, Central and SW Asia, Europe
Dhori	Fever	*Hyalomma* sp.	Europe
Dugbe	Fever	–	Africa
Ehrlichiosis	Fever	*Ixodes* and *Amblyomma* sp.	USA, Asia Europe
Hanzalova	Fever	*Ixodes* sp.	Europe, Russia
Issyk-Kul	Fever	–	Central Asia
Karshi	Fever, encephalitis	–	Central Asia
Kemerovo	Fever	–	Russia
Kumlinge	Fever	*Ixodes* sp.	Europe, Russia
Kyasanur Forest disease (Section 16.10.1)	Haemorrhagic fever and encephalitis	*Haemophysalis* sp.	India
Lipovnik	Meningitis	Several species	Europe
Louping ill	Encephalitis	*Ixodes* sp.	Western Europe
Lyme disease (Section 16.8)	Erythematous migrans, meningitis	*Ixodes* sp.	USA, Canada, Europe, Asia
Nairobi sheep	Fever	–	Africa, India
Omsk haemorrhagic fever (Section 16.10.1)	Haemorrhagic fever	*Dermacentor* sp.	Russia
Powassan	Encephalitis	*Ixodes*	USA, Canada, Russia
Quaranfil	Fever	–	Africa, Arabia
Rocky Mountain spotted fever (Section 16.7)	Fever and rash	*Dermacentor* and *Amblyomma*	North, Central and South America
Tamdy	Fever	–	–
Thogoto	Encephalitis	Several species	Europe, Africa
Tick-borne encephalitis (Section 16.9)	Fever, myelitis, encephalitis, post-encephalitic	*Ixodes*	
– European	syndrome	*I. ricinus*	Europe
– Far-Eastern	(neuropsychiatric)	*I. persulcatus*	China, Japan
– Siberian		*I. persulcatus*	East Russia
Tick-borne relapsing fever (Section 16.4)	Periodic fever, mainly in children	*Ornithodorus* sp.	Africa, Asia, Central and South America
Tick typhus (Section 16.6)	Fever and rash	*Rhipicephalus* and *Amblyomma*	Europe, Africa
Tularaemia (Section 19.6)	Lymphadenopathy, systemic lesions	*Ixodes* and *Dermacentor*	Africa, Europe, Asia, Australia
Wanowrie	Fever and bleeding	–	Europe, Asia, Africa

Clinical features. Generally a mild illness of a few days, infection is characterized by an eschar (small ulcer with black centre) at the site of the tick bite and regional lymphadenopathy. There is fever and a generalized maculopapular rash, which resolves spontaneously after about a week.

Diagnosis is usually made on clinical appearance following history of a tick bite, but can be confirmed with serological tests or PCR.

Transmission. The reservoir of infection is the dog tick (*Rhipicephalus sanguineus* in the Mediterranean

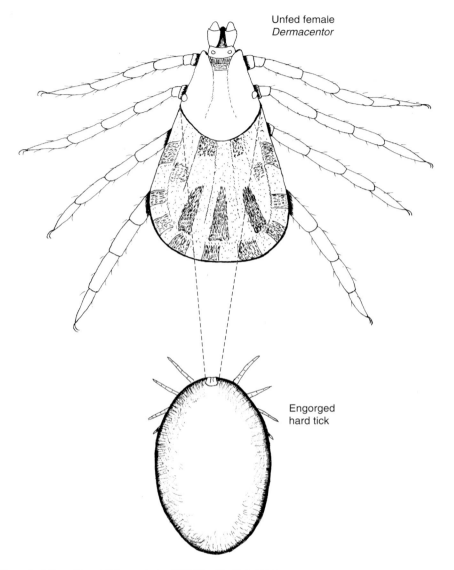

Chapter 16

Unfed female
Dermacentor

Engorged
hard tick

Fig. 16.5. Characteristics of hard ticks as exemplified by *Dermacentor*.

area, and *Amblyomma hebreum* in Africa), which inadvertently moves from the dog to its human handler during their close association. Alternatively, humans acquire infection from passing through scrub forest inhabited by rodents and their ticks (*Ixodes holocyclus* in Australia, *Dermacentor* and *Haemaphysalis* in Siberia), the rodent serving as a secondary reservoir.

Incubation period. 1–15 days (generally 5–7 days).

Period of communicability. Not transmitted from human to human, the tick remaining infected for life.

Occurrence and distribution. Found in slightly different forms in the Mediterranean region, Africa, Indian subcontinent, Australia and North-east Asia.

Control and prevention. Where dogs are the carrier of ticks they should wear tick-repellent collars and be inspected regularly to ensure that animals are tick free. In Australia, Siberia, Mongolia and northern China, where rodents and small marsupials are mainly responsible, then repellents and insecticide-treated socks and trousers should be worn. As it takes the tick about 2 h to fully attach itself it is always a good practice to examine the body carefully after going through 'tick' country. When camping, people should sleep off the ground, e.g. on camp beds, and dogs should be kept away.

Treatment is with tetracycline, doxycycline or chloramphnicol.

Surveillance. Make a regular habit of examining the body after walking through countryside.

16.7   Rocky Mountain Spotted Fever

Organism. Rickettsia rickettsia.

Clinical features. The illness commences suddenly with onset of high fever, headache, malaise, muscle pains and rash. The characteristic maculopapular rash which develops from numerous petechial haemorrhages appears on about the third day and covers the whole body, including the palms and soles. The disease is fatal in up to 25% of untreated cases, but is reduced to 3–5% in treated cases.

Diagnosis is made clinically with the additional help of enzyme immunoassay (EIA) and immunofluorescence tests containing the specific antigen. PCR can detect rickettsiae in blood.

Transmission. Humans are infected by the bite of a tick (*Dermacentor* or *Amblyomma*), although infection can also be acquired by scratching in tick faeces or crushing the tick on the skin or mucous membranes. Larval and nymphal stages, as well as adult ticks, can transmit the infection. Rickettsial infection is maintained by transovarial transmission, so the tick is the reservoir.

Incubation period. 3–14 days.

Period of communicability. Because the tick is the reservoir of infection it is not spread from person to person.

Occurrence and distribution. First described in the Rocky Mountains of North America, the disease is now more common in Oklahoma and North Carolina. It is also found in Mexico, Panama, Costa Rica, Brazil, Colombia and Argentina.

Control and prevention. Prevention is by avoiding any known tick country or wearing protective clothing, treated with repellents or insecticides. The common vector in North America is the dog tick, *D. variabilis*, or the wood tick, *D. andersoni*, so the control of dogs and their ectoparasites with tick-repellent collars is effective. *A. cajennense* is the main vector in the rest of the Americas.

Treatment is with doxycycline, tetracycline or chloramphenicol.

Surveillance. Dogs and other animals should be checked regularly for ticks.

16.8   Lyme Disease (Borreliosis)

Organism. Borrelia burgdorferi, B. garinii and B. afzelii.

Clinical features. The herald sign is an annular expanding erythematous skin lesion, called erythematous migrans (EM), often accompanied by fever, muscle pain, arthralgia and signs of meningeal irritation. The EM lesion will reach or exceed 5 cm in diameter and can be single or multiple. Infection may develop over weeks or months into aseptic meningitis, cranial nerve signs including facial palsy and optic nerve damage, peripheral nerve signs (both motor and sensory), cardiac irregularities and polyarthritis.

Diagnosis is mainly clinical, with the EM lesion exceeding 5 cm, and aided by serological tests. Immunofluorescence and ELISA, followed by Western immunoblot, are more useful in the latter stages of the disease.

Transmission is from the bite of an infected deer tick (*Ixodes scapularis* or *I. pacificus*) in North America, or the sheep tick (*I. ricinus*) in Europe. In Asia, *I. persulcatus* is the vector. The reservoir of infection is in the tick, which can transmit the *Borrelia* transovarially. Adult ticks largely feed on deer (sheep in Europe), while the nymphal stage is responsible for transmitting the infection to humans and other animals, such as dogs, which will often develop similar symptoms to humans.

Incubation period. 3–32 days (generally 7–10 days).

Period of communicability. Not transmitted from person to person.

Occurrence and distribution. Found in well-defined areas of the USA and Canada, the disease distribution is largely related to the deer population. It is similarly found in areas of Russia, China and Japan. Foci of infection can be delineated by looking for the vector tick. In Europe, *I. ricinus* is the main vector of Lyme disease (and also of tick-borne encephalitis). Due to global climate change *I. ricinus* has extended its range into higher latitudes (Scandinavia) and higher altitudes (mountainous areas of the Czech Republic), so there is likely to be an increase in the spread of these two diseases. The rise in temperature could prolong the season as well, thereby intensifying transmission in areas where infection is already prevalent. A similar scenario is likely to take place with the vector ticks of Lyme disease in North America.

Control and prevention is similar to that in the other tick-borne diseases mentioned above, with the use of repellents and insecticide-treated clothing when passing through known infected areas. As transmission of infection takes in excess of 24 h after the tick has attached, careful search of the body should be made after walking through countryside. The nymphal stage is the main transmitter to humans so small black spots should be looked for, possibly with the aid of a lens (see Fig. 16.5).

A vaccine has been developed against Lyme disease in North America, but it is not effective in other parts of the world. It is only useful for persons at constant risk of infection, such as game wardens or camp attendants, but other precautionary measures should also be taken.

Treatment is effective with doxycycline 100 mg twice daily or amoxicillin 500 mg four times daily for 2 weeks in the early EM stage of the disease. In the late arthritic, cardiac or neurological stages of the disease treatment is with benzylpenicillin or ceftriaxone for up to 21 days.

Surveillance. Infected areas should be delineated and warning signs posted.

16.9 Tick-borne Encephalitis

Organism. A flavivirus related to dengue virus, yellow fever virus and Japanese encephalitis virus.

Clinical features. The first signs of infection are non-specific, such as headaches, fatigue and a low-grade fever. Only about a third of clinical cases enter a second phase, with a high fever, meningitis, myelitis and encephalitis. The encephalitis can produce cerebellar ataxia and paralysis, particularly involving muscles of the shoulder region. Less than half of the encephalitic cases develop the post-encephalitic syndrome, which includes psychiatric problems.

Diagnosis during the initial infection is with PCR, while once neurological symptoms have developed serodiagnostic techniques such as ELISA and haemagglutination inhibition (HI) can be used. False positives can occur with other flaviviruses, including from yellow fever vaccination.

Transmission. There are three main types of tick-borne encephalitis: European, transmitted by *I. ricinus*; and Far-Eastern and Siberian, mainly transmitted by *I. persulcatus*. Larvae, nymphs and adult ticks can all be infected and transmit the infection. Transovarial infection can take place in these ticks. Small rodents are the main reservoirs, but many other animals, including cows, goats and sheep can also maintain the infection, so that people can become infected by drinking unpasteurized milk or milk produce. However, most infections occur through working or in recreational activities outdoors, particularly in forested areas, where people come into contact with ticks.

Incubation period. 2–28 days (normally 7–14).

Period of communicability. The infection is not transmitted from person to person.

Occurrence and distribution. The European form of the disease is mainly found in the Baltic States and Slovenia, and the Far-Eastern in China, Mongolia, Japan and the eastern part of the Russian Federation, which is also the endemic area of the Siberian subtype. Climate change is allowing the tick to extend its range so that infection is found in areas where it formally did not occur – in Germany, Scandinavia and Switzerland.

Control and prevention. Personal protection as previously described is the main method of prevention, paying particular attention to examining the body after passing through sheep-rearing areas and forests. All milk should be pasteurized.

Vaccination is effective and should be offered to persons at risk through their occupation or recreation, while in highly endemic areas (>5 cases/100,000 population per year) vaccination should be offered to all ages, including children. The 50–60 year age group tends to get more serious disease so should be targeted. Three doses of vaccine (1 month interval between the first and second dose and 6–12 months between the second and third) are required, with booster doses every 3–5 years for those at continued risk. Post-exposure vaccination is not recommended.

Treatment. There is no specific treatment.

Surveillance. Tick-borne encephalitis is a focal disease so foci should be delineated and warning notices posted, bearing in mind that the range of the tick is extending and new areas developing.

16.10   Arboviruses

16.10.1   Kyasanur Forest disease and Omsk haemorrhagic fever

Kyasanur Forest disease (KFD) is named after the forest in Karnataka, south India, where an epidemic was first identified in 1983. A very similar disease is Omsk haemorrhagic fever (OHF), which is restricted to western Siberia. The organisms and clinical features are described with the other arbovirus haemorrhagic fevers in Section 15.2.

Transmission is by *Haemaphysalis spinigera*, with a reservoir in rodents and monkeys in KFD and in *Dermacentor reticulatus* and *D. marginatus* in OHF. The muskrat is the reservoir so hunters, which are the main victims, can acquire the infection either directly from the muskrat or the bite of the tick.

Incubation period. 3–8 days.

Control is the same as that of the other tick-borne diseases. Experimental vaccines are under trial.

16.10.2   Crimean–Congo haemorrhagic fever

Crimean–Congo haemorrhagic fever (see also Section 15.2.3) is related to dengue and yellow fever with which it shares a similar clinical presentation (Sections 15.4 and 15.5, respectively). It is found in a wide area stretching from west and southern Africa through central and North-east Africa into the Arabian Peninsula, to west and central Asia (Iraq, Iran, Pakistan, Afghanistan, Russia and west China) and westwards into the Balkans and Greece.

Transmission is by *Hyalomma marginatum* and *H. anatolicum* ticks, which also serve as reservoirs, although birds, rodents and hares may be involved. Person-to-person infection can also occur from exposure to blood and other body fluids. The ticks feed on domestic animals (cattle, sheep and goats) so the disease is an occupational hazard of farmers and shepherds, who can also contract the illness by contact with animal tissues and fluids.

Incubation period. 1–3 days, but can be up to 12 days.

Period of communicability. During the entire period of illness the patient is highly infectious from urine, blood and other body fluids.

Control and prevention. All the precautions mentioned above should be taken to prevent being bitten by ticks, including insecticide treatment of domestic animals. Strict barrier nursing should be observed with all cases. Gloves and overalls should be worn when working with animals. People in high-risk areas can be vaccinated.

16.10.3   Other arbovirus diseases

Hard ticks can also be responsible for spreading other arbovirus diseases normally transmitted by mosquitoes, such as Japanese encephalitis (JE; Section 15.3), and St Louis, Eastern and Western equine encephalitis (see Section 15.2).

Arboviruses are further discussed as new and emerging diseases in Section 19.4.

Summary

- The close proximity of humans and their ectoparasites, particularly fleas, lice and ticks, can be a cause of several important illnesses.

- These ectoparasites often live in close association with small mammals in delineated areas and when humans accidentally enter these foci, infection takes place.
- Knowledge of their ecology and vector characteristics is essential in understanding the nature of these infections.
- Avoiding endemic foci and taking precautions against ectoparasites are the main preventive actions.
- Personal hygiene, especially in situations of overcrowding such as occurs in cold weather, or in emergency situations such as refugee camps, will prevent ectoparasite infestation.

Further Reading

Ergonul, O. and Whitehouse, C.A. (2007) *Crimean–Congo Hemorrhagic Fever: A Global Perspective*. Springer, Dordrecht, The Netherlands.

Githeko, A.K., Lindsay, S.W., Confalonieri, U.E. and Patz, J.A. (2000) Climate change and vector-borne diseases: a regional analysis. *Bulletin of the World Health Organization* 78, 1136–1147. Available at: www.who.int/bulletin/archives/78(9)1136.pdf (accessed 22 February 2012).

Goddard, J. (2008) *Infectious Diseases and Arthropods*, 2nd edn. Humana Press/Springer Science, Totowa, New Jersey.

Service, M.W. (2001) *The Encyclopedia of Arthropod-transmitted Infections of Man and Domesticated Animals*. CAB International, Wallingford, UK.

Service, M.W. (2008) *Medical Entomology for Students*, 4th edn. Cambridge University Press, Cambridge, UK.

World Health Organization (1999) *Plague Manual: Epidemiology, Distribution, Surveillance and Control*. Document No. WHO/CDS/CSR/EDC/99.2, WHO, Geneva.

World Health Organization (2006) *Pesticides and Their Application*, 6th edn. Document No. WHO/CDS/NTD/WHOPES/GCDPP/2006.1, WHO, Geneva.

World Health Organization (2007) *Long-lasting Insecticidal Nets for Malaria Prevention*, 3rd edn. WHO, Geneva.

World Health Organization (2009?) *Frequently Asked Questions: Scrub Typhus*. WHO Regional Office for South-East Asia, New Delhi, India. Available at: www.searo.who.int/LinkFiles/CDS_faq_Scrub_Typhus.pdf (accessed 9 March 2012).

Web resource

Plague vaccines. WHO Initiative for Vaccine Research (IVR), Zoonotic Infections, Plague. Available at: www.who.int/vaccine_research/diseases/zoonotic/en/index3.html (accessed 9 March 2012).

17 Domestic and Synanthropic Zoonoses

A zoonosis is an infection that is naturally transmitted between vertebrate animals and humans. In the last chapter a group of infections that were mainly zoonoses, but also involved a vector were covered, while this chapter includes infections in which a vector is not involved. Most of these infections are due to the close association humans have with their domestic animals, but there are also some zoonoses in which animals that live close to humans but are not welcomed, such as rats, are involved in the transmission of disease – these are synanthropic zoonoses (see Section 1.3.5). Some zoonotic infections have been covered in earlier chapters – diseases in which the means of transmission and control are similar to those in other allied conditions, e.g. the pork and beef tapeworms covered in Section 9.8, under food-borne diseases.

The most important source of infection from which humans suffer is that from other humans, but the animals on which people depend for their livelihood and companionship are responsible for many others. Paramount among these is the dog, which is either involved directly in a number of diseases, or acts as a reservoir for many others (Table 17.1). Less important, except to people who have close association with them, are cats, cattle and other domestic animals (Table 17.3). The principal synanthropic vector is the rat, already covered in some detail in Section 16.1 on plague, but also involved in several other infections mentioned in this chapter. Control depends upon an understanding of the contact with the animal and how best to reduce it.

17.1 Rabies

Organism. Rabies virus (RABV) belongs to the genus *Lyssavirus.* There are 11 related viruses, including Mokola and Duvenhage (found in Africa) that produce rabies-like illness. The virus withstands freezing temperatures for considerable periods of time, but is killed by boiling, sunlight and drying. It is not easily destroyed by disinfectants.

Clinical features. The initial symptoms are often fever with pain or paraesthesia at the wound site, but then continue with malaise, fever, sore throat lack of appetite and abnormal muscle movements. The patient then enters the excitable stage, when they become anxious, there is difficulty in swallowing and hydrophobia with generalized convulsions takes place. The patient either dies in the convulsive stage or enters progressive paralysis as the terminal symptom. In the bat-transmitted form of the disease there is no excitable stage and the patient dies from respiratory paralysis.

Diagnosis. The clinical picture following a history of an animal bite is usually sufficient to make the diagnosis, but the virus may be isolated from saliva, tears, cerebrospinal fluid (CSF) or urine and grown in mouse tissue or cell culture. Immunofluorescent antibody (IFA) staining of tissue smears, e.g. skin biopsy, is of value.

Transmission. Virus enters the body through a bite or abrasion of the skin. Classically this is a dog bite, but if an infective dog, cat or cow licks the abraded skin then transmission can occur in this manner. The vampire bat also transmits rabies, but mainly to cattle, with humans only occasionally infected this way. People have contracted rabies from entering bat-infested caves, where it is thought that fine particles of bat faeces contaminate the conjunctiva or enter the respiratory mucosa.

The virus has a special affinity for brain and mucus-secreting tissue, travelling along peripheral nerves to the central nervous system (CNS) and salivary glands. Large quantities of virus particles are present in the saliva from 1 to 10 days before the development of symptoms, right up until an infected animal dies.

Table 17.1. Infections transmitted to humans from dogs and cats or in which the dog or cat is the reservoir. (**Bold** mentioned in the text.)

Organism	Dogs	Cats
Viruses	**Arboviruses**	
	Nipah	Nipah
	Rabies	**Rabies**
Bacteria	**Anthrax**	**Anthrax**
	Brucella canis	*Bartonella benselae* (cat-scratch disease)
	Clostridium tetani	*Chlamydia psittaci* (**conjunctivitis**)
	Campylobacter jejuni	*Campylobacter jejuni*
	Capnocytophaga	
	Escherichia coli	
	Leptospira canicola	
	Mycobacterium	
	Pasteurellosis	
	Salmonella	*Salmonella*
	Spirium minus	
	Tularaemia	
	Yersinia pestis (plague)	*Yersinia pestis*
Rickettsiae	*Coxiella burnetii* (Q fever)	*Coxiella burnetii*
	Rickettsia rickettsii, R. conorii, R. africae,	*Rickettsia typhi*
	R. australis, R. siberica, R. typhi	
	(murine typhus)	
Fungi	**Dermatophytosis (tinea)**	**Dermatophytosis (tinea)**
	Microsporum canis	*Microsporum canis*
		Sporothrix schenkii
Protozoa	**Chagas' disease**	
	Cryptosporidiosis	**Cryptosporidiosis**
	Isospora belli	*Isospora belli*
	Leishmaniasis	*Toxoplasma gondii*
Helminths	*Ancylostoma braziliense, A. caninum,*	*Ancylostoma braziliense, A. caninum,*
	A. ceylonicum (larva migrans)	*A. ceylonicum*
	Brugia malayi, B. pahangi, B. patei	*Brugia malayi, B. pahangi, B. patei*
	Capillaria aerophilia	*Capillaria aerophilia*
	Diphylobothrium latum	*Diphylobothrium latum*
	Dipylidium canium	
	Dirofilaria immitis, D. repens	*Dirofilaria immitis, D. repens*
	Dracunculus medinensis	
	Echinococcus granulosus,	
	E. multilocularis, E. vogeli	
	Echinostoma	
	Gnathostoma spinigerum	*Gnathostoma spinigerum*
	Heterophyes heterophyes	*Heterophyes heterophyes*
	Metagonimus yokagawi	*Metagonimus yokagawi*
	Multiceps multiceps	
	Clonorchis sinensis	*Clonorchis sinensis*
	Opisthorchis felineus, O. viverrini	*Opisthorchis felineus,*
		O. viverrini
	Paragonimus westermani, P. africanus,	*Paragonimus westermani, P. africanus,*
	P. calensis, P. heterotremus,	*P. calensis, P. heterotremus, P. kellicotti,*
	P. kellicotti, P. mexicanus,	*P. mexicanus, P. philippensis,*
	P. philippinensis, P. polonaise,	*P. polonaise, P. uterobilateralis*
	P. uterobilateralis	
	Schistosoma japonicum	*Schistosoma japonicum*
	Strongyloides stercoralis	*Strongyloides stercoralis*

Continued

Table 17.1. Continued.

Organism	Dogs	Cats
Arthropods	***Toxocara canis*** ***Trichinella spiralis*** **Fleas** Pentastomids (*Linguatula*) Ticks	***Toxocara cati*** ***Trichinella spiralis*** **Fleas**

The disease in the dog occurs in two forms, the furious and the dumb. In furious rabies, the animal becomes restless, wanders away from home and bites anybody or anything that comes in its way. It is unable to bark, may attempt to eat sticks and stones, but is foiled in the attempt by a difficulty in swallowing. It foams at the mouth and suffers from the progressive paralysis of dumb rabies and is dead within a few days. Sometimes the furious course is not followed and only dumb rabies is manifest.

While the disease is invariably fatal in domestic dogs, cats and cows, it would appear to have a more variable effect in wild dogs such as foxes and wolves. Certainly, rabies controls fox populations, but individuals do recover from the disease. There is little evidence to support the finding of a reservoir in such canines, but this may not be the case in rodents and bats. Rabies virus has been found in the mongoose and in the multimammate or grey rat, *Mastomys natalensis*. These animals suffer from rabies, but subclinical infections may occur. When canines feed on small mammals then they can acquire rabies. Vampire bats have been shown to recover from the disease, and rabies virus has also been isolated from insectivorous bats, which do not take blood meals. This suggests that rabies may exist in a mild and asymptomatic form for most of the time in these mammals, but that when they bite or people enter their virus-contaminated habitat, they are at risk of losing their life.

Incubation period. This depends upon the proximity of the point of introduction of the virus to the brain and the size of the infective dose. It is usually 2–12 weeks, but can be years in young children with a minor bite.

Period of communicability. Theoretically, person-to-person infection is possible, so barrier nursing should be instigated. Animals are infectious from 3 to 14 days before clinical signs start until they die or are killed, but their saliva remains infectious.

Some 60% of persons bitten by a known rabid animal do not contract the disease.

Occurrence and distribution. A disease that strikes terror into people, it is widely spread throughout the world, as important in temperate as in tropical countries. It is common in Russia, Africa, Asia and South America. It is estimated that there are 20,000 deaths per annum in India and 24,000 for the whole of Africa. It is particularly dangerous to children aged 5–15 years, especially males, who are the main victims.

In industrialized countries and urban areas of South America, rabies is largely eliminated. Developing countries that have undertaken mass vaccination of dogs, such as Thailand, now have very low rates. The majority of post-exposure rabies vaccinations are given in China and India.

In South America, the vampire bat transmits rabies, particularly to cattle, but insectivorous and fruit-eating bats have also been found infected. Other animals that have transmitted rabies are wolves, foxes, jackals, hyenas, mongooses, skunks and racoons.

Control and prevention. Control measures can be aimed against the domestic dog and the reservoir in wild animals, and also in protecting the human.

Domestic dogs should be licensed and vaccinated, destroying all strays. Vaccination of all domestic animals with an approved vaccine should be mandatory in all endemic areas.

Control of the wild animal reservoir is a massive undertaking but alteration of habitat and local destruction around dwellings or place of work can be practised. As rabies follows a natural cycle in many wild animals, their total destruction over large areas may upset this balance and produce a rebound increase, so it is preferable to try and maintain this balance by using vaccination. This has been effectively used in Europe and Canada by leaving vaccine baits for wild animals to take. With bat rabies, control of bats is largely unsuccessful and it is preferable to vaccinate cattle, which are the main victims.

People who are at special risk, such as veterinarians, animal handlers and those working with bats, can be vaccinated with human diploid cell vaccine (HDCV), purified Vero cell vaccine (PVRV) or purified chick embryo cell vaccine (PCEV). Adverse reactions do occur so the vaccine should only be administered to those at risk of exposure to rabies. The vaccine is given on days 0, 7 and 21 or 28. Antibody monitoring, if available, is preferable to giving booster doses, but if the rabies-virus neutralizing antibody titre falls to >0.5 IU/ml then booster doses at 1 year and then every 5 years can be given. However, with HDCV and PVRV, protection is probably maintained for 10 years.

Because children 5–15 years old are the group most at risk of dying from rabies, some countries may consider vaccinating children with three doses of 0.1 ml (HDCV) given intradermally at 2, 3 and 4 months of age.

The criteria generally applied to visitors entering a rabies area are: if they can reach a vaccination centre within 24 h then there is no need to have prophylactic vaccination, otherwise they should receive a course of vaccination before they enter the area.

Treatment. Fortunately, rabies virus can be inactivated on its passage along the peripheral nerves and this is the main method of protecting the individual bitten by a rabid dog. The first procedure is to wash out the wound thoroughly with soap or detergent under running water, followed by a quaternary ammonium compound or 0.1% iodine. Any alcohol, such as whisky or gin, can be used if there is nothing else available. If there is a high suspicion of infection then rabies antiserum should also be injected locally around the wound. Tetanus toxoid and penicillin should be administered, as tetanus is often a greater danger from a bite than rabies.

If the biting animal can be caught then it should be tied up and observed for 10 days. After this time it will either have died from the disease or remained well. If it has died or was killed, then the head is severed with aseptic precautions (as the saliva is highly infectious), packed in ice and sent to a laboratory for viral antigen testing or histological studies. Sections of the brain will show characteristic Negri bodies.

Post-exposure vaccination can be given with HDCV, PVRV or PCEV immediately and on days 3, 7, 14 and 28, into the deltoid muscle in adults and the thigh in children (do not give in the gluteal region). An alternative is to give two doses immediately, one into the left deltoid and the other into the right, followed by one dose on day 7 and another on day 21. If pre-exposure immunization was given, then give one dose immediately and a second in 3 days. The normal dose is 1 ml intramuscularly (or 0.5 ml with some preparations), but because of the high cost money can be saved by giving much smaller doses (0.1 ml HDCV) intradermally.

Post-exposure vaccination must be given as soon as possible and definitely within 24 h of the bite. Every effort should be made to reach a vaccination centre within this period, but if this becomes impossible or the nature of the animal contact is uncertain then it is still worth giving a course of vaccination as soon as this can be done (see Table 17.2).

Hyperimmune antirabies serum is given as soon as possible, half around the wound and the rest intramuscularly. Human immune globulin is preferable, but if horse serum only is available then a test dose must first be given. The doses are:

- human immune globulin 20 IU/kg body weight; or
- animal immune globulin 40 IU/kg body weight.

Table 17.2 summarizes the procedure to be followed in treating a person who has been attacked by an animal that could have rabies.

Surveillance. Cases of rabies should be reported to the World Health Organization (WHO) which has been collecting information on its Rabnet site (see Further Reading). Countries should work towards a system of vaccine certification of dogs using microchip implants or permanent collars containing vaccination details.

17.2 Hydatid Disease

Organism. *Echinococcus granulosus*, a cyclophyllidean tapeworm of canines.

Clinical features. Infection is normally acquired in childhood, but clinical manifestations do not appear until middle age. There may be vague epigastric pain in the early stages but it is normally only when cysts develop in specific organs that symptoms related to that organ develop.

Hydatid cysts, the intermediate stage of the parasite, have been recorded from all parts of the human body. The commonest site is the liver,

Table 17.2. Post-exposure and antirabies guide. This is only a guide and should be used in conjunction with local knowledge of rabies endemicity and the animal involved.

Type of animal	Status of animal	Type of exposure	Treatment
Domestic			
Dog, cat, cow	Healthy and remains so for 10 days	Category 1: touching, feeding or licks on intact skin	None
Dog, cat, cow	Signs suggestive of rabies. Retain animal for 10 days	Category 2: minor scratch, abrasion or lick on broken skin, nibbling of uncovered skin	Rabies vaccine (can be discontinued if animal not rabid by day 5)
Dog, cat, cow	Rabid or becomes so during retention	Category 3: single or multiple transdermal bite, scratch or lick of mucous membrane with saliva	Immunoglobulin plus vaccine
Domestic or wild			
Fox, wolf, racoon, mongoose, bat, etc.	Unprovoked attack, escaped, killed or unknown	Category 3: bite, scratch or contamination of mucous membrane with saliva (lick)	Immunoglobulin plus vaccine

followed by the lung, abdomen, kidney and brain in descending order of frequency. As the cysts increase in size they can cause serious problems, sometimes fatally. The cyst contents are infective so if they rupture either accidentally or at operation, then numerous new cysts are formed. The liberation of so much foreign protein into the body can result in a severe anaphylactic reaction.

Diagnosis of the disease is clinically, from enlargement of liver, or from the discovery of a cyst on chest X-ray. Ultrasound scanning of suspect cases is a simple method in rural areas. Immunological methods are useful. A diagnostic aspiration of the cyst must never be made.

Transmission. Eggs passed in dog faeces contaminate pasture land and when eaten by sheep, pigs, goats, cattle, camels and horses develop into hydatid cysts (Fig. 17.1). The hydatid cyst is a fluid-filled sack containing enormous numbers of scolices, any of which can become an adult worm in the dog. The common means of infection is for dogs to be fed the offal of domestic animals. In the wild, jackals, wolves and wild dogs become infected by killing and eating infected herbivores.

Humans enter this cycle accidentally by swallowing the eggs either:

- through food items, e.g. fruit or vegetables contaminated by dog faeces;

- drinking water contaminated by dog faeces;
- close contact with dogs, e.g. by touching their fur or being licked by them (when a dog licks itself it can spread eggs all over its body as well as them sticking to its tongue).

Primary infection commonly occurs in childhood, with symptoms developing in adult life.

Incubation period. Generally a period of several years.

Period of communicability. Dogs are often repeatedly infected so continue to be a source of infection, especially to children.

Occurrence and distribution. The disease is widespread, but occurs in concentrated pockets, such as sheep-rearing areas or where dogs live in close proximity to humans. A very high rate of infection is found in the Turkana people of northern Kenya where dogs are trained to care for young children.

Control and prevention can be implemented at several points in the life cycle. Infected material should not be fed to dogs or, if this cannot be avoided, it must be well cooked. Dogs can be treated with praziquantel to remove any adult worms. Measures should be taken to reduce faecal contamination, such as fencing water sources and food gardens, or the general training of dogs.

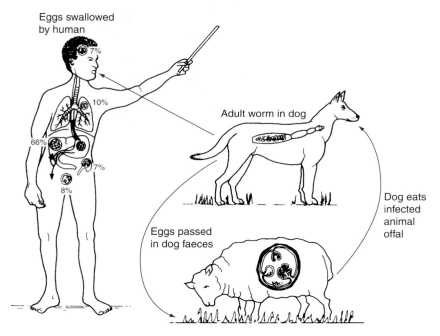

Fig. 17.1. Hydatid disease, the life cycle of *Echinococcus granulosus*.

Ultimately though, control will depend upon human attitudes to dogs – by keeping them to their proper place, not touching them or feeding them at mealtimes, destroying unwanted animals and observing personal hygiene. Children, in particular, should be taught to wash their hands before eating and after touching dogs.

Treatment. Albendazole and mebendazole are effective but, where necessary, surgical removal may be required, taking care to remove the entire cyst or, if rupture seems likely, to sterilize the contents with formalin. Praziquantel will prevent the development of secondary cysts if rupture of a primary cyst has taken place, so is a useful precaution during surgery.

A similar, but rarer, infection is with *E. multilocularis*, which as its name suggests forms multiloculated lesions rather than single cysts. These invade the body in much in the same way as a neoplastic growth, including producing metastases. *E. multilocularis* is found in the colder regions of the world (Siberia, Alaska and northern Canada), and is a parasite of foxes and dogs, with voles, lemmings and mice being intermediate hosts.

Another variety of the disease, found in Colombia, Ecuador and Brazil is that from infection with *E. vogeli*, and is caught by dogs eating agoutis, pacas and spiny rats. A polycystic hydatid cyst results.

Surveillance. Sheep carcases can be inspected in abattoirs to detect hydatid cysts. Ultrasound scans can be used in high prevalence areas to detect cases.

17.3 Toxocariasis

Organism. The roundworms of dogs, *Toxocara canis* and less commonly that of cats, *T. catis*.

Clinical features. Finding themselves in an abnormal host, larvae are unable to complete their development in the human body and wander until they die. The body responds to this invasion by the production of eosinophils but, more serious, is the tissue to which the larvae go. While much of the time this is not serious, they have an unfortunate predilection for the eye, which can result in blindness. In heavy infections there is fever, a cough, an urticarial rash and enlargement of the liver.

Pneumonitis, chronic abdominal pain and focal neurological lesions may also develop.

Diagnosis can be made with larval antigen ELISA.

Transmission. Eggs are accidentally ingested from the dog's fur, from contaminated soil or from vegetables contaminated by dog faeces. The typical picture is of the young child playing with soil frequented by pet dogs and putting their fingers in their mouth. The eggs are resistant to desiccation and remain in the soil for many months so that the soil in parks and other areas where dogs are taken for walks can be heavily contaminated.

Larvae are also found in the livers of chickens, cattle and sheep, and if these are not adequately cooked infection can result from their consumption.

Incubation period. Transient infection may occur after a few weeks, but more serious eye complications will probably not present until the child is 5 years or older.

Period of communicability. Although the infection itself is not transferred from one human to another, the eggs may be so from unhygienic habits.

Occurrence and distribution. Distribution is worldwide wherever dogs and cats are found living in close association with humans, especially as pets. There is a high seroprevalence rate in the Caribbean, indicating heavy contact with infected dogs in early childhood.

Control and prevention. Dogs should be prevented from promiscuous defecation in playgrounds, streets, parkland and vegetable gardens. Owners of pets should scoop up faeces and dispose of them safely. Stray animals, especially unwanted puppies, should be destroyed. Dogs and cats should be dewormed at 6 monthly intervals, starting when the animal is 3 weeks old. Young children should not play with pets and be taught personal hygiene from a young age.

Treatment. Albendazole and mebendazole are used in treatment of the acute case, but will not cure eye damage.

Surveillance. Warning signs should be erected, particularly in urban areas, to instruct people to collect their pet's faeces and dispose of them

properly. Checks can be made regularly to see that this is being done. School health programmes will detect children with damaged eyes and indicate an area where further investigation is required.

17.4 Larva Migrans

Organism. The larval forms of several animal parasites wander aimlessly in the human body if they enter it by mistake. Examples are the cat and dog hookworms, *Ancylostoma brasiliense*, *A. stenocephala* and *A. canium*, which produce a condition called creeping eruption; and the cat and dog filariae, *Dirofilaria immitis*, *Brugia pahangi* and *B. patei*, which cause the more serious disease of visceral larva migrans. *Bayliscaris procyonis*, a roundworm of racoons, can result in fatal encephalitis.

Clinical features. Creeping eruption is often visible as serpiginous tracks just underneath the skin, which contain wandering larvae. These are painful and red at the advancing end, and cause intense pruritus. They advance a little each day, sometimes continuing for several years.

In larva migrans, the body reacts to the wandering parasites, especially when they pass through the lungs, with a profound eosinophilia, one of the causes of the condition known as pulmonary eosinophilia. Symptoms are a paroxysmal cough, not unlike asthma, with the production of large quantities of sputum, sometimes streaked with blood. A diagnosis of tuberculosis can mistakenly be made.

Diagnosis is largely made on clinical grounds but the filaria antigen of *D. immitis* can be used as a skin test in larva migrans.

Transmission. The animal hookworm larvae are contracted in the same way as human *Ancylostoma* infection (Section 10.3): walking without adequate foot covering in an area of soil contaminated by dog and cat faeces. The filarial worms are transmitted by culicine mosquitoes, but as with human disease, repeated infection is required. The racoon roundworm is deposited in frequently used defecation areas, which can be associated with urban structures such as rooftops, attics and woodpiles, and found in gardens close to trees, where humans, especially children, inadvertently pick up the eggs and swallow them.

Incubation period. Variable, weeks to months.

Occurrence and distribution. Found in the tropical and temperate regions of the world in areas where dogs and cats are kept as pets or for hunting. Racoons are progressively moving into urban areas where they pose a risk to children in particular.

Control and prevention. Infection with animal hookworms is prevented in the same way as human infection with *Ancylostoma*, through the wearing of adequate footwear (Section 10.3). Efforts can be made to reduce cat and dog fowling by restraining the animals and keeping them to designated parts of the village. Children should be taught to wash their hands before eating.

The same methods as are used to reduce mosquito bites in lymphatic filariasis (Section 15.7) are applicable to the prevention of infection by dog and cat filariae, especially the use of repellents and insecticide-treated nets.

Treatment. Larva migrans responds dramatically to diethylcarbamazine, while albendazole or ivermectin can be used in creeping eruptions.

Surveillance. *D. immitis* skin test surveys can be used, but there is a cross reaction with other filarial infections. Regular surveys can be made of dog populations and unwanted animals destroyed.

A localized form of visceral larva migrans occurring in Thailand and China results from *Gnathostoma spinigerum*, an intestinal parasite of cats and dogs. People are infected by the larval stage through eating raw fish. The infection presents as a single migratory swelling, either superficially or in the deeper tissues. Cerebral lesions are not uncommon, while generally there is intense itching and eosinophilia. If the larva comes near the surface of the body it can be removed surgically, otherwise albendazole, mebendazole and diethylcarbamazine have been reported to have some effect. Ensuring that fish are properly cooked is the easiest method of control.

17.5 Toxoplasmosis

Organism. The coccidian protozoan *Toxoplasma gondii*, found in the cat.

Clinical features. The toxoplasmas which develop from the oocysts disperse to many parts of the body, including the CNS, where they form small inflammatory foci (pseudocysts). They result in surprisingly little pathology to their host, only occasionally producing lymphadenopathy and a low-grade fever. The lymph nodes are discrete, firm and persist for some time. A maculopapular rash may develop and hepatosplenomegaly, and hilar and mediastinal lymphadenopathy may develop. The illness is generally self-limiting but if primary toxoplasmosis is acquired during pregnancy congenital infection of the foetus will develop. The infant may have hepatosplenomegaly, chorioretinitis or mental retardation and quite often dies. Hydrocephaly, microcephaly, jaundice and convulsions can suggest infection in the infant that survives. Toxoplasmosis can also become reactivated in the immunocompromised, e.g. in the human immunodeficiency virus (HIV)-infected individual, causing pneumonia, a maculopapular rash, chorioretinitis, myocarditis or fatal cerebral toxoplasmosis.

Recent evidence has suggested that far from the pseudocysts causing little pathology when they attach to the brain of the non-neonate, an alteration in human response time may result. Experiments in mice show that by the parasite selectively attacking the brain, it disables the animal's response to the presence of a predator, so making that animal more easily caught and the parasite therefore transmitted. In the human, the effect is to prolong reaction time, making the victim more likely to have a road-traffic accident.

T. gondii has also been linked to neurosis and schizophrenia, the innocent pseudocyst being a causal factor in these conditions. Of more serious consequences is a recently discovered correlation between this parasite and brain cancer, but a cause and effect has not yet been established.

Diagnosis can be made by finding the specific IgM or a rise in IgG in sequential sera. The characteristic pseudocysts can be found in the blood, in enlarged lymph nodes or in post-mortem material. These consist of cells distended with the characteristic nucleated crescent shaped bodies of *T. gondii* filling the cavity. PCR can be used but is not specific enough to recommend termination of pregnancy.

Transmission. Oocysts are passed in cat faeces and, if accidentally swallowed by humans, the humans acquire the disease. Children are commonly infected when playing with pets, or in sand and soil in which cats defecate. Adults are more commonly infected from swallowing pseudocysts in undercooked meat (generally mutton or pork). Congenital infection occurs when the mother becomes infected during the early course of her pregnancy. Oocysts can be inhaled or drunk in contaminated water, and toxoplasma tachyzoites are passed in cow and goat milk. They can also be dispersed into the air from dried material, e.g. cat faeces.

Incubation period. 10–20 days.

Period of communicability. Mothers can pass on infection to their fetus anytime during pregnancy, but the more serious disease results from infection in the first few months. Oocysts remain viable in moist soil or water for at least a year, and in raw meat until it is cooked.

Occurrence and distribution. Exposure to toxoplasmosis is common and widespread, with up to 40% of people seropositive in some countries. Infection is also found in birds and other mammals, including sheep, cattle, goats, pigs, chickens and rodents. All members of the cat family can produce oocysts, and often become infected from eating rodents or birds.

Control and prevention is by personal hygiene, especially hand washing after touching cats. Cats should be banished at mealtimes and when food is being prepared. The habit of giving cats scraps of food during the course of a meal should be strongly discouraged. All meat should be properly cooked and milk pasteurized. Children's play areas, especially sandpits, should be protected from cats.

Treatment. Sulfadiazine plus pyrimethamine plus folinic acid can be used for treatment and also as prophylaxis in the HIV-infected person.

Surveillance. In high-incidence areas, pregnant women can be asked questions on contact with cats or eating undercooked meat during antenatal visits. Seroprevalence surveys can be undertaken in households and neighbourhoods of a case and in areas of high prevalence.

17.6 Brucellosis

Organism. A Gram-negative bacillus, *Brucella melitensis* (biovars 1–3), *B. abortus* (biovars 1–6), *B. suis* (biovars 1, 3 and 4) and *B. canis*. *B. melitensis*

causes the disease in goats that was first investigated in Malta (Melita was the Roman name for the island). *B. abortus*, as its name implies, causes abortion in cattle. *B. suis* is an infection of pigs. Both pigs and sheep are often infected with *B. melitensis* and *B. abortus*. *B. canis* is restricted to dogs.

The organism is killed by heating at 60°C for 10 min and by treating with 1% phenol for 15 min. It survives well in milk and cream cheeses that have not fermented or gone hard. In places contaminated by the faeces and urine of infected animals, survival can be for months and even years, especially at lower temperatures. With temperatures above 25°C, survival time is reduced.

Clinical features. The severity and duration of the disease is very variable and it may go undiagnosed for a considerable period of time. Characteristically, there are intermittent or irregular fevers (undulant fever) with generalized aches and pains. The patient is unduly weak and tired, often retiring in the second half of the day. There may be depression, a cough, lymphadenopathy and splenomegaly. Recovery may occur spontaneously or the disease may become chronic, with the undulant pattern of fever and fatigue more pronounced. If not treated, this can continue for 6 months to 1 year, after which 80% of patients fully recover. A wide range of complications can occur, including large joint destruction, depression, deafness, meningitis, endocarditis and glaucoma. Changes in vessel walls can lead to a propensity to deep vein thrombosis and pulmonary embolus.

Diagnosis is difficult, but isolation of the organism from blood, bone marrow or urine should be attempted. A test for serum agglutinating antibodies (the Rose Bengal test, RBT; or the serum agglutination test, SAT) combined with the detection of non-agglutinating antibody test using ELISA IgG or Coombs IgG is confirmatory. PCR can be used where facilities exist.

Transmission. Humans are infected by drinking raw milk or consuming milk produce. *B. melitensis* is mainly spread by unpasteurized goat's milk or in cream cheeses prepared from it. *B. abortus* has less invasive power and virulence when consumed in cow's milk and so asymptomatic infection can occur. Infection can also be transmitted by blood,

Table 17.3. Infections transmitted to humans from cattle and pigs or in which cattle and pigs are the reservoir. (**Bold** mentioned in the text.)

Organism	Cattle	Pigs
Viruses	**Cowpox** **Crimean–Congo** **haemorrhagic fever** **Hepatitis E** **Rabies** **Rift Valley fever**	**Avian influenza** **Crimean–Congo** **haemorrhagic fever** **Influenza** **Hepatitis E** **Japanese encephalitis** La Crosse encephalitis Manangle Nipah **Severe Acute Respiratory** **Syndrome (SARS)**
Prion	**Creutzfeldt–Jakob (variant)**	
Bacteria	**Anthrax** *Brucella abortus* *Campylobacter jejuni* *Clostridium perfringens* *Escherichia coli* O157 *Leptospira interrogans* Hardjo **Lyme disease** *Mycobacterium bovis* *Salmonella* **Staphylococcal food poisoning** **Streptococcal infection** **Tetanus**	**Anthrax** *Brucella suis*, *B. melitensis*, *B. abortus* *Campylobacter jejuni* *Clostridium perfringens* *Leptospira interrogans* Pomona *Salmonella* Yersiniosis **Tetanus**
Rickettsia	Q fever	
Fungi	Coccidioidomycosis Cryptococcosis *Trichophyton verrucosum*	Coccidioidomycosis
Protozoa	Babesiosis **Cryptosporidiosis** **Toxoplasmosis**	*Balantidium coli* **Cryptosporidiosis** **Toxoplasmosis** *Trypanosoma brucei gambiense*
Helminths	*Fasciola hepatica* *Fasciolopsis buski* *Schistosoma japonicum* *Taenia saginata*	*Fasciolopsis buski* *Heterophyes heterophyes* *Metagonimus yokogawai* *Clonorchis sinensis*, *Opisthorchis viverrini* *Paragonimus westermani*, *P. africanus*, *P. calensis*, *P. heterotremus*, *P. kellicotti*, *P. mexicanus*, *P. philippinensis*, *P. pulmonalis*, *P. uterobilateralis* *Schistosoma japonicum* *Taenia solium* *Trichinella spiralis*, *T. nelsoni*, *T. nativa*
Arthropods	Pentastomids (*Linguatula*) **Ticks**	**Ticks**

placental tissue or uterine secretions from cattle, sheep, goats and camels when they are slaughtered, during delivery of their young or through close contact. Those whose occupations brings them into close proximity to infected animals can acquire infection through abraded skin, mucous membranes, the conjunctiva, or by an aerosol of organisms through the respiratory tract. Such persons as farmers, shepherds, goatherds, vets and abattoir workers are at greatest risk. Animal handlers can contract the much rarer *B. canis* infection from dogs.

Incubation period is from 7 to 60 days (usually 2–4 weeks) but can be up to 7 months.

Period of communicability. Not transmitted from person to person.

Occurrence and distribution. The disease is mainly one of animals, resulting in economic losses to society and ill health to those involved in looking after animals. Brucellosis is common in South and Central America, Africa, the Mediterranean and South, South-west and Central Asia. It is often not recognized, but is found in a large number of animals if it is looked for. In the Sudan and Nigeria 60% of cattle were found to be infected.

Cattle become infected from eating placentae, licking a dead fetus or close contact with contaminated surroundings, such as cattle paddocks, barns or shelters. The young can obtain infection through the milk of their mothers.

Control and prevention is by pasteurization or boiling of cow's and goat's milk. Where pasteurization is not a legal requirement then people should be told of the risks of drinking raw milk and advised to boil it.

Anybody working with animals, especially those concerned with the slaughter of animals, or coming into contact with products of abortion, should wear overalls and gloves that are frequently washed and sterilized. Proper animal husbandry reduces areas of contaminated pasture land that perpetuates infection.

Where facilities permit, animals can be rendered *Brucella* free by diagnosis and slaughter of infected animals. A useful test for this purpose is the milk ring test on cow's milk. Haematoxylin-stained *Brucella* antigen is added to a sample of cow's milk and, if positive, a blue ring appears at the interface.

By removing infected animals from a herd and preventing them from coming into contact with others, whole areas of land, and even complete countries, have been made *Brucella* free. This is a large and expensive undertaking and beyond the means of many developing countries. An alternative is to vaccinate herds. The live attenuated vaccine Rev-1 or the recombinant vaccine RB51 can be given to calves at 6–8 months. Vaccination can also be given to adult animals but should not be administered if an eradication programme is envisaged as it then becomes impossible to tell whether an animal is infected or not.

Treatment is with doxycycline 100 mg twice a day for 45 days + streptomycin 1 g daily for 15 days. Alternatively, doxycycline 100 mg twice daily for 45 days + rifampicin 600–900 mg daily for 45 days can be given. Gentamycin can be used instead of streptomycin in the event of side effects.

Surveillance of cattle is by using the milk-ring test (see above). Brucellosis is a notifiable disease in countries in which it has been eliminated, such as in northern Europe, the USA and Japan.

17.7 Anthrax

Organism. *Bacillus anthracis* is a rod-shaped organism occurring in pairs or chains and staining positively with Gram stain. In the vegetative state in the animal, or where there is a low oxygen content, the bacillus is surrounded by a capsule. If the dead animal's tissues become exposed to the air or the organism is cultured aerobically then spores develop. Spores have the appearance of round filling defects within the stained rods.

The vegetative form is killed by heat at 55°C for 1 h, or if the carcass is not opened, putrefaction will raise the internal temperature sufficiently (30°C for 80 h) to render it free of organisms. However, if the carcass is butchered or a post-mortem performed then exposure to the air encourages the development of the highly resistant spores, which are one of the most persistent forms of life known. They have survived 160°C for 1 h and −78°C despite thawing and refreezing, while in pastures they have been found viable after 12 years and possibly up to 60 years.

Clinical features. Essentially an infection of cattle, anthrax ranks with rabies and plague as a much-feared and fatal disease. Infection commences with a small papule at the site of inoculation. By the second day, a ring of vesicles surrounds the lesion; these are at first clear, but then become bloodstained. The central papule then ulcerates and enlarges to form a depressed dark eschar, which increases in size and darkens to the black coal colour that gives the disease its name (anthrax is Greek for coal). Pus is never present despite the development of oedema around the lesion. The oedema is extensive and may cause respiratory difficulty if around the neck. The associated lymph nodes are often enlarged, but must be left to resolve spontaneously. The primary lesion commonly occurs on the head or face, while the neck and forearm are also often affected. Surprisingly, the fingers are rarely involved.

As well as the primary lesion and its surrounding oedema, there are systemic symptoms of varying severity. The patient feels unwell although the temperature is normal or only slightly raised. A high temperature or weak pulse are serious signs, generally indicating pulmonary disease which results from the inhalation of a large dose of spores. Illness sets in rapidly with cough, dyspnoea and cyanosis. Lymph nodes enlarge and there is splenomegaly. This passes into a stage of cardiovascular collapse and the patient is dead within 2–3 days.

Intestinal anthrax is another uncommon but severe form of the disease resulting from people eating infected meat. The primary lesion occurs in the intestines and the massive oedema that results produces intestinal obstruction as well as systemic symptoms. However, cutaneous anthrax is the commonest form of the disease, even in people who butcher and subsequently eat an animal that has died from anthrax.

Diagnosis is made by examining fluid from the vesicle in a person who gives a history of contact with an animal that recently died. A smear is made on to two slides, one being stained by Gram and the other fixed by heat and stained with methylene blue or Giemsa. The first shows Gram-positive rods and the second demonstrates the red capsule surrounding the blue bacilli. This finding can be confirmed by culture on selective media.

Transmission. Anthrax spores are ingested or become accidentally inoculated through the skin, such as by thistle scratches around the muzzle or legs of an animal close grazing in an infected pasture. Biting flies have also been incriminated. The spores germinate into the vegetative form, which rapidly invades, increasing in virulence. A local lesion grows at the point of inoculation and extensive oedema develops around it. The capsulated bacilli produce a lethal factor which causes anoxic hypertension or cardiac collapse, resulting in sudden death of the animal. After death the animal appears black from tarry blood that is slow to clot.

People are infected by contact with the deceased animal, either in butchering and handling of the infected meat, or at a place far removed from the death of the animal from spores in its hide, hair or bones.

Incubation period is from 2 to 7 days, but can be up to 60 days.

Period of communicability. Not transmitted from person to person.

Occurrence and distribution. The disease commonly affects cattle, sheep, goats and horses, but has occurred in dogs and cats. It is probably widespread in the wild and has been found in elephants and hippopotami and on the claws and beaks of vultures and other scavenger birds. Widespread in the bovine populations of the world, its persistence in the environment and in the produce of cattle makes it an ever-present threat both in the developing and developed world. It is a particular problem in Africa, South-west Asia, Russia, South and Central America.

Control and prevention are difficult owing to the persistence of the organism in the environment, but once an outbreak starts it should be possible to bring it to an end by vigorous control of animals and their slaughter. No animal that dies from anthrax should be allowed to be butchered and sold for meat. Its hide and bones are also infectious, so should be deep buried with lime or burnt. Anthrax is a common disease in pastoralists. For fuel, these people often conserve dried cow dung, which also makes an ideal material to incinerate the carcass as it burns slowly but continuously.

The animal should not be cut open to obtain specimens or perform autopsy; cutting off an ear is quite sufficient for diagnostic purposes.

Once anthrax is recognized then all animals should be vaccinated with a live attenuated vaccine. Due to the persistence of the organism in the soil, especially at a site where an infected animal has been buried, anthrax is likely to recur year after year at the same site, so called anthrax districts. Hot, moist areas are particularly liable to offer the right conditions for continuous sporulation and germination, leading to a steady infectious state throughout the year. In contrast, hot arid areas encourage spore formation and when the vegetation dries out, close grazing brings the animal into proximity with the spores in the dust, so a dry season outbreak is more common. This can be anticipated and cattle vaccinated prior to the anthrax season.

Anthrax is an occupational disease in those persons who deal with the hides, hair (including wool) and bones of animals. The spores can persist almost indefinitely in these animal remains and when tested are found to be present in a large proportion. Pastoralists in particular will not waste an animal that dies, and taking off its skin and leaving the bones to dry in the sun encourages formation of spores which remain with these products when they are shipped all over the world. It is an impossible task to identify these infected animal products and because of the high proportion of them involved, an uneconomic process to destroy them. Quite surprisingly, people who handle infected hides and other animal products only rarely develop anthrax but they should be warned and provided with facilities for examination and treatment. Protective clothing should be provided and a ventilation system installed to remove spores in facilities where animal products are handled. Many industrial processes disinfect the animal products; hypochlorite effectively kills spores. With persons at increased risk of developing anthrax, then vaccination can be offered. The vaccine is from a sterile filtrate of *B. anthracis* and is given in 0.5 ml doses at 6 weeks after the initial dose, then at 6 months and thereafter at annual intervals. Modified anthrax can occur in vaccinated persons.

Treatment is with penicillin, to which the organism is very sensitive. Benzylpenicillin 4 million IU every 4–6 h for 7 days or, if still available, procaine penicillin 1 mega unit daily for 3 days can be used. No local treatment is required and surgical removal of the eschar or incision of oedema only leads to unpleasant scarring and the development of intractable sinuses. Ciprofloxacin or doxycycline can be used for respiratory and intestinal cases. Supportive measures need to be given for shock and tracheostomy may be required when there is severe oedema of the neck.

Surveillance. Anthrax is a notifiable disease in many countries. Where no animal source can be shown then bioterrorism should be considered (Section 19.6).

17.8 Leptospirosis

Organism. Leptospira interrogans, which has a large number of serovars, the most important of which is Icterohaemorrhagiae. It is passed in the urine of rats and can contaminate any area that they frequent. For the survival of the organism, there must be moisture, such as a canal or sewer, or else damp soil, the washings of abattoirs or similar conditions. The pH of the soil or water is important and the *Leptospira* cannot survive in an acid environment. Leptospirosis is therefore commoner in places where the soil is alkaline. Salt water and chlorine solutions rapidly kill the organism.

Clinical features. Commencing with fever, malaise, vomiting and myalgia, jaundice subsequently develops and there may be haemorrhages into the skin, mucous membranes and internal organs (including the lungs). The disease may progress to a more serious form with liver failure, renal failure or meningitis. However, many people only have mild infections and the vast majority do not exhibit any symptoms at all. In endemic areas, children are probably the most commonly infected.

Diagnosis is by finding the motile organism by dark field microscopy in a wet blood film during the first week of the disease. After this time, serological tests or animal inoculation can be used; *Leptospira* may be found in the urine from the third week onwards. Culture of the organism can take up to a month. Rapid tests that give a presumptive diagnosis are IgM ELISA, latex agglutination and lateral flow. A confirmatory test is a fourfold rise in the microscopic agglutination test (MAT) in paired samples taken at least 2 weeks apart, but because of the large numbers of serovars it is difficult to prepare the MAT for the specific infection. PCR can also be used.

Transmission. The *Leptospira* enters the skin of humans through minor abrasions or mucous membranes, although it does appear to be able to enter unbroken skin as well. Infection results from exposure to contaminated moist areas, such as during swimming in canals or walking barefoot over damp rat-infested soil. A direct rat bite can also transmit the disease, as can an aerosol of contaminated fluid or ingestion of contaminated food.

Other animals can become infected with different serovars, cattle and water buffalo with the Hardjo serovar, dogs with Canicola and pigs with Pomona. These domestic animals subsequently excrete *Leptospira* in their urine, thus contaminating the surroundings.

Incubation period is 4–19 days, usually 10.

Period of communicability. Leptospira are excreted in the urine for several months, but person-to-person spread is rare.

Occurrence and distribution. Where rats are common and conditions are favourable then the infection is widespread. In many areas that have been surveyed, *Leptospira* antibodies have been found in a large percentage of the population, and the disease is endemic in the community, with the occasional severe case. It is common in the tropics, particularly where the soil is alkaline or irrigation is used for agriculture. Infection is therefore common in rice paddy areas and sugarcane estates. This association of the disease with certain occupations is helpful in making the diagnosis. Such occupations as mine workers, farmers, canal cleaners, sewer workers, and people employed in the cleaning and preparation of fish or in abattoirs are at greatest risk.

Flooding can widen the area of contamination, leading to outbreaks in people not normally at risk. Disasters and any alteration in conditions that leads to an increase in the rat population will have a similar but more long-term effect.

Leptospirosis is a very widespread zoonotic infection of animals, endemic in many rodents, but especially rats. The organism has been found in a variety of wild animals, opossums, mongooses, skunks, hedgehogs, squirrels, deer and bats, but the two domestic rats *Rattus rattus* and *R. norvegicus* are by far and away the most important reservoirs. Domestic animals, dogs, cattle, water buffalo and pigs can become infected by wild animals and provide a ready source of infection to their attendants.

Control and prevention involves the avoidance of areas contaminated with rat and animal urine, often a difficult thing to achieve. Various measures are:

- the reduction of rats by extermination and the protection of buildings, especially those used for preparing meat and fish and housing domestic animals (see rat control in Box 16.1);
- the burning of sugarcane fields after harvest and the drying out of rice fields;
- the wearing of protective clothing to reduce abrasions and contamination;
- avoiding canals, lakes and bodies of water known to be infected;
- controlling the number of dogs;
- providing proper pens with drainage for domestic animals so that urine does not collect and make the surroundings sodden; and
- washing down food premises with a solution of chlorine or salt water.

Vaccination of persons at risk has been achieved in some countries using the specific serovar (this is available in China, Japan and Vietnam). Doxycycline prophylaxis can be used where short-term exposure is expected (e.g. in troops).

Treatment is with benzylpenicillin 2 million IU every 6 h or doxycycline 100 mg for 7 days, preferably within the first week of the illness.

Surveillance. Leptospirosis is a notifiable disease in many countries. Where outbreaks occur the cause should be investigated and specific control measures instituted.

17.9 Lassa Fever

Organism. Lassavirus, an arenavirus.

Clinical features. There is a gradual onset with fever, malaise, sore throat, cough, vomiting, diarrhoea and general aches and pains. By the second week, lymphadenopathy, pharyngitis and a maculopapular rash on the face or body develop. In severe cases, pleural effusion, encephalopathy, and cardiac and renal failure can occur, with a mortality of 15–20%.

In endemic areas, 80% of cases are mild or asymptomatic, so that serological investigation will find a large number of people with a past history of infection.

Diagnosis is often made on clinical criteria once the first case has been identified, in particular from inflammation of the throat and white tonsillar patches. Confirmatory diagnosis is made by testing for IgM or IgG in urine, blood or throat washings, with ELISA, PCR or IFA, and using extreme care.

Transmission is primarily through contact with the excreta (urine and faeces) of infected rodents, deposited on floors, beds or other surfaces, or through rat contamination of food or water. The main reservoir is the multimammate rat, and this is probably the method of spread in the endemic area, resulting in a large number of asymptomatic cases. However, in the severe case, all human body fluids are highly infectious so that secondary spread commonly occurs through contact with blood, urine, throat secretions and the aerosol produced by a coughing bout. The semen remains infectious for a considerable period of time so transmission via the sexual route can occur long after the person has recovered from their clinical illness.

Incubation period is 6–21 days.

Period of communicability. All body fluids are infectious from the start of the illness and for up to 9 weeks for urine and 3 months for semen.

Occurrence and distribution. Lassa fever is found in West and Central Africa, including the countries of Guinea, Sierra Leone, Liberia, Nigeria and Central African Republic (CAR), but serological testing has also found evidence of infection in Senegal, Mali, Guinea Bissau and the Democratic Republic of the Congo (DRC).

All ages and both sexes are susceptible, but pregnant women have a severe infection with high mortality and loss of the fetus.

Control and prevention is by control of the rats and careful isolation of patients. The multimammate rat lives in close proximity to humans in the home, in fields where people tend their crops, and in mines and similar industrial sites. Rats should be controlled (see Box 16.1) and prevented from entering the home. Food and drinking water should be protected with covers and a state of cleanliness observed to minimize contamination by rat excreta.

All cases must be hospitalized and:

- The patient should be rigorously isolated by the most secure means possible.

- Syringes, needles and all reused equipment should be carefully sterilized with 0.5% sodium hypochlorite, 0.5% phenol with a detergent, or by autoclaving or boiling.
- Extreme precautions should be taken with any oral secretions, blood, faeces and urine. Blood must be handled with the utmost precaution, using as a minimum hole-less rubber gloves. Faeces and urine should be placed in plastic bags, which are boiled or burnt.
- All articles used by the patient should be terminally disinfected with formaldehyde fumigation.

Treatment is with ribavirin intravenously for 10 days within the first 6 days of illness.

Surveillance. All close contacts of a case should be identified and followed up for 3 weeks with the temperature taken twice daily, with hospitalization if it rises above 38.3°C. Air travel makes it possible for an incubating case to travel to another country before showing symptoms, so if there is any indication, such as coming from an infected area, then the person should be admitted to hospital with strict barrier-nursing procedures. Any known or suspected case should be reported to WHO and neighbouring countries.

Summary

- Zoonoses are infections that are transmitted between animals and humans with dogs, cats, cattle and pigs as the main source, while the domestic rat is inadvertently involved.
- Understanding the nature of these diseases and, particularly, of the keeping of animals that transmit them, particularly pets, are necessary precautions.
- Proper animal husbandry and good personal hygiene are general preventive measures.
- Unwanted animals should be destroyed, vaccinated or controlled, and rats actively eliminated.

Further Reading

Eckert, J., Gemmell, M.A., Meslin, F.-X. and Pawlowski, Z.S. (2001) *WHO/OIE Manual on Echinococcosis in Humans and Animals: a Public Health Problem of Global Concern.* WHO, Geneva and World Organization for Animal Health, Paris.

Macpherson, C.N., Meslin, F.-X. and Wandeler, A.L. (2000) *Dogs, Zoonoses and Public Health.* CAB International, Wallingford, UK.

World Health Organization (2003) *Human Leptospirosis: Guidance for Diagnosis, Surveillance and Control.* WHO, Geneva.

World Health Organization (2005) *WHO Expert Consultation on Rabies, First Report, Geneva 5–8 October 2004.* Technical Report Series No. 931, WHO, Geneva.

World Health Organization (2008) *Anthrax in Humans and Animals*, 4th edn. WHO, Geneva.

Web resource

Rabies 'Rabnet', an interactive information system able to generate interactive maps and graphs using human and animal rabies data. Available at: www.who.int/rabies/rabnet/en/ (accessed 12 March 2012).

18 Pregnancy and Infection

Communicable diseases can have a major effect on a woman before, during and after pregnancy. She will be subject to any of the communicable diseases affecting the community but, in addition, there are certain infections that have particular importance to her and her offspring. Many of these have already been mentioned, but the full burden of the problem does not become apparent until they are all covered together. This chapter also includes rarer infections that have particularly damaging effects on the developing fetus.

Maternal mortality is a very sad cause of death and one of the most preventable of health problems. While the place of infection in this tragedy is not properly defined, some 358,000 women die each year in pregnancy and childbirth.

Communicable diseases affecting maternal and perinatal health are discussed here according to the timescale of a woman's life (Fig. 18.1).

18.1 Before Pregnancy

Any disease process that causes disfigurement, reduces the woman's general health or leads to infertility will handicap her likelihood of getting married. This group of diseases includes filariasis, leprosy and the sexually transmitted infections (STIs).

18.1.1 Filariasis

Infection with lymphatic filariasis, in its worst manifestations, leads to elephantiasis, gross disfiguring swellings of the legs, arms and, occasionally, breasts. The young woman with an elephantiasis limb, particularly in the Indian subcontinent, has almost no chance of getting married although the disease has no effect on her ability to become pregnant and successfully produce a child.

The World Health Organization (WHO) programme to eliminate filariasis using mass drug administration (MDA) excludes pregnant women and nursing mothers as well as children less than 1 year old, owing to the unwanted side effects of the medicines. Unlike malaria, it is the total number of mosquito bites that results in infection (probably in the order of tens of thousands), so methods of reducing the number of mosquito bites with mosquito nets, clothing, repellents, etc. all have their place in preventing this disfiguring disease. (See further in Section 15.7.)

18.1.2 Leprosy

Fortunately, with the availability of effective treatment, leprosy has lost much of the stigma that it had in the past. However, its presence has always been a reason for a man not to take a woman in marriage, unless that man also had leprosy. This has resulted in leprosy communities in many parts of the world where many of the members have or have had the disease and, with prolonged close contact, most of their children were subsequently afflicted. In more enlightened societies, the newly discovered leprosy patient, once started on treatment, can be fully integrated into ordinary life.

There has been considerable progress in the detection and treatment of leprosy cases, with the result that the disease is decreasing in all parts of the world. Only Brazil, Nepal and Timor-Leste (East Timor) have not yet reached the elimination target of one new case per 10,000 population; these three countries have 17% of all new cases detected globally. (See further in Section 12.6.)

18.1.3 Gonorrhoea

Gonorrhoea is one of the commonest STIs and is showing an increase in all parts of the world. It results in a mucoid or purulent urethral discharge in the male, but often goes unnoticed in the female unless it produces urethritis or acute salpingitis. It is the latter, or more commonly in an undetected

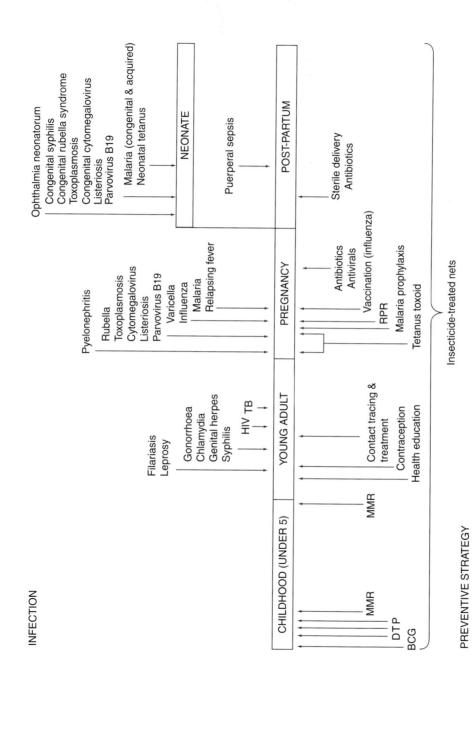

Fig. 18.1. Infections that impinge on the woman at different stages in her life and preventive measures that can be taken. BCG, Bacillus Calmette–Guérin vaccine; DTP, diphtheria, tetanus, pertussis vaccine; HIV, human immunodeficiency virus; MMR, measles, mumps, rubella vaccine; RPR, rapid plasma reagin test (for syphilis); TB, tuberculosis.

chronic form of salpingitis, that can lead to pelvic inflammatory disease and subsequently sterility in the female.

Some societies, particularly in Africa, and also Afro-Caribbean communities, prefer the woman to demonstrate her fertility by producing a child before she marries, while in others infertility can be grounds for divorce. Active infection while the mother is delivering can result in ophthalmia neonatorum in the newborn.

Diagnosis and adequate treatment are particularly difficult in developing countries and, as a result, it is estimated that there are some 62 million cases in the world. Gonorrhoea is more a problem of the sexually active under 25s than the existence of a reservoir in the commercial sex worker. Where possible, cases presenting at STI clinics should be encouraged to bring their partners (or provide information so that they might be traced) for counselling and treatment. Alternatively, contact cards can be sent anonymously to all contacts of a case. Any treatment regime may be ineffective in certain parts of the world and local expertise should be consulted to develop routines that are compatible with the resistance pattern and the availability of resources. (See further in Section 14.2 and Box 14.1.)

18.1.4 Chlamydia

Infection with chlamydia may present as a cervical discharge or urethritis in the female, but is usually asymptomatic and is often indistinguishable or present at the same time as gonorrhoea. Undiagnosed and untreated it can lead to salpingitis and pelvic inflammatory disease, which can result in ectopic pregnancy and chronic pelvic pain. In pregnancy, *Chlamydia trachomatis* infection of the cervix can cause ophthalmia neonatorum and neonatal pneumonia.

Chlamydia is probably one of the commonest of the STIs, but because it so often goes undiagnosed the full burden of infection is unknown. Local policy needs to be decided as to whether to attempt diagnosis or to routinely treat it if infection is suspected. (See further in Section 14.3.)

18.1.5 Genital herpes

Infection with herpesvirus simplex type 2 (HSV-2) produces painful vesicles on the genitalia, which can ulcerate. After apparent healing they recur at frequent intervals, often brought on by stress or menstruation. If the woman has a primary outbreak in late pregnancy, this can cause fetal infection, resulting in encephalitis, liver damage or lesions to the eye, mouth or skin. HSV-2 infection also carries an increased risk of the woman developing human immunodeficiency virus (HIV) infection.

Genital herpes is found worldwide and is becoming an increasing problem in the sexually active. As there is no cure, there is an increasing reservoir of infection, especially in developed countries. (See further in Section 14.8.)

18.1.6 Syphilis

The primary lesion of syphilis is the chancre (a painless ulcer with serous discharge), but pregnancy may mask its appearance, so it is often not noticed. It may look just like an abrasion or be on the cervix or extragenitally. Should syphilis not be discovered in the pregnant woman, the consequences for her fetus will be serious. If in early pregnancy, the child is likely to be stillborn, while in the later stages it will be born with a range of abnormalities, including deafness, sabre tibia, Hutchinson teeth and central nervous system (CNS) involvement. The use of antenatal screening tests (see Section 14.1) is therefore of the utmost importance where circumstances permit.

Syphilis is predominantly a disease of urban areas and where there is a sexual imbalance, such as mines, military establishments and among seamen. The increase in urbanization has resulted in migrant labourers who take the infection back home with them and pass it on to their wives or established partners. The main reservoir of syphilis is generally in the commercial sex worker or woman forced into prostitution to support her children. It is estimated that there are some 12 million cases of syphilis in the world, with a large proportion of these in tropical countries.

The main method of prevention is health promotion, which should start at school, encouraging the delay of first sexual experience and the benefits of a monogamous relationship. Programmes to support single mothers, divorced women and others forced into prostitution should be encouraged. Regular testing of commercial sex workers is often difficult unless their confidence is first obtained and treatment facilities made widely available on a walk-in basis. (See further in Section 14.1 and Box 14.1.)

18.1.7 Human immunodeficiency virus (HIV)

HIV infection threatens the mother and child at all stages of life, from the young sexually active adult, to infection in pregnancy and in the neonate.

After exposure to infection there is a latent period of 2–4 weeks, followed by an acute febrile illness, generally with lymphadenopathy, pharyngitis and a maculopapular rash. There is then a dormant period of several months after which there is a persistent and generalized lymphadenopathy, moderate weight loss and a number of other problems, including recurrent respiratory infections, chronic diarrhoea and unexplained anaemia. The disease progresses through a range of more serious symptoms, including HIV wasting syndrome and Kaposi's sarcoma; these are listed in Section 14.10. In addition, any infection with tuberculosis, leishmaniasis and American trypanosomiasis (Chagas' disease) will progress and become more severe.

Exposure is generally by sexual contact with an infected person, but can also be by inoculation with infected blood or blood products, and from an infected mother to her child before or during delivery or for up to 2 years after, if breastfed. Unprotected sexual contact is the most common method of transmission and the migrant worker acquiring infection from a commercial sex worker and returning to his home village to subsequently infect his wife is a very common pattern in many countries. The use of unsterile needles in the treatment of a range of conditions is also thought to be the manner in which infection has been widely disseminated in many developing countries. The infected mother can pass on infection congenitally to her fetus, but it more commonly occurs at the time of delivery due to contamination by the mother's blood. One of the commonest opportunistic infections in the severe case of HIV infection, Kaposi's sarcoma, can also be transmitted transplacentally. HIV virus is found in the mother's milk, with breastfeeding accounting for almost 50% of children infected.

HIV infection is found worldwide with an estimated 2.5 million people acquiring infection each year and 2.1 million dying from it. The worst affected area is sub-Saharan Africa, where the rates in young women are three times those in young men due to women's lack of socio-economic independence, and lack of education and access to health information and health services. The Caribbean is the second most affected area in the world, with some islands having very high incidence rates due to the lax attitude to promiscuity. The wide availability of treatment has resulted in a reduced fear of infection, leading to more risky behaviour, despite there still being no cure.

The contribution of HIV infection to maternal mortality is considerable, with an estimate of 61,400 extra maternal deaths due to HIV in 2008. Maternal mortality had been declining at a rate of 2.2% until 1980, but with the onset of the HIV epidemic in the early 1980s the rate of decline dropped to 1.8% between 1980 and 1990, and to 1.4% from 1990 to 2008. Southern Africa bore the greatest burden, with maternal mortality rates increasing in 2008 in Botswana, Lesotho, Malawi, Mozambique, Namibia, South Africa, Swaziland, Zambia and Zimbabwe.

The main method of control is health promotion, stressing monogamous relationships, safe-sex practice and the use of contraceptives (see Box 14.1). Contraceptive practice to reduce unintended pregnancies not only reduces the number of HIV-infected children, but the barrier effect of male and female condoms also decreases the risk of infection. Vaginal microbicides have recently been shown to provide a safe and effective method of preventing HIV.

Commercial sex workers should be identified and offered regular HIV testing and contraceptives, rather than making them illegal and driving the practice underground. HIV testing and counselling should be available at all special and general clinics and all mothers encouraged to be tested when attending antenatal clinic. An HIV mother should be advised on the risks to her and her infant during and after pregnancy and whether to breastfeed or artificially feed her child. Generally the risk of a child dying from diarrhoea resulting from contaminated bottles is greater than that of contracting HIV infection from breastfeeding, but local circumstances will dictate the best policy. Good obstetric practice should be promoted to reduce unnecessary interference, such as artificial rupture of the membranes and fetal scalp monitoring. There is no urgency to cut the umbilical cord, delaying this until it has stopped pulsating, or if the infant has taken its first breaths the placenta can even be delivered with the cord still intact. Disposable gloves, syringes, needles, scissors, etc. should be used or proper sterilization of these ensured. All blood for transfusion should be screened. Caesarean section should not be encouraged in developing countries as a way to reduce the risk of HIV transmission, as the dangers in subsequent pregnancies are considerably increased, but this might be the strategy of choice in developed countries. Treatment must be accompanied by preventive methods, as viral shedding can still occur.

When a pregnant woman is found to be HIV positive at antenatal clinic she should be counselled or else there is a strong possibility that she will not return. Her positive test should be confirmed using different antigens or confirmatory tests and her CD4 level (the level of T-lymphocytes bearing the CD4 receptor) determined. If the CD4 level is less than 350 or she has clinical stage 3 or 4 HIV she can be given cotrimoxazole prophylaxis for opportunistic infection and started on long-term antiretroviral therapy (ART). However, efavirenz should not be started in the first trimester. If the CD4 level is greater than 350 the woman should be given zidovudine (AZT) from 28 weeks until delivery and a single dose of nevirapine to take when she goes into labour. AZT and lamivudine are given during the course of labour and continued for 7 days after delivery. (For treatment regimes and details of the clinical staging of HIV see Section 14.10 and WHO, 2005 and 2010.)

The mother's CD4 level will determine the risk of transmitting the virus while breastfeeding, as shown in Table 18.1. The infant is given a single dose of nevirapine as soon after birth as possible (within the first 72 h) and a course of AZT depending on how long its mother took AZT for; if less than 4 weeks, then give a course of 4 weeks and if 4 or more weeks then AZT is prescribed just for 1 week. At 4 weeks, the infant should be given cotrimoxazole/trimethoprim prophylaxis.

Table 18.1. CD4 levels in HIV infection and the risk of a mother passing on infection to her child during delivery, by breastfeeding and the risk of maternal death as a result of her pregnancy. (From Kuhn *et al.*, 2009.)

CD4 level	Transmission (%)	Breast-feeding (%)	Maternal death (%)
>500	10	2	–
350–500	13	7.4	–
200–250	28	13	–
<200	44	21	55

18.1.8 Tuberculosis

Pregnancy, by lowering the immunological defences of the woman, makes her more liable to contract tuberculosis (TB) when she becomes pregnant and increases the severity of the disease if she is not adequately treated. Her problems are only compounded if she should have both TB and HIV.

Diagnosis can be difficult as lassitude and chronic anaemia are also found in pregnancy, but if there is a chronic cough then a sputum smear should be taken. Full treatment should be given, except for streptomycin which can be toxic to the fetus. It is unclear to what extent TB affects pregnancy outcome, although if treatment is not started until late pregnancy prematurity and neonatal mortality are increased. Even on treatment, there are more low-birth-weight and small-for-gestational-age infants.

In co-infection with HIV, combination ART should be started after but within 8 weeks of starting treatment for TB. (See further in Sections 13.1. and 18.1.7.)

18.2 During Pregnancy

Pregnancy is a dangerous time for the woman as she is burdened with an additional strain on her normal physiology and her immunity is decreased, making her more susceptible to infection, yet she is expected to continue to work and perform as she has always done. She also has to look after her children from previous pregnancies.

In many countries where there is a seasonal climatic pattern, conception generally takes place during the harvest when there is opportunity to reap the rewards of the year's labour, but this means that late pregnancy coincides with the rains when the greatest work effort is required but the mother's physical reserves are at their lowest. The rainy season is also the time for many seasonal illnesses, such as diarrhoea and malaria, increasing even more the burden of ill health on the woman and her children.

The pregnant woman's lowered immunity, a physiological process to prevent her rejecting her growing fetus, is probably due to high levels of adrenal steroids as well as to placental chorionic gonadotrophin and alpha-fetoprotein during the second half of pregnancy. There may also be a depression of lymphocyte activity. This makes her more susceptible to infections such as malaria, chickenpox and influenza. She also becomes more likely to contract common infections such as crypt-osporidiosis, although these are not more serious illnesses in the pregnant woman. With any infection, the extra strain placed on her body and her lowered immunity will increase her chance of developing more serious disease and a pregnant woman unfortunate enough to contract Lassa fever is more likely to die from it. Similarly hepatitis E (HEV), which normally occurs in epidemics with a low mortality rate, has an increased fatality rate of up to 20% if the pregnant woman is infected in the third trimester.

Early pregnancy is also a dangerous time for the developing fetus. Certain infections, such as rubella, toxoplasmosis and cytomegalovirus can cause severe damage, leading to disability or death of the developing infant. Mumps contracted during the first trimester is a cause of abortion but not of congenital abnormality.

18.2.1 Pyelonephritis

During pregnancy, there is an increased urinary flow and stasis due to atonia of the ureters as a result of the action of progesterone and of obstruction caused by the enlarging uterus. Asymptomatic bacilluria is also more common so that urinary tract infection ranging from a mild inconvenience in early pregnancy to severe renal disease can occur. Seventy five per cent of infections are due to *Escherichia coli*, with the remainder due to streptococci, staphylococci or the Proteus group of organisms. Acute pyelonephritis is the most common infection, affecting 1–2% of all pregnant women.

Clinically, there is pain on micturition (dysuria), the desire to pass urine even though the bladder is empty, with the small amounts of urine passed causing scalding. There is pain radiating from the bladder area around to the kidneys with a rapidly rising temperature. Pus cells will be found on microscopy and the incriminating organism can be cultured from a midstream specimen of urine.

Pregnant women should have a routine urine test and bacilluria, even if asymptomatic, should be treated. Early and adequate treatment with antibiotics will prevent the infection becoming chronic, which can result in renal failure and hypertension. Asymptomatic bacilluria during pregnancy is also associated with an increase in prematurity, and the endotoxin of *E. coli* can be toxic to the fetus. Renal failure is a sad cause of death in many women several years after their pregnancy, but is often not included in any statistics on maternal mortality.

18.2.2 Rubella

Infection with rubella virus is generally mild, presenting with a maculopapular rash of short duration, fever, conjunctivitis and cervical lymphadenopathy. Some 20–50% of infections are asymptomatic. However, if the woman is pregnant, especially in the first 10 weeks of pregnancy, her developing fetus will be afflicted with congenital rubella syndrome (CRS). The earlier in pregnancy, the more severe the effects, and they result in stillbirth in the first few weeks. Common congenital defects are cataracts, glaucoma, deafness, heart defects and microcephaly. Between the 11th and 16th week of pregnancy the defects will be milder, and after the 20th week there is no further risk.

The infection is found worldwide, but its importance in developing countries has not been fully appreciated. It occurs in epidemics, generally in children aged 2–8 years in urban areas and 6–12 years in rural areas. The main method of control is to vaccinate children and adults, depending on the most suitable strategy for each particular country. The target population is adolescent girls and women of childbearing age, although this strategy will never eliminate infection so ideally all children of both sexes should be vaccinated. Unfortunately, if the vaccination programme is only partially carried out this will have the effect of raising the age of infection to older and more dangerous age groups in the population, including women likely to be pregnant. Developing countries therefore need to decide between protecting adolescent girls and women of childbearing age or to vaccinate all children of 9–15 months old as part of the routine vaccination programme. If the vaccination programme is considered sufficiently efficient to embark on the latter strategy, then an extra campaign to target all women and girls over 12 years of age should be run at the same time for the first few years of the programme. Rubella vaccine, if part of the childhood vaccination programme, is best administered with measles and mumps as MMR vaccine. (See further on vaccination in Section 3.2.)

18.2.3 Toxoplasmosis

A mild infection in adults, toxoplasmosis can cause severe damage to the developing fetus if the mother becomes infected in early pregnancy. She may not know that she has even been infected, or else just has a mild fever and lymphadenopathy, the lymph nodes being discrete and firm, and persisting for some time. However, the infant may have hepatosplenomegaly, chorioretinitis or mental retardation, and often dies. Hydrocephaly, microcephaly, jaundice and convulsions can suggest toxoplasmosis in the infant that does survive. Toxoplasmosis can also become reactivated in the immunocompromised adult, e.g. in the person with HIV, causing pneumonia, a maculopapaular rash, chorioretinitis, myocarditis or fatal cerebral toxoplasmosis.

The infection is transmitted from cats, with oocysts passed in the cat's faeces. These can be accidentally swallowed by humans, such as by stroking a cat while eating. Children are commonly infected while playing in sand or soil in which cats have defecated. Oocysts can also be inhaled from desiccated cat faeces or drunk in contaminated water. Exposure is common and widespread, with up to 40% of the population testing seropositive (specific IgM or a rise in IgG) in some countries. All members of the cat family can produce oocysts.

Control is by the reduction of contact with cats, such as banning them at mealtime and when food is being prepared. Simple procedures, such as washing the hands before eating and after touching cats should be practiced, extra precautions being taken by the newly pregnant woman. Children's play areas should be protected from cats. Sulfadiazine plus pyrimethamine plus folinic acid can be used for treatment and also as prophylaxis in the HIV-infected person.

N.B. Another similar infection from animals, brucellosis does not produce any different disease in the pregnant woman. Although one of the infecting organisms *Brucella abortus* causes abortion in cattle, there is no evidence to show that it does so in humans.

18.2.4   Cytomegalovirus infection

Cytomegalovirus (CMV) is found widely in the human population and is transmitted through mucosal contact with urine, saliva, breast milk, semen and cervical secretions. Infection can occur in adults, e.g. through sexual intercourse, but is more commonly acquired in childhood at the time of delivery, from breast milk and from close contact with other children. However, the most important

consequence is infection of the mother in early pregnancy or the reactivation of an earlier infection at this time, resulting in damage to the developing fetus. The damage is mainly to the liver and CNS, resulting in jaundice, hepatosplenomegaly, chorioretinitis, and intracerebral calcifications. Microcephaly, mental retardation, motor dysfunction and hearing loss may occur or the infant may die *in utero*. Infection is probably the cause of many cases of stillborn infants, and in those that survive without gross effects, of later neurological disability. The HIV-infected or immunocompromised individual can also suffer from reactivated infection, resulting in pneumonitis, hepatitis, severe gastritis and retinitis.

This infection is widespread in the world, with up to 1% of pregnancies resulting in intrauterine infection in some countries. Serum antibodies are 100% in some developing countries and 40% in developed countries, but this varies considerably according to socio-economic status. There is no animal reservoir of human CMV.

The woman likely to become pregnant or in early pregnancy should take extra precautions when dealing with young children, especially in the toilet and changing nappies, washing her hands frequently. She should be particularly cautious of, or if possible avoid, working with mentally retarded people and in hospital paediatric wards at this time.

18.2.5   Listeriosis

The food-borne infection produced by *Listeria monocytogenes* is a dangerous infection in the pregnant woman as it can result in abortion, stillbirth or perinatal infection. Listeriosis often occurs in epidemics from a common source of infection such as unpasteurized milk or cheese, vegetables contaminated from manure and meat produce. Asymptomatic infection can happen, still with serious consequences to the neonate. Abortion can occur at any stage of pregnancy, but mainly in the second half, while perinatal infection may develop in the last trimester. This may be acquired during delivery with signs of septicaemia, pulmonary infection or meningoencephalitis, with a case fatality rate of up to 50%.

There is a worldwide distribution of listeriosis, especially in areas where domestic animals are reared. The organism is found in silage, water and mud in close proximity to animals. The seasonal use of fodder can bring about an increased incidence of infection in animals during the late winter and spring, while human infection is commoner in the summer and early autumn. Asymptomatic passage of *L. monocytogenes* can occur in farmers, abattoir workers and others working with animals. It has also been isolated from human as well as cow's milk, so breastfeeding cannot be discounted as a means of transmission.

All milk and milk produce must be pasteurized before consumption and food fads such as fresh milk straight from the cow or cheeses made from unpasteurized milk should be avoided, especially by the pregnant woman. All meat and meat products should be well cooked and items such as pâté and pastes avoided. All vegetables must be thoroughly washed and untreated manure not used for the growing of vegetables. All utensils used in the preparation of meat should be washed with a chlorine solution and contact with infective animal material, such as aborted foetuses, avoided. Penicillin or ampicillin can be used in treatment.

18.2.6 Parvovirus B19 (fifth disease)

Infection with parvovirus B19, also called erythema infectiosum or fifth disease, presents as an erythematous eruption, commonly seen on the cheeks, giving the appearance of the person having been slapped on the face. There may also be a recurring rash, mainly on the limbs, often brought on by heat or sunlight. Joint pain, especially in women, may also be a feature. A quarter of all infections are asymptomatic. Infection in the first trimester of pregnancy may result in intrauterine damage to the fetus, predominantly producing anaemia and hydrops fetalis, with a 10% death rate.

The infection is found mainly in children, with epidemics occurring in the winter in temperate climates. Although the infection is found worldwide its extent and significance in the developing world is not known. Transmission is from respiratory droplets or blood transfusion, or is intrauterine.

Diagnosis can be confirmed by specific IgM antibodies against parvovirus B19 which should be offered to the pregnant woman suspected of having acquired the infection. Pregnant women should avoid contact in epidemic situations and common sources of infection such as hospitals and schools. Washing hands and good personal hygiene will go a long way to reducing the risk of acquiring fifth disease.

18.2.7 Chickenpox (varicella)

Chickenpox (varicella) is predominantly an infection of children, presenting as a skin rash of macules, papules, vesicles, pustules and dried crusts, following a prodromal fever. The lesions occur in groups, appearing over several days, resulting in pocks of different stages present at the same time. This is a characteristic feature of the rash, as is its central distribution, mainly on the chest and abdomen.

The majority of people contract chickenpox as children and this should be encouraged as infection in the adult can be a serious matter, producing pneumonia, encephalitis and cardiomyopathies, with fatalities in the elderly. This is a particular problem in developing countries, especially in isolated island communities. The pregnant woman is at risk of developing severe generalized varicella, with a 30% mortality. Also, chickenpox in early pregnancy may result in congenital malformation of the fetus. The neonate acquiring infection within the first 10 days of life is also liable to serious infection.

Chickenpox is found worldwide in epidemic form, spreading serially from one place to another. A common pattern is for an epidemic to develop in a school, and then when it is almost over to spread to another school or community and start a fresh epidemic there. It is transmitted by both skin contact, predominantly by the fluid from vesicles, but also by droplet infection, often before the rash appears. Articles soiled by discharges, such as cloths, towels and soft toys can readily spread infection.

Children with chickenpox should be isolated as far as possible, not go to school and, unless seriously ill, be kept at home rather than go to a clinic or hospital. Every effort should be made to keep them from coming into contact with a pregnant woman or neonate. A vaccine is available and can be used for vaccinating high-risk groups such as women of childbearing age who have not had varicella as a child (but not in pregnant women). However, it should not be used in the general population as it will shift the age of developing naturally acquired infection to an older and more dangerous age group. Acyclovir and vidarabine can be used for treatment if started soon after the rash appears. Human varicella-zoster immunoglobulin (VZIG) is available in some centres and can be given to the pregnant woman or neonate within 4 days of exposure. It will reduce the severity of infection in the mother but may not prevent congenital malformation of the fetus.

18.2.8 Influenza

Seasonal influenza occurs at regular, generally annual, intervals, but owing to the changing antigenic type of the virus pandemics can develop which have a global coverage. These two stages of influenza need to be considered separately in terms of protecting the mother.

Influenza presents as a fever with malaise, muscle aches and upper respiratory symptoms of sudden onset. There is initially a dry cough but this can be complicated by secondary infection, with the production of sputum. It is this severe respiratory infection that can be fatal in the very young, the elderly and the immunocompromised.

Influenza is highly contagious, and is spread by droplets and contact with surfaces that have been contaminated from coughing bouts. It spreads rapidly through the community, facilitated by close contact, so in urban areas and institutions such as schools almost everyone is affected in a short space of time, while in rural areas spread is slower. In temperate climates, seasonal influenza mainly occurs in the winter months, while in the tropics it is predominantly in the rainy season. Two recent major concerns have been the spread of avian influenza H5N1 and of so-called 'swine flu', an H1N1 variant.

As influenza is so infectious, the majority of the population will become infected during an epidemic, but any reduction of social contact, such as in markets and meetings, will reduce the risk. Young children in particular should not be carried around and exposed to crowded places if they can be safely left in the care of someone at home. Spitting should be outlawed and people encouraged to cough into a tissue that is then placed in a bin or burnt. Frequent hand washing, especially before meals, will reduce spread from contaminated surfaces.

Influenza vaccine is prepared each season depending on the expected composition of antigenic subunits. The influenza vaccine has been given to thousands of pregnant women at various stages of pregnancy with no evidence of any effect on the developing fetus, so it should be given to pregnant women that are at risk of complications from influenza before the flu season, whatever the stage of pregnancy. In seasonal influenza, vaccination is not essential to the pregnant woman who has no at-risk medical conditions, although she should receive vaccination against an outbreak of A(H1N1) swine flu.

Pregnant women are at increased risk of severe disease from A(H1N1), the risk increasing with the stage of pregnancy, so those in the third trimester are at greatest risk. Pregnant women were ten times more likely to need care in an intensive care unit compared with the general population. Of the two vaccines available, Pandemrix is recommended for pregnant women as it gives good levels of antibodies after a single dose. The pregnant woman can have both the seasonal vaccine and the swine flu vaccine.

There has also been recent concern over A(H5N1) avian influenza. People working closely with infected poultry have contracted the more serious disease, which has a high mortality. So far there has been no sustained human-to-human transmission, but there is concern that co-infection with seasonal human influenza could produce a new strain that is more easily transmitted between people. Anybody working with poultry should therefore be vaccinated against seasonal influenza, and women when pregnant should avoid poultry as far as possible. (More on influenza can be found in Sections 13.3 and 19.2.)

18.2.9 Malaria

Malaria is one of the most important diseases in the world and is particularly serious in the pregnant woman owing to her lowered immunity. Even if she has lived in an endemic area for some time and built up her immunity, this is decreased during pregnancy, making her more susceptible to infection and contracting serious disease. This is greater in the first pregnancy than in subsequent ones.

Infection commences with fever and headache, which takes on a series of peaks of fever followed by sweating and profound chills. Classically, these develop into a pattern of either 3 days (tertiary malaria) or 4 days (quaternary malaria) but often, this pattern, especially in falciparum malaria, proceeds rapidly to severe disease. This can be cerebral malaria (encephalopathy and coma), acute shock, haematuria (blackwater fever) and jaundice. The higher the parasitaemia the more severe the illness and the greater the mortality. Diagnosis is with a thick blood smear (to detect parasites) and a thin smear (to determine the species). A rapid diagnostic test (RDT) using a dipstick has been developed and is progressively replacing blood slide diagnosis.

Malaria is transmitted by *Anopheles* mosquitoes, the efficiency of the vector depending upon the species and feeding habits, with *A. gambiae* (the main vector in Africa) being the most efficient, and *A. culicifacies* (an important vector in the rural Indian subcontinent) an inefficient vector for human transmission. (For a list of vectors and more details about malaria see Section 15.6.)

Maternal immunosuppression occurs during the second half of pregnancy and, as well as these physiological mechanisms, malaria infection will also depress the existing immunity to various antigens of the different species of parasite. Immunity in malaria is acquired by repeat infections, and when a mother becomes pregnant it is possible that this will unmask an infection, for which she must be treated. Acute renal insufficiency as a complication of falciparum malaria is more likely in pregnant women and can often be confused or superimposed on toxaemia of pregnancy. Treatment should not be withheld because the mother is pregnant as her chance of dying is far greater than any risk to the developing fetus.

Transplacental transmission of malaria can occur, more commonly in the non-immunes than in mothers who have built up a high level of immunity (such as in Africa). Massive infections of the placenta are commonly seen, but congenital malaria is rare due to antibody transfer from the mother to her developing fetus. This, unfortunately, only provides passive immunity for a few months, and antibody is not transmitted through breast milk.

Epidemic malaria is an important cause of abortions and stillbirths, especially in communities with little immunity. Low birth weight is a feature of endemic malaria and a control programme or preventive measures to the individual will increase birth weight.

Prevention of malaria in pregnant women and in children under 5 years of age in seasonal areas of transmission of Africa should be by a combination of seasonal malaria chemoprevention (SMC), insecticide treated nets (ITNs) and access to treatment facilities. SMC is with 2 doses of sulfadoxine-pyrimethamine plus amodiaquine given 1 month apart after quickening or one dose at 20–24 weeks and a second at 28–32 weeks. In other areas, the same overall strategy should be used, but different SMC regimes maybe appropriate, such as the use of chloroquine in areas where Plasmodium vivax is the predominant species and chloroquine resistance does not occur. This can be combined with proguanil. In other areas, mefloquine may be appropriate, but local advice should be sought.

Pregnant women with HIV infection are more likely to have an increased prevalence and intensity of infection, with the multigravida responding in a similar way to a primigravida. These women should have a course of prophylactic AZT (see HIV above) plus sulfadoxine-pyrimathamine plus amodiaquine SMC unless they are on ART in which case the cotrimoxazole prophylaxis will give them protection against malaria.

The main method of preventing malaria is with ITNs, and pregnant women and children should always be given priority in the use of nets. Conscientious use of mosquito nets by the mother and her newborn child is the most effective way of preventing malaria.

The effectiveness of a mosquito net is improved by treating the net with synthetic pyrethroids which repel mosquitoes and kill those that come in contact with the net. When used on a community scale, the concentration of ITNs can produce a mass effect, reducing the mosquito population, the sporozoite rate and the number of microfilariae in filariasis. (For the use and treatment of nets see Box 3.1.)

Nets for infants consist of a metal frame supporting the net that can be placed over the child, rather like a food cover. Children should be put to bed before mosquitoes start to bite, or where the mother and child sleep together the mother should also retire early. Every effort should be made to reduce mosquito biting by using clothing which covers exposed parts of the body and repellents. Items of clothing (such as socks and shawls) can be treated with repellents which retain activity for some time, especially if stored in plastic bags when not in use. There are often naturally occurring plants which have repellent properties, such as *Tegetes minuta* in East Africa.

Other methods of malaria control and treatment are detailed in Section 15.6.

18.2.10 Relapsing fever (tick-borne)

Tick-borne relapsing fever is a common infection in babies and young children in Central and Eastern Africa, but the lowered immunity in the pregnant woman makes her susceptible to infection. Congenital infection can occur, resulting in abortion, stillbirth and premature delivery.

Infection commences with a fever which develops into a recurring pattern, the period of fever lasting for a few days and then recurring 2–5 days later. Ten or more relapses may occur in the untreated case. Complications are bronchitis, nerve palsies, hepatosplenomegaly and signs of renal damage. The disease is particularly serious in the young child. Its similarity to malaria might cause initial confusion, but on examining a blood film, spirochaetes rather than malaria parasites are found. The blood slide should be taken during febrile periods and the spirochaete *Borrelia duttonii* can be seen in stained films or moving around in dark field illumination.

There are two patterns of tick-borne relapsing fever, endemic in Africa and epidemic in other parts of the world. In Africa, the vector is the soft tick *Ornithodorus moubata* which lives in and around the house in cracks in the walls or floor in the traditional dried mud building. Once infected, the tick remains so for life and can transmit infection transovarially to its offspring. People are infected both from the bite of the tick and from its coxal fluid when this is accidentally rubbed into a scratch or mucous membrane.

The epidemic form of the disease is found in Asia, North Africa, Central and South America where the reservoir is maintained in rodents living in caves, temporary shelters or campsites. It is then more commonly an infection of adults setting up temporary camp in a rodent-infected area. Relapsing fever can also be transmitted by the louse, overlapping in much of its area with the endemic form of the disease in Africa, but this tends to be less severe and without major complications. (See Sections 16.3 and 16.4 and Fig. 16.4.)

Prevention of tick-borne relapsing fever is by improved housing or the use of insecticides sprayed around the house, paying particular attention to any cracks or crevices. When houses are constructed, repaired or replastered (an annual event in parts of the Indian subcontinent), an insecticide such as benzene hexachloride can be mixed with the plaster. Infants and adults can be protected by sleeping under mosquito nets (see Box 3.1) or by using repellents such as diethyltoluamide or dimethyl phthalate smeared on to skin or clothing. Ticks are also deterred from entering a room in which a night light is glowing.

Treatment is with a single dose of 300,000 units of procaine penicillin followed the next day by tetracycline 500 mg four times a day for 10 days. Destruction of large numbers of spirochaetes can cause a reaction if just penicillin is used, so judgement has to be made in the treatment of the pregnant woman if it is decided not to use tetracycline because of its effect on the fetus.

18.3   Post-partum

The post-partum period can be a problem time obstetrically from the complications such as a retained placenta and bleeding, while damage done to tissues and interference in the delivery process, especially if not sterile, can lead to infection. A clean delivery is also important to prevent a number of infections to the newborn, such as ophthalmia neonatorum and neonatal tetanus.

18.3.1   Ophthalmia neonatorum

Ophthalmia neonatorum can be due to gonococcal or chlamydial infection (see Sections 18.1.3 and 18.1.4) and presents in the infant as a 'sticky eye' – conjunctivitis due to contamination of the conjunctiva as the infant passes through the birth canal. Untreated, it is an important cause of blindness in developing countries. Prevention is by detecting the discharge in the infected woman and actively treating it, while at delivery all babies eyes should routinely be wiped and a 1% aqueous solution of silver nitrate instilled. Wiping both eyes at delivery alone can reduce the incidence of infection if silver nitrate is not available and should always be practised. A 2.5% solution of povidone–iodine, tetracycline 1% or erythromycin 0.5% eye ointment can be used as an alternative to silver nitrate or for treatment of the established eye infection.

18.3.2   Neonatal tetanus

Neonatal tetanus is normally due to infection of the umbilical cord, often by the use of traditional poultices, which often incorporate cow dung. It can also result from unclean deliveries, such as cutting the umbilical cord with a rusty knife or covering the stump with an unsterile dressing. Some 5–10 days after birth the infant has difficulty in sucking, then rigidity of muscles and generalized convulsions develop, with nearly always a fatal outcome.

Neonatal tetanus is predominantly a problem in Africa, where birth practices are rudimentary, but in any community where rigid ideas of dressing the cord stump prevail neonatal tetanus can be a serious problem. On the isolated island of St Kilda, off the Western Isles of Scotland, the insistence in using a traditional way of treating the cord stump with an unsterile preparation of fulmar oil is thought to be the reason why nearly all newborn children died of tetanus and the community became unsustainable.

Neonatal tetanus is entirely preventable by ensuring that the mother has been vaccinated and the delivery conducted in a clean manner using sterilized instruments and dressings. The WHO policy is to give all women a lifetime total of five doses of tetanus toxoid. This is preferable to waiting until the woman becomes pregnant because many women do not attend antenatal clinic, especially those likely to have an unsterile delivery. The initial vaccination is given to a woman at first contact or as early as possible during pregnancy. The second is given 4 weeks later, and the third 6–12 months after the previous dose or during the next pregnancy. Doses four and five are given at yearly intervals. Where a woman has a certificate to show she received vaccination as a child then she only needs to have two doses during the first pregnancy and one more before or during the second pregnancy. (See also Section 10.5.)

18.3.3 Puerperal sepsis

Puerperal sepsis used to be an all-too-frequent outcome of the mother delivering in hospital in 19th century Europe, and is still a problem in some developing countries where unclean deliveries take place. Symptoms commence with fever and abdominal pain, and there is a foul vaginal discharge. Bloodstream spread can also occur, leading to obstetric shock and a high death rate.

Puerperal sepsis is responsible for at least 75,000 maternal deaths a year, mainly in low-income countries, and is caused by a range of organisms, including staphylococci and coliforms, and generally due to operative intervention or remnants of the placenta still remaining. Indeed, Caesarean section is now the commonest cause of infection in the post-partum period. Puerperal sepsis ranges in incidence from 5.2 per 100 live births in the WHO Region of the Americas to 2.7 per 100 live births in the Western Pacific Region and European Region,

with Caesarean section rates ranging from 26.1 per 100 live births in the same region of the Americas (mainly South America) to 10.2 per 100 live births in the other two regions mentioned above. Interestingly, the Africa Region had an estimated puerperal sepsis incidence of 4.1 per 100 live births and the lowest Caesarean section rate of 4.2 per 100 live births. Antibiotic prophylaxis coverage was a feature in all regions, ranging from 20 to 80 per 100 Caesarean section births.

Prevention is by a proper sterile delivery using sterilized instruments, masks worn by birth attendants, the wearing of gloves, minimal interference and the maintenance of as sterile surroundings as possible. Treatment is with antibiotics and will depend upon the resistance pattern in the country, but an active regime given intravenously is ampicillin 2 g every 6 h, gentamycin 5 mg/kg every 24 h and metronidazole 500 mg every 8 h.

Induced abortion is also an important cause of puerperal sepsis, with unsafe induced abortion responsible for 50% of maternal deaths in India. Strict conditions of sterility need to be observed where termination of pregnancy is to be undertaken and every effort made to reduce unsafe abortion with, if necessary, legalization.

Septic abortion in the second trimester of pregnancy is also an important cause of acute renal failure.

Summary

- Before pregnancy, disfiguring diseases such as filariasis and leprosy will reduce the woman's chance of marrying, while the STIs can cause infertility and damage to the fetus.
- HIV infection is a serious disease in the woman in all stages of her life, the severity of infection measured by the CD4 level determining her chance of surviving pregnancy and the likelihood of transmitting infection to her offspring.
- It is while the mother's immunity is compromised during pregnancy that the most serious threat is posed to her from chickenpox, influenza and malaria, while there are threats to her fetus from syphilis, genital herpes, rubella, toxoplasmosis, cytomegalovirus, listerosis and parvovirus B19. Also at this time are the risk of contracting pyelonephritis, which if untreated can lead to renal failure, and of relapsing fever which can cause abortion and stillbirth.

- During delivery, ophthalmia neonatorum due to maternal gonococcal or chlamydial infection can cause blindness to the infant, and unhygienic delivery practices can cause neonatal tetanus and puerperal sepsis.
- Seeing the mother antenatally is crucial in detecting and treating infections early and ensuring that she is adequately protected by vaccination to give her and her infant the best chance of a successful outcome to her pregnancy. The use of ITNs by the mother and child will do much to prevent all the consequences of malaria, filariasis and relapsing fever.

Further Reading

Berg, C., Daniel, I., Atrash, H., Zane, S. and Bartlett, L. (eds) (2001) *Strategies to Reduce Pregnancy Related Deaths: From Identification and Review to Action.* Centers for Disease Control and Prevention, Atlanta, Georgia.

Dolea, C. and Stein, C. (2003) *Global Burden of Maternal Sepsis in the Year 2000.* WHO, Geneva.

Duffy, P.E. and Fried, M. (2001) *Malaria in Pregnancy: Deadly Parasite, Susceptible Host.* Taylor & Francis, London/Informa Healthcare, New York.

Family Planning New South Wales (2011) *Reproductive and Sexual Health: An Australian Clinical Practice Handbook,* 2nd edn. Family Planning New South Wales, Sydney.

Hogan, M.C., Foreman, K.J., Naghavi, M., Ahn, S.Y., Wang, M., Makela, S.M., Lozano, R. and Murray, C.J.L. (2010) Maternal mortality for 181 countries, 1980–2008: a systematic analaysis of progress towards Millennium Development Goal 5. *The Lancet* 375, 1609–1623. Published online 12 April doi:10.1016/S0140-6736(10)60518-1.

Hussein, J., McCaw-Binns, A. and Webber, R. (eds) (2012) *Maternal and Perinatal Health in Developing Countries.* CAB International, Wallingford, UK.

Kuhn, L., Aldrovandi, G.M., Sinkala, M., Kankasa, C., Semrau, K., Kasonde, P., Mwiya, M., Tsai, W.Y. and Thea, D.M. (2009) Zambia Exclusive Breastfeeding Study (ZEBS). Differential effects of early weaning for HIV-free survival of children born to HIV-infected mothers by severity of maternal disease. *PloS One* 4(6):e6059.

Mayani, C.N. and MacIntyre, J.A. (2010) Tuberculosis in pregnancy. *BJOG: An International Journal of Obstetrics and Gynaecology* 118(2), 226–231.

Mullick, S., Watson-Jones, D., Beksinka, M. and Mabey, D. (2005) Sexually transmitted infections in pregnancy; prevalence, impact on pregnancy outcomes, and approach to treatment in developing countries. *Sexually Transmitted Infections* 81, 294–302.

Prakash, A., Swain, S. and Seth, A. (1991) Maternal mortality in India: current status and strategies for reduction. *Indian Pediatrics* 28, 1395–4000.

Tiono, A.B., Ouedraogo, A., Bongouma, E.C., Diarra, A., Konaté, A.T., Nébié, I. and Sirima, S.B. (2009) Placental malaria and low birth weight in pregnant women living in a rural area of Burkina Faso following the use of three preventive regimes. *Malaria Journal* 7, 224. Published online 2009 October 7. doi: 10.1186/1475-2875-8-224.

van Dillen, J., Zwart, J., Schutte, J. and van Roosmalen, J. (2010) Maternal sepsis: epidemiology, etiology and outcome. *Current Opinion in Infectious Diseases* 23, 249–254.

World Health Organization (2004a) *Integrating Care for Reproductive Health, Sexually Transmitted Infections in Pregnancy: A Guide to Essential Practice.* WHO, Geneva.

World Health Organization (2004b) *Strategic Framework For Malaria Control During Pregnancy in the African Region,* Document No. AFR/MAL/04/01, WHO Regional Office for Africa, Brazzaville, Congo. Available at: http://www.afro.who.int/index.php?option=com_docman&task=doc_download&gid=147 (accessed 12 March 2012).

World Health Organization (2005) *Interim WHO Clinical Staging of HIV/AIDS and HIV/AIDS Case Definitions for Surveillance, African Region.* Document Ref. No. WHO/HIV/2005.02, WHO, Geneva. Available from: http://www.who.int/hiv/pub/guidelines/clinicalstaging.pdf (accessed 12 March 2012).

World Health Organization (2010) *Antiretroviral Therapy for HIV Infection in Adults and Adolescents: Recommendations for a Public Health Approach, 2010 Revision.* WHO, Geneva. Also available at: http://whqlibdoc.who.int/publications/2010/9789241599764_eng.pdf (accessed 6 March 2012).

Web resource

Swine flu (H1N1). Available at: www.nhs.uk/Conditions/Pandemic-flu/Pages/Introduction.aspx (accessed 29 March 2010).

19 New and Emerging Diseases

Biology is not static; evolutionary forces will always look for opportunities to exploit new situations and no more so than in the field of communicable diseases. Humans have always waged a continuing war against organisms that attack them and although many of these might now be prevented, new organisms will seek to exploit any weakness in our defences. This chapter therefore looks at new and emerging diseases, infections that have appeared in recent times and others that have not fully developed into the serious problem that they could become.

The terminology of conflict has been used above not only because our battle with parasitic organisms is like an arms race but also because the horror of using infectious organisms by terrorist organizations in a purposeful way to attack people is now a possibility. This will probably be with organisms that are known to us, but in a way that would ensure that they are particularly potent. So the last section of this chapter looks at these possible bioterrorist-instigated diseases.

This chapter, more than any other in this book, will change and need updating, which can be done with much useful information now freely available on the World Wide Web. The best source of information on epidemics and new diseases, with good updates on major health problems, is the *Weekly Epidemiological Record* (*WER*), produced simultaneously in English and French by the World Health Organization (WHO) and available at www.who.int/wer/2012/en/. To find a particular copy, change the year in the address to the one required and look through the index. Also available, from the US Centers for Disease Control (CDC), is the *Journal of Emerging Infectious Diseases*, at www.cdc.gov/ncidod/eid/index.htm, which publishes research and general articles. In the UK, the Health Protection Agency has a section on emerging diseases on its helpful web page at www.hpa.org.uk. A good resource of public health and practice is the Global Health archive operated by CABI, which can be found at www.cabi.org/globalhealth.

19.1 The Animal Connection

In the 1970s, it seemed as though the battle against the communicable diseases was won, we had all the weapons we needed to control most of them, and all that was required was to have sufficient resources to combat the diseases in the developing world. Smallpox had been eradicated and the development of vaccines promised a similar fate for polio and other immunizable diseases; but in 1981 there was a rude shock.

In June 1981, the CDC reported five cases of *Pneumocystis jiroveci* pneumonia. In the following month, 15 more cases of this normally rare disease were reported as well as 26 cases of Kaposi's sarcoma, an unusual tumour. The common feature was that all these cases were in homosexual men. By the end of 1981, acquired immune deficiency syndrome (AIDS), as it was called, was also being reported from countries in Europe. In Belgium and France, an AIDS-like illness was noted among people originating from Africa. These observations led to investigations in Rwanda and Zaire (now the Democratic Republic of Congo, DRC), where many AIDS patients were found. At the same time, an aggressive form of Kaposi's sarcoma was reported from Zambia and a new disease, called slim disease, was described in Uganda. These were all found to be manifestations of AIDS. The African infection was transmitted heterosexually, starting its relentless course, which has continued unabated until the present time.

There had previously been the new diseases of Lassa fever, Ebola haemorrhagic fever and Marburg disease, but it was the appearance of human immunodeficiency virus (HIV) infection – the causative agent of AIDS – that really alerted the world to new communicable diseases. Where had they come from and why were they appearing at this time? The first clue came with the discovery of a virtually identical retrovirus to HIV in simian monkeys (called SIV), which suggested that HIV originated from a monkey source.

Then, in 1986, a disease appeared in cattle in England called bovine spongiform encephalopathy (BSE), which was shown to be have been caused by cattle being fed with feed containing the remains of sheep, some of which had the similar sheep disease of scrapie. The disease had not been transmitted from sheep before so somehow the organism had crossed the species barrier, and if this had happened from sheep to cattle then why not from cattle to humans, when they ate infected meat. Sure enough, the first case of a new variant of Creutzfeldt–Jakob disease (vCJD) appeared in 1995, and this condition was linked to the consumption of beef. Because BSE had a 4–5 year incubation period, the potential for human infection was enormous and there was much speculation as to what would happen.

CJD is one of the group of transmissible spongiform encephalopathies (TSEs) which, as well as BSE in cattle and scrapie in sheep, is also found in other animals such as mink, elk and North American mule deer. The only other human TSEs are kuru, Gerstmann–Sträussler–Scheinker syndrome (in which there is a hereditary predisposition) and fatal insomnia (which occurs in a familial and sporadic form). Kuru is found in the Fore people of Papua New Guinea who traditionally eat the brains of the recently dead in the belief that they will obtain the wisdom and prowess of their ancestors.

The TSEs have been shown to be due to a new kind of organism, a self-replicating protein called a prion, which produces a clinical picture in humans of depression, followed by organic brain disease, including cerebella ataxia, cortical blindness, localized weakness and progressive intellectual deterioration. Speech is lost, swallowing becomes difficult and a rigidity of limbs develops as the patient sinks further into a hopeless state of debility and death. Unfortunately, in the case of vCJD, it is difficult to confirm the diagnosis until after death. There were three cases confirmed on death in 1995, after which there was a gradual increase to 28 cases in the year 2000, followed by a steady decline to one death in 2008, three in 2009 and three in 2010. Four cases remain alive. As well as the 174 cases in the UK, there were six cases in France and one each in Ireland, Italy, Canada and the USA; however,

three of the French cases as well as those in Canada and the USA were considered to be due to exposure in the UK. All offal-based ruminant feeds were banned in Europe in 1994 (from 1989 in UK), so it is hoped that this is the end of the tragic epidemic.

While the public health profession was recovering from BSE and vCJD, another new communicable disease, severe acute respiratory syndrome (SARS) was reported from Vietnam in February 2003. A businessman who had been travelling in China was admitted to hospital in Hanoi with a history of high fever, cough and difficulty in breathing. His condition worsened so he requested to be transferred to Hong Kong where, despite ventilatory support, he died. In the hospital in Hanoi several health care workers contracted a similar illness and the attending doctor and a nurse died. Search was made for the organism, which at first was thought to be a new strain of influenza, but subsequently was identified as a coronavirus. An incubation period of 1–14 days, but more commonly of 3–5 days, and period of communicability of 3–14 days from the start of symptoms was worked out. Fortunately, the household secondary attack rate was between 6 and 15% in Singapore and Hong Kong, contrasting with a much higher rate in hospitals, especially if barrier nursing was deficient.

Tracing the case back, it was discovered that there had been a number of cases of a severe and highly contagious pneumonia in Guangdong Province (Canton), southern China, in which 1 in 30 people had died. The attending specialist travelled to Hong Kong for a wedding where, in the early stages of the illness himself, he infected all the people in a lift in the hotel in which he was staying. One of these persons was the case that came to Hanoi, another was a person from Singapore and the third a lady returning to her home in Toronto, Canada. Hong Kong, southern China, Singapore, Vietnam and Canada then became the centres of epidemics, which demanded strict quarantine measures to contain them. After draconian measures, especially in China, the last case recovered at the end of July 2003. By that time there had been 8422 cases and 916 deaths.

Coming back to the original question of what was the link between the three epidemics of HIV, BSE/vCJD and SARS, it seems likely that the organism, originally in animals, had crossed the species barrier into humans: HIV from simian monkeys and BSE from scrapie-infected sheep and subsequently via beef to humans, while SARS possibly also had an animal connection. Southern China enjoys a culinary custom of eating any kind of animal, often held in cages or fish tanks, until required for the table. Such is the close proximity of people to all these animals and the general poor state of hygiene that all possible methods of transmission are possible. As well as the respiratory route, the SARS virus was found to be excreted in the faeces and urine of patients, possibly up to 23 days after symptoms first started. The original cases in southern China were in food handlers, 66 of which were found to have antibodies, while of the animals tested, masked palm civets, racoon dogs, ferret badgers, cynomolgus macaques, fruit bats, snakes and wild pigs were all found to test positive. Transmission in humans was through close human contact as the infection was in large droplets rather than aerosol, and possibly also via sewage contamination in one area of Hong Kong. Several of the animals listed are regarded as delicacies and kept in cages, so it seems quite possible that either of these methods could have been how the food handlers were infected. After the main epidemic had finished, a new case was found to be strongly associated with the masked palm civet, so it seems likely that this could have been how the epidemic started. The close proximity of humans to animals, and modifications of animal feeds, may be the way in which new diseases could develop in the future, so precautions need to be taken.

19.2   Avian Influenza and its Implications

The so-called Asian flu epidemic of 1957 was found to have originated in chickens in Guangdong province in China as a genetic shift. This was followed in 1968 by the Hong Kong influenza epidemic, which also originated from the same area. Although the 1918 epidemic was termed Spanish flu, it is thought that this too might have started originally in southern China as a genetic drift (bird flu variant).

There were influenza pandemics in 1889–1892, 1918–1920, 1957–1958, 1968–1969 and 1977–1978, and in 2009 there was the so-called swine flu A(H1N1), originating in Mexico, which predominantly affected younger age groups and pregnant women. It would appear that the same virus had circulated reasonably widely in the past as older age groups were not susceptible. The swine flu

pandemic continued into 2011 during the winter season in the northern hemisphere.

A recent cause for concern was the appearance of avian influenza A(H5N1) in January 2004. This is an infection predominantly of chickens and ducks, is highly infectious and results in an almost 100% mortality of domestic fowls. The infection is maintained in wild waterfowl, predominantly ducks and geese, which can spread the infection over long distances when they migrate. The virus circulates asymptomatically, with individual birds remaining infected for about a month and excreting large quantities of virus in their droppings. Congregations of large numbers of birds prior to migration provide ideal conditions for the transmission and mixing of avian influenza virus.

While migrating wildfowl might have been the initiating cause of the outbreak of A(H5N1), the main method of continued transmission was probably by the transport of birds, contaminated clothing and equipment. Bird excrement is highly infectious, so humans coming into contact with sick birds or their droppings are at risk of infection. In Hong Kong in 1997, as well as the domestic fowl outbreak of the disease there were 18 human cases (six of which died). The same virus was identified in fowls in 2002, resulting in mass slaughter of chickens, but despite this action there were four more human cases (all of which died). In 2004, there was a more serious epidemic in Thailand (five human cases, all died) and Vietnam (18 cases, 13 died) that spread to domestic fowl in other countries in South-east and East Asia (Cambodia, China, Indonesia, Japan, Laos and South Korea). Initially, there was a very marked clustering of cases as shown in Fig. 19.1, which also maps the course of the epidemic. Clusters peaked during 2005 and 2006, although the highest proportion of cluster-associated cases was in 2003. This demonstrates the benefit of actively dealing with any cluster rather than when the cases become more sporadic.

The initial symptoms are very similar to ordinary influenza – malaise, myalgia, cough and sore throat – but then develop within a few days to pneumonia. This can be severe, with progress to respiratory failure, resulting in a 50–60% death rate. Other serious complications are multi-organ failure, sepsis-like syndromes and, rarely, encephalopathy.

Infection is due to close proximity to infected poultry and places contaminated with their droppings. Greatest exposure probably occurs

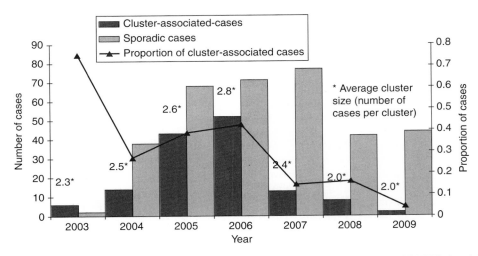

Fig. 19.1. Worldwide distribution of sporadic and cluster-associated cases of human influenza A(H5N1) virus infections, January 2003–March 2009. (Reproduced by permission of the World Health Organization, Geneva.)

when the bird is killed, plucked and prepared for cooking, but once it is cooked, transmission does not result from eating the meat. There is considerable concern that A(H5N1) (or, less commonly, H7 or H9) could acquire the necessary characteristics to allow it to be transmitted from human to human. Even more worrying is that it could interact with an established human influenza strain and produce a potent infection that nobody would have any resistance to. Fortunately, neither of these possibilities has so far happened, but they remain a considerable cause for concern.

The close proximity of humans to animals of all types for culinary purposes in Asia and, particularly in south China, has already been mentioned in Section 19.1 above. This continues as a dangerous source of infections that could cross from animal to human and then continue as human-to-human transmission. Considerable effort needs to be made to control this trade, with the implementation of good practices, including the wearing of protective clothing, use of antiseptics to clean out cages and all other methods of prevention of disease spread. Also, any dead migratory bird should be treated with caution and reported to the appropriate authority for protected handling and examination for H5N1 infection. In circumstances where people have come into contact with an infected bird then they can be given a neuraminidase inhibitor (oseltamir, zanamivir, etc.) as a prophylactic. An A(H5N1) vaccine has been developed which could be used to protect persons in high-risk occupations involved with poultry or their preparation, and will also be valuable should an epidemic begin.

19.3 Other Animal-related Emerging Infections

19.3.1 Animal poxes

Like the diseases already mentioned, there is a possibility that one of the animal pox diseases could become serious in humans. Smallpox vaccination (against the variola virus) provided protection for 10 years, possibly up to 30, and would have been effective against other animal pox diseases, but since smallpox vaccination was stopped in 1979 there is probably nobody with any remaining immunity.

Monkeypox is a rare zoonosis, significant because it produces a disease similar to smallpox. It is localized to tropical rainforest areas of West and Central Africa. Most cases have been reported from the DRC, and although a disease of monkeys, it occasionally also affects humans. It has a comparable case-fatality rate to smallpox although the secondary attack rate is much lower (15%).

The characteristics of smallpox and monkeypox are:

- clear-cut prodromal period of sudden onset of fever, headache and prostration;
- peripheral distribution of the rash (including soles and palms);

- lesions pass through the same stages at the same time;
- fever intensifies as the rash progresses to the pustular stage; and
- lesions are deeply seated, flat topped and centrally depressed.

These features should be compared with those of chickenpox (see Section 12.1).

There has been much speculation that monkeypox could develop in humans as vaccination against smallpox has now stopped (see above), and any pre-existing immunity will by now have waned; however, so far this has not happened. The possibility always remains though, and the development of a suspicious rash within the monkeypox geographical area should be reported to WHO. Fortunately, the low secondary attack rate in close contacts makes it unlikely that this would develop into a serious epidemic and smallpox vaccination can (still) be used to prevent it.

There are also other animal pox virus diseases which have or could infect humans. Examples are cowpox, camelpox, tanapox, yabapox, buffalopox, sheep pox and goat pox. There is very little evidence to suggest that any of these diseases can cause an infection in people that is likely to be spread from one person to another to any marked extent, but their importance is to recognize that they can occur and to differentiate them from smallpox.

19.3.2 Bat-transmitted diseases

The bat was first considered as a reservoir of infection for rabies during work in Trinidad in the 1930s. Transmission of the disease involves both vampire bats that inflict a wound, and insectivorous bats – from virus in their droppings. In 1999, a new viral infection appeared in pig farmers in Malaysia; this was subsequently found to also have a reservoir in bats. Nipah, as it was called, is a henipavirus and it was soon discovered that another similar illness, Hendra, was transmitted by a related virus found in bats.

Nipah presents as an encephalitis, with headaches, muscle pains and sore throat, progressing to drowsiness and neurological signs; it has a case fatality rate of 40–70%. Diagnosis is by ELISA or PCR and there is an incubation period of 4–45 days.

Fruit bats of the family Pteropodidae are natural hosts of the Nipah virus without there being any apparent disease among them. Bats of the genus *Pteropus* are mainly responsible for the infection, and serological studies have shown that wherever the *Pteropus* genus is found the Nipah virus is also present. This includes the countries of India, Bangladesh, Thailand, Malaysia, Indonesia, Cambodia, China, Timor-Leste (East Timor), Papua New Guinea and Australia. The same genus of bats and the virus are found in Madagascar, but recently bats of another genus (*Eidon*) belonging to the same family and which are widely spread in Africa also tested positive for antibodies to the virus.

Pigs become infected in a manner similar to humans, although many of them do not show such severe symptoms, while other animals – horses, goats, sheep, cats and dogs – can also acquire infection. Transmission is predominantly from droplets, so contact with sick pigs or their tissues could result in infection and all precautions need to be taken when handling them. In outbreaks of Nipah virus in Bangladesh and India, infection resulted from the consumption of fruit or fruit products contaminated with saliva or urine of bats. This was particularly from date palms and the juice made from them, so this must be boiled before consumption and all fruit that cannot be protected from fruit bats avoided.

Hendra virus is similar in distribution and species of bat to Nipah virus, but it is predominantly an infection of horses with serious economic consequences; only a few humans have contracted the disease and all of these have so far been in Australia. Human infection has resulted from close contact with horses and although the virus is found in bats there have been no human cases resulting from this source. The mechanism of infection appears to be due to bats contaminating pasture land with fetal tissues and fluids during delivery, and horses subsequently grazing these pastures. The clinical symptoms are similar to Nipah but with a fatal respiratory disease in one case while in another it was an encephalitis. There seems to be a worrying trend towards an encephalitis, rather than a respiratory disease, both in horses and humans.

The main method of control is the destruction of infected horses and the quarantine and protected handling of all horses when cases occur. Horse feeds and water troughs should be protected or moved so that bat contamination does not take place.

Virus infections are not the only danger from bats; histoplasmosis, a fungal disease, has also been contracted from bat-inhabited caves (as has Ebola haemorrhagic fever, see Section 14.14).

19.3.3 Rodents as disease reservoirs

Rodents are well-established reservoirs of infections that can be transmitted to humans. Many of these are mentioned in Chapter 16, but one that is emerging in a number of countries is the hantavirus. This causes two differing clinical syndromes, haemorrhagic fever with renal syndrome found in the Balkans, Eastern Russia, China and Korea, and hantavirus pulmonary syndrome found in North and South America. The mode of transmission is thought to be respiratory, from an aerosol of rodent excreta, so precautions need to be taken in areas where rats and field rodents are commonly found.

19.3.4 Food-borne diseases of animal origin

Another concern has been the increase of food-borne diseases of an animal origin, particularly salmonellosis and *Campylobacter*. Fish-transmitted trematodes have also increased in South-east Asia and Latin America.

The globalization of food production means that an infected animal source can be transmitted to another country in a short space of time, bypassing protection measures that the home country might have in place for the control of the infection at source. Sadly, the opportunity for profit has led to the unscrupulous production of food at less than acceptable standards of quality, or breakdowns in the production process have resulted in the manufacture of unsafe food. Owing to sourcing by wholesalers on an international basis, and the availability of air transport, foods in one country can be rapidly carried to another. Once an associated disease outbreak takes place, it can be a complex problem tracing the food back to its original source, and by then the same batch might have been distributed to many countries.

Salmonellosis has become a particular problem because of the indiscriminate use of antibiotics in animal husbandry to improve meat yields, as this practice provides the opportunity for drug-resistant organisms to develop. These have then contaminated the meat in the production process and if this is not adequately cooked then serious drug-resistant *Salmonella* infection can result. It is estimated that 50–60% of chickens are infected with *Salmonella*, and infected chickens produce infected eggs. If it is not the infected food source that is imported then it can be the traveller visiting a foreign country and bringing the infection back with them. It is estimated that 90% of all cases of salmonellosis in Sweden are imported. (See further in Section 9.1.2.)

It is globalization that has made the problem of food-borne diseases more serious and several countries have made efforts to rely more on home production which, although it has cost implications, also reduces dependence on international transport and the unwanted production of atmospheric carbon dioxide.

19.4 Arboviruses

The arboviruses (Section 15.2) have a propensity for producing new diseases that is unmatched by any other organism. New arboviral diseases appear at quite regular intervals, or those normally restricted to small areas of the world spread to new areas or become more important as human diseases. Examples are West Nile virus (Section 15.2.1) which has appeared for the first time in North America, Rift Valley fever which was normally confined to Africa, but has now spread to Asia (Section 15.2.3) and Crimean–Congo haemorrhagic fever which now has a worldwide distribution (Sections 15.2.3 and 16.9.2).

Chikungunya, normally a disease of East Africa, (see Section 15.2.1) took on a worldwide distribution between 2001 and 2007 with outbreaks in India, Indonesia, Malaysia and Gabon, and the Indian Ocean islands of Madagascar, Comoros, Mayotte, Seychelles, Mauritius and La Réunion, where it had a particularly devastating effect. From here, cases were carried back to Europe and in August 2007 indigenous transmission took place in the Emila-Romagna region of north-east Italy, originating from a person that had been to the Kerala region of India. This was due to transmission by *Aedes albopictus*, which is widespread and numerous in Italy, but it is the invasion of parts of the world by this mosquito, especially North and South America, within recent times that makes the threat of spread of a number of serious arbovirus infections a great concern.

The number of arbovirus infections in the world is enormous (Chapter 20) and new ones are likely to appear at any time. Although they are mainly transmitted by mosquitoes or ticks, it is likely that the reservoir will be in birds or mammals, as new-species adaptations, similar to the diseases mentioned above, arise in the human population.

19.5 Antimicrobial Resistance

With the introduction of penicillin in 1940, the use of antibiotics reduced the dependence on antisepsis to control infection. Unfortunately, soon after, antibiotic resistance developed, and it has been a continuous process of developing new antibiotics to combat organisms that are no longer killed by existing ones. *Staphylococcus aureus* has been problematic from the start, developing resistance to each of the penicillins (and other types of antibiotics) soon after they were developed, leading to methicillin-resistant *S. aureus*, commonly known as MRSA. (This is a general term used to signify resistance to all penicillins and cephalosporins, not only methicillin.) MRSA is now a serious hospital infection and, although many people carry this organism as a commensal, it is in hospital that serious wound infections result.

Recently, a strain of MRSA identical to that in humans has been found in cattle and especially in cow dung, indicating that there may be an additional source of infection. As yet it is uncertain whether the strain in cattle developed from contact with humans or the other way round, but in any case the cattle infection now provides an additional source. Once again, the animal connection in emerging diseases is demonstrated.

Methods to combat MRSA have revolved around cleanliness and the use of antiseptics, especially by attendant staff and visitors. A return to the methods of Semmelweis and Lister, with less dependence on ever more potent antibiotics, may be the best approach. When a similar problem arose in the 1960s, and the armamentarium of antibiotics available at the time was exhausted, the brave decision was taken to stop the use of antibiotics and rely entirely on cleanliness and antisepsis. In time, the resistant organisms were overcome by stronger strains that were able to return once the blanket of antibiotics had been removed. Perhaps it is necessary to use the same strategy again.

A new procedure, similar to sterilization, actually coats the surfaces of walls and surgical instruments with a nano-coating that kills any MRSA bacteria that land on it. It is made from lysostaphin, a naturally occuring enzyme, packaged into carbon nanotubes. This has been found to work when mixed with paint and applied to walls and could be formulated to coat instruments in a similar way.

As well as resistant organisms resulting directly from the pressure of antibiotics, they can also develop as a result of the utilization of antibiotics for other uses. When respiratory and other infections are treated with broad-spectrum antibiotics they also kill off the normal gut flora, making the person susceptible to intestinal infections, particularly with *Salmonella* and *Campylobacter*. As many of these *Salmonella* are resistant (as mentioned above) serious infection can result.

Many other resistant organisms have already been mentioned, multi-drug-resistant *Mycobacterium tuberculosis*, the continually evolving strains of resistant *Escherichia coli*, problems associated with treating *Neisseria gonorrhoea*, and intestinal infections due to *S. typhi* and *Vibrio cholerae*. Fortunately, there is now an effective vaccine against *Streptococcus pneumoniae*, but children will still present with resistant infection that requires more expensive and perhaps unobtainable antibiotics.

The excessive use of antibiotics in treating infections, or the more questionable practice of giving antibiotic cover where no infection has actually occurred, has allowed organisms that are not normally serious pathogens to develop, such as *Clostridium difficile*. This infection produces a pseudomembranous colitis with prolonged diarrhoea and fulminating toxic megacolon. Patients in hospital with other conditions are particularly susceptible to infection, and reducing the use of hospitals to all but the most serious cases may be the main strategy to eliminate this intractable problem.

Other unexpected infections that have developed, particularly in a hospital environment, have been due to *Acinetobacter baumanii*, *Pseudomonas aeruginosa*, *Stenotrophomonas maltophilia*, *Enterococcus faecium* and *E. faecalis*. Expanded-spectrum β-lactamase (ESBL) producing Gram-negative bacteria, including *Klebsiella pneumoniae* (which produces *K. pneumoniae* carbapenemase, KPC), have been particularly difficult as they have developed new ways of disabling antibiotics. Most of these infections take advantage of the debility of the person and are not serious problems outside hospital or in the fit person.

As if these problems were not enough, a new superbug that produces New Delhi metallo-β-lactamase (NDM-1), which was first identified in 2008, is resistant to nearly all known current treatments. The β-lactamase enzyme that it produces destroys antibiotics, making it immune to all but colistin and tigecycline, one of which is only partially effective and the other of which has unpleasant side effects. What is worse is that its resistance gene can be picked up by other bacteria, transforming them into totally resistant organisms. This has already happened to *E. coli* and is likely to happen with other bacteria, rendering the administration of antibiotics a useless strategy.

If this does become the case, then other methods of combating bacteria will be required, such as the use of bacteria to attack other bacteria. Much in the same way as *Bacillus thuringiensis* attacks mosquito larvae, it may be possible to use bacteria that do not harm humans to attack these super-resistant bacteria. In a similar manner, bacteriophages have been used for some time in typing organisms, but they could be used to destroy the bacteria if a safe means of using them can be developed. The bacteriophage attaches itself to a bacterium and injects its DNA, making the bacterium produce so many viruses that it finally explodes, and the viruses go on to infect more bacteria. It may also be possible to engineer bacteria to destroy themselves, just as cells are programmed to commit suicide after a certain period of time. For example, exposing bacteria to hydoxyurea induces bacteria to produce molecules to which they are themselves toxic.

Other methods that are being tried give hope that the conundrum of hospital infection could be beaten provided that sufficient resources are given to their development and the wanton use of antibiotics, as happened in the past, is not allowed to happen again. For example, existing antibiotics could be coated with aptamers that prevent bacteria from disabling them. Normally, bacteria disable an antibiotic by developing enzymes that metabolize it, so an aptamer coating will make the antibiotic effective again. Also, it may be possible to block the attack mechanism that bacteria use. When they invade a new host they wait until there are sufficient numbers before mounting their assault. A chemical signal is used to initiate this, so if it was possible to block this, invasion of the host would not occur. However, all of these methods are very much at the experimental stage, and although they give considerable hope that hospital infection can be overcome, for the time being caution and simple methods of extreme cleanliness will be required.

19.6 Bioterrorism

The idea of using biological substances for warfare is not a new one. In 1347, when the Mongols laid siege to the port of Caffa (now part of the Ukraine, but established as a Genoese port in 1266) they catapulted the bodies of plague victims over the walls at the Genoese defenders. After escaping in their ships, the soldiers accidentally carried the bacillus back with them to Mediterranean ports, so starting the devastating epidemics of plague that became known as the Black Death. Since then, there has been such a horror of biological warfare that treaties and understandings, even in the midst of world wars, have prevented their use to any large extent. Sadly, unscrupulous persons have now resorted to these methods to terrorize people in this modern age. So what are they likely to use and with what results?

The most highly infectious disease of humans is smallpox and this would be the disease of choice if one wanted to produce the most devastating effect. The last two remaining colonies of variola virus left in the world, one in the USA and the other in Russia, were due to be destroyed in 2002, but this plan has now been changed to one of regular inspections. So unless the virus is stolen or obtained in any other way from either of these sources, the risk is minimal. Even if an outbreak did occur, then the means to control it, by vaccination, is readily available, so would then just depend upon the time it took to produce enough vaccine and vaccinate people. As mentioned above, anyone born before 1979 is likely to have been vaccinated and even though their immunity will have waned, they would probably have a milder form of the disease.

Plague is a more likely contender, as the bacillus is readily obtainable and, as shown above, can be spread with devastating results. However, it is an infection that is well known and reasonably easy to contain within well-circumscribed areas, as outlined in Section 16.1. To make an effective weapon, the bacillus would need to be formulated in such a way that it was spread by the respiratory route which, without first passage through a human as septicaemic or pneumonic plague, might not be possible. A vaccine is available which could be utilized in an emergency and treatment is effective if given soon after symptoms develop.

Similar to plague and easy to obtain would be *Francisella tularensis*, the organism that produces the disease tularaemia. Found in the northern part of the world (Russia, China and the USA) it is transmitted by almost every conceivable method: from the bites of ticks, mosquitoes and the biting fly *Chrysops*; in contaminated water or uncooked meat; by the inhalation of dust and hay from contaminated areas; and through handling small animals, either by their bite or contact with their tissues. The disease presents as an ulcer at the site of introduction of the organism, with localized lymphadenopathy, then spreads to many sites in the body, including the lungs. It is this respiratory form, like pneumonic plague, that would make it a possible weapon. Sprayed as an aerosol, the cause would probably go unrecognized. Fortunately, tularaemia can be treated with streptomycin or gentamicin and a vaccine has been used in Russia, so providing that the cause could be identified reasonably quickly, preventive action could be taken.

Anthrax is probably the most likely candidate and was used in the USA in 2001 in an attempt to target certain individuals through the postal system. A special formulation, probably obtained illegally from a biological warfare establishment, was used and this would be necessary if this attack was to be tried again. Cutaneous anthrax is generally a non-fatal disease, readily responding to treatment, and is the commonest form of the disease (Section 17.7). For anthrax to be a deadly weapon, the organism needs to be inhaled or swallowed without first touching the skin. In natural infections, where people consume meat from an animal that has died of anthrax, nearly all of them develop cutaneous rather than intestinal disease. To be effective, anthrax would therefore need to be administered as a fine powder or in an aerosol.

Probably the easiest biological substance to use as a terrorist weapon is botulinum toxin. The toxin is produced by *Clostridium botulinum* in foods that have been poorly processed in any preserving method, particularly in home-preserved fruit and vegetables that have not been held at a high enough temperature for a sufficient length of time. When these foods are eaten, the patient, after a brief incubation period of 12–36 h, develops a dry mouth, followed by blurring of the vision, difficulty in swallowing, weakness and, in the severe case, a flaccid paralysis, with mortality of about 10%. It would, therefore, be quite easy to produce the toxin and introduce it as a foodstuff to the unsuspecting recipients or administer it as an aerosol in a direct attack. So if there is no obvious source of botulism in a food source then bioterrorism should be suspected.

Any case of botulism should be reported to the local medical authority responsible and the suspect food item sent for analysis prior to destruction by prolonged boiling or incineration. The patient should be purged, the stomach washed out and if seriously ill should be given polyvalent botulinum antitoxin. The usual cause of death is respiratory failure, so facilities, including intubation, should be made ready in case of need. Everybody else who might have eaten from the same food source must be contacted and observed.

With any biological weapon, it is the preparation and means of administration that are the key factors, so unless the terrorist has resource to laboratories and some sophisticated equipment it is likely to be by theft or purchase that substances will be obtained. It is to be hoped these are being carefully guarded against.

Summary

- New infections will continue to appear and organisms that have caused us illness will continue to evolve into different forms.
- Our close association with animals, both domestic and wild, has led to species transfer and several new diseases appearing in humans. This has been the commonest cause of new communicable diseases and is likely to be their main source in the future.
- More stringent methods need to be used to prevent this animal–human contact, and to modify feeding and husbandry practices of domestic animals that might have an effect on human health.
- Sadly, several serious infections have resulted from the excessive use – and often misuse – of antimicrobials, while terrorists have used disease organisms to attack people.
- Basic methods of cleanliness, antisepsis and careful control of organisms and treatments will go a long way to reducing these threats, but new methods are required.

Further Reading

This section includes general works relevant to many of the preceding chapters as well as specific titles that may be useful in this one.

Childs, J.E., Mackenzie, J.S. and Richt, J.A. (eds) (2007) *Wildlife and Emerging Zoonotic Diseases: The Biology, Circumstances and Consequences of Cross-Species Transmission.* Current Topics in Microbiology and Immunology Vol. 315. Springer, Berlin, Heidelberg, New York.

Cook, G.C. and Zumla, A.I. (eds) (2008) *Manson's Tropical Diseases*, 22nd edn. Saunders Elsevier Health Sciences, Philadelphia, Pennsylvania. Online access at Expert Consult.

Eddleston, M., Davidson, R., Brent, A. and Wilkinson, R. (2008) *Oxford Handbook of Tropical Medicine*, 3rd edn. Oxford University Press, New York.

Emond, R.T., Welsby, P.D. and Rowland, H.A. (2003) *Colour Atlas of Infectious Diseases*, 4th edn. Mosby-Wolfe, London.

Gilles, H.M. and Lucas, A.O. (2002) *Short Textbook of Public Health Medicine for the Tropics*, 4th edn. Hodder Arnold, London.

Guerrant, R.L., Walker, D.H. and Weller, P.F. (eds) (2011) *Tropical Infectious Diseases: Principles, Pathogens and Practice*, 3rd edn. Saunders Elsevier Health Sciences, Philadelphia, Pennsylvania. Online access at Expert Consult.

Hawker, J., Begg, N., Blair, I., Reintjes, R. and Weinberg, J. (2005). *Communicable Disease Control Handbook*, 2nd edn. Blackwell Publishing, Malden, Massachusetts/Oxford, UK/Carlton, Victoria, Australia.

Heymann, D.L. (ed.) (2008) *Control of Communicable Diseases Manual*, 19th edn. American Public Health Association, Washington, DC.

Noah, N.D. (2006) *Controlling Communicable Disease*. Understanding Public Health Series. Open University Press/McGraw-Hill Education, Maidenhead, UK.

Parry, E.H., Godfrey, R.T., Mabey, D. and Gill, G. (eds) (2004) *Principles of Medicine in Africa*, 3rd edn. Cambridge University Press, Cambridge, UK.

Peters, W. and Pasvol, G. (2006) *Atlas of Tropical Medicine and Parasitology*. 6th edn. Mosby-Wolfe, London.

Van-Tam, J. and Sellwood, C. (eds) (2010) *Introduction to Pandemic Influenza*. CAB International, Wallingford, UK.

Warrell, D.A., Cox, T.M. and Firth, J.D. (eds) (2010) *Oxford Textbook of Medicine*, 5th edn. Oxford University Press, New York.

Web resources

Emerging Infections Monthly Summaries (from the UK Health Protection Agency). Available at: www.hpa.org.uk/Topics/InfectiousDiseases/InfectionsAZ/EmergingInfections/EmergingInfectionsMonthlySummaries/ (accessed 13 March 2012).

Global Health Archive (from CAB International, Wallingford, UK). Available at: www.cabi.org/globalhealth (accessed 13 March 2012).

Journal of Emerging Infectious Diseases (from the US Centers for Disease Control). Available at: www.cdc.gov/ncidod/eid/index.htm (accessed 13 March 2012).

MedlinePlus (with links to journal articles; from the US National Library of Medicine, National Institutes of Health). Available at: www.nlm.nih.gov/medlineplus/ (accessed 13 March 2012).

Weekly Epidemiological Record (*WER*). Available at: www.who.int/wer/2012/en/ (accessed 13 March 2012).

List of Communicable Diseases

Communicable diseases are listed in alphabetical order by the most commonly used name. Other names will be found in the index. Diseases printed in **bold** are covered in the text.

Incubation periods are the usual range, but exceptions to these limits do occur. Agents are: arboviruses (A); bacteria (B); ectoparasites (E); fungi (F); helminths (but not nematodes) (H); nematodes (N); prions (O); protozoa (P); rickettsiae (R); spirochaetes (S); toxins (T); and other viruses (V). Methods of control are: animal elimination, vaccination and the wearing of gloves and protective clothing (An); testing of donors and treatment of blood for transfusion (Bl); chemotherapy where this is used as a method of control (Ch); food hygiene, cooking and refrigeration (Fo); personal hygiene (Hy); vaccination/immunization (Im); sterilization of needles, instruments and blood giving sets (Ne); rat control (Ra); sanitation (Sa); water supply (Wa); vector control (Vc); and methods for controlling sexually transmitted infections (Xe).

Disease/causative organism	Clinical features (agent)	Means of transmission (control method)	Incubation period
Absettarov virus	Fever (A)	*Ixodes* ticks (Vc)	–
Acanthamoebiasis	Granulomatous amoebic encephalitis (P)	Through skin lesion or conjunctiva	Weeks
Actinomycosis	Sulphur-granule lesions in jaw, thorax or abdomen (F)	Oral–oral (dental hygiene)	Months–years
Acute respiratory infections	Fever, cough, pneumonia (B, V)	Airborne and oral (Ch, Im)	1–3 days
Aeromonas gastroenteritis	Diarrhoea, vomiting (B)	Contaminated food or water (Fo, Hy, Wa)	–
Alenquer virus	Sandfly fever (A)	*Phlebotomus* sandfly (Vc)	3–6 days
Amoebiasis	Diarrhoea and systemic abscesses (P)	Faecal contaminated water and food (Sa, Wa)	2–4 weeks
Angiostrongylus	Meningeal, CNS[a] and abdominal signs (N)	Uncooked snails and slugs; rat reservoir (Fo, Ra)	1–3 weeks
Anisakiasis	Intestinal abscess (N)	Uncooked fish (Fo)	Hours
Anthrax	Skin, intestinal or respiratory lesions (B)	Contact with infected animal tissues (An, Ch)	2–7 days
Apeu fever	Fever (A)	*Aedes* and *Culex* mosquitoes; rodent reservoir (Vc)	3–12 days
Apoi virus	Encephalitis (A)	Vector (unknown)	5–15 days
Armillifer disease	Calcified nodules (E)	Eating raw snakes or snake-contaminated water (Fo, Wa)	–
Ascaris	Malnutrition, intestinal symptoms (N)	Ingestion of soil or food (Fo, Hy, Sa)	10–20 days
Aspergillosis	Bronchial obstruction and eosinophilia (F)	Airborne from compost, hay or stored grain	Days–weeks
Babesiosis	Fever and haemolytic anaemia (P)	*Ixodes* ticks, blood transfusion (Bl, Vc)	1–8 weeks

Continued

Disease/causative organism	Clinical features (agent)	Means of transmission (control method)	Incubation period
Bacillary dysentery	Diarrhoea with blood (B)	Faecal–oral, water, milk, flies (Hy, Sa, Wa)	1–7 days
Balantidiasis	Diarrhoea (P)	Faecal–oral, food, water (pig reservoir) (Fo, Hy, Wa)	Days
Bangui virus	Fever and rash (A)	Vector (unknown)	4–5 days
Banzi virus	Fever (A)	*Culex* mosquito (Vc)	5–15 days
Barmah Forest virus	Fever, arthritis (A)	Culicine mosquito (Vc)	–
Bartonellosis	Fever or skin sore (B)	*Lutzomyia* sandflies (Bl, Vc)	16–22 days
Batai virus	Fever (A)	Culicine mosquito (Vc)	4–5 days
Benign myalgic encephalomyelitis	Muscle weakness and headache (V)	Airborne (Hy)	–
Bhanja virus	Fever, encephalitis (A)	Tick (Vc)	–
Blastomycosis	Pneumonia, skin lesions, (F)	Airborne in spore-laden dust	Weeks–months
Bluetongue	Fever (A)	*Culicoides* midge (Vc)	3–12 days
Botulism	Paralysis (B, T)	Preserved food (Fo)	12–36 hours
Brazilian purpuric fever	Conjunctivitis, meningitis (B)	Contact with conjunctival discharges (Hy)	1–3 days
Brucellosis	Undulant fever (B)	Milk, cheese and contact with animal fluids (An, Fo)	7–60 days
Bunyamwera virus	Fever (A)	*Aedes* mosquito (Vc)	3–12 days
Burkitt's lymphoma	Lymphoma (V)	Associated with malaria (Vc)	–
Buruli ulcer	Skin and tissue loss (B)	Inoculation of organism possibly by aquatic insect	–
Bussuquara virus	Fever (A)	Culicine mosquito (Vc)	5–15 days
Bwamba fever	Fever and rash (A)	Culicine mosquito (Vc)	3–12 days
California encephalitis	Encephalitis (A)	*Aedes* mosquito (Vc)	5–15 days
***Campylobacter* enteritis**	Diarrhoea (B)	Food, milk, water or contact with animals (Fo, Wa)	1–10 days
Candidiasis	Thrush (F)	Contact with secretions (Ch)	2–5 days
Candiru virus	Fever (A)	*Phlebotomus* sandfly (Vc)	3–6 days
Capillariasis, hepatic	Hepatitis and eosinophilia (N)	Uncooked liver (Fo)	3–4 weeks
Capillariasis, intestinal	Malabsorption syndrome (N)	Uncooked fish (Fo)	Months
Capillariasis, pulmonary	Pneumonitis (N)	Ingestion of foods contaminated by soil (Fo)	3–4 weeks
Capnocytophaga	Fever, meningitis (B)	Dog bite, scratch or lick (An)	1–5 days
Caraparu fever	Fever (A)	Culicine mosquito, rodent reservoir (Vc)	3–12 days
Cat-scratch fever	Fever, lymphadenitis (B)	Cat scratch, bite or lick (An)	3–14 days
Catu fever	Fever (A)	Culicine mosquito (Vc)	5–15 days
Chagas' disease	Carditis and megacolon (P)	Reduviidae bug, blood transfusion (An, Bl, Ra, Vc)	5–14 days
Chagres fever	Fever (A)	*Phlebotomus* sandfly (Vc)	3–6 days
Chancroid	Genital ulcer (B)	Sexual contact (Ch, Xe)	3–14 days
Chandipura virus	Fever (A)	*Lutzomyia* sandfly (Vc)	1–6 days
Changuinola fever	Fever (A)	*Phlebotomus* sandfly (Vc)	3–6 days
Chickenpox	Rash (V)	Skin or airborne contact	2–3 weeks
Chikungunya	Fever, rash, arthritis (A)	*Aedes* mosquito; reservoir in baboons and bats (Vc)	3–12 days
Chlamydia	Urethral discharge (B)	Sexual contact (Ch, Xe)	7–14 days

Continued

Disease/causative organism	Clinical features (agent)	Means of transmission (control method)	Incubation period
Cholera	Watery diarrhoea (B)	Faecal contamination of water or food (Hy, Sa, Wa)	1–5 days
Chromomycosis	Skin growths (F)	Penetrating wound, e.g. splinter of wood	Months
Clonorchis sinensis	Liver damage (H)	Uncooked freshwater fish (Fo)	4 weeks
Clostridium difficile	Diarrhoea, colitis (B, T)	Faecal–oral (Hy, and reduce antibiotic use)	2–5 days
Coccidioidomycosis	Disseminated abscesses (F)	Airborne from soil in endemic areas (dust control)	1–4 weeks
Cold, common	Respiratory infection (V)	Airborne droplets through nose, conjunctiva or swallowed (Hy)	1–3 days
Colorado tick	Fever (A)	*Dermacentor* tick; reservoir in small mammals (Vc)	4–5 days
Congenital cytomegalovirus	CNS and liver abnormalities (V)	From genital secretions or breast milk; adults infected by sexual contact or blood transfusion (Bl, Xe)	3–12 weeks
Conjunctivitis	Sore eyes (B, V)	Contact with eye discharges, airborne, flies (Hy, Sa, Wa)	1–3 days
Creeping eruptions	Urticaria and eosinophilia (N)	Soil contaminated by dog and cat faeces (An, Hy, footwear)	Weeks–months
Creutzfeldt–Jacob disease	Encephalopathy and paralysis (O)	Infected meat and tissue contact (Fo)	4–5 years
Crimean–Congo haemorrhagic fever	Haemorrhagic fever (A)	*Hyaloma* ticks and body fluid contact with humans and animals (An, Vc)	1–12 days
Cryptococcosis	Meningitis and skin lesions (F)	Airborne from pigeon droppings? (An)	–
Cryptosporidiosis	Diarrhoea (P)	Faecal–oral and from animals and water (An, Hy, Sa, Wa)	1–12 days
Cyclospora	Diarrhoea (P)	Water and fruit (Fo, Hy, Wa)	5–10 days
Cytomegalovirus infection	Mononucleosis and congenital CNS lesions (V)	Contact with body fluids and congenital; blood transfusion or transplant (Bl, Xe)	3–12 weeks
Dakar bat virus	Fever (A)	Vector, unknown	5–15 days
Dengue	Haemorrhagic fever (A)	*Aedes* mosquito (Vc)	3–15 days
Dermatophagoides	Asthma (E)	Inhaled dust mites (reduce dust)	–
Dhori virus	Fever (A)	Tick vector (Vc)	3–12 days
Dicrocoelias	Liver damage (H)	Eating ants and uncooked liver (Fo)	–
Dipetalonematosis	Fever and swellings (N)	*Culicoides* (Vc)	1 year
Diphtheria	Pharyngitis, Cutaneous lesions (B)	Airborne or skin contact from case or carrier (Im)	2–5 days
Diphyllobothrium	Macrocytic anaemia (H)	Eating uncooked freshwater fish (Fo, Sa)	3–6 weeks
Dipylidium	Tapeworm (H)	Swallowing infected flea (An, Hy, Vc)	3–4 weeks
Dirofilariasis	Pulmonary eosinophilia (N)	Culicine mosquito (Vc)	Weeks–months
Dugbe virus	Fever (A)	Tick vector (Vc)	4–5 days
Duvenhage virus	Rabies-like illness (V)	Animal saliva or bite (An)	–
Eastern equine encephalitis	Encephalitis (A)	*Aedes* mosquito; bird and rodent reservoir (Vc)	5–15 days
Ebola haemorrhagic fever	Haemorrhagic fever (V)	Contact with body fluids or tissues (barrier nurse)	2–21 days

Continued

Disease/causative organism	Clinical features (agent)	Means of transmission (control method)	Incubation period
Echinococcus	Hydatid cysts (H)	From dog via licking, or contaminated food or water (An, Fo, Hy, Wa)	Months–years
Echinostoma	Diarrhoea (H)	Food (raw snails, fish or freshwater plants) (Fo)	–
Edge Hill virus	Fever, arthritis (A)	Culicine mosquito (Vc)	–
Ehrlichiosis	Fever (R)	*Ixodes* and *Amblyomma* ticks (Vc)	1–3 weeks
Encephalitis lethargica	Fever, encephalitis (V)	Airborne	–
Enteritis necroticans	Gangrene of bowel (B)	Uncooked pork and beef (Fo)	6–12 hours
Enterobius	Anal pruritis (N)	Faecal–oral and in dust (Hy)	2–6 weeks
Enteroviral carditis	Fever and myocarditis in neonates (V)	Faecal–oral or airborne (mucus or faecal material) (Hy)	3–5 days
Entomophthoramycosis	Granuloma in skin or nasal passage (F)	Organism found in soil and rotting vegetation	–
Epidemic haemorrhagic conjunctivitis	Conjunctivitis and conjunctival haemorrhages (V)	Contact with eye discharges, airborne and in water (Hy)	1–3 days
Epidemic keratoconjunctivitis	Keratoconjunctivitis (V)	Contact with eye discharges or shared treatments (Hy)	5–12 days
Epidemic myalgia	Fever and pain in chest or abdomen (V)	Faecal–oral or airborne (Hy)	3–5 days
Erysipelas	Cellulitis of tissue (B)	Contamination of abraded skin, flies (Hy, Sa)	1–3 days
Erysipaloid	Skin infection (B)	Handling fish (Hy)	–
Erythema infectiosum	Rash, fetal damage (V)	Airborne, congenital, blood transfusion (Bl, Hy)	4–20 days
***Escherichia coli* O157**	Haemorrhagic colitis (B)	From uncooked beef, milk, faecally contaminated water or vegetables (Fo, Hy, Wa)	2–8 days
Everglades virus	Fever, encephalitis (A)	Culicine mosquito (Vc)	5–15 days
Exanthem subitum	Fever, rash (V)	Salivary contact (Hy)	5–15 days
Fascioliasis	Liver damage (H)	Uncooked freshwater plants (Fo)	–
Fasciolopsis	Intestinal ulceration (H)	Uncooked freshwater plants (Fo)	2–3 months
Filariasis, lymphatic	Lymphoedema (N)	Anopheline and culicine mosquitoes (Ch, Vc)	1 year +
Fish poisoning	Vomiting and paraesthesia (T)	Eating toxic fish (Fo)	0.5–3 hours
Food poisoning	Diarrhoea and vomiting (B, T)	Contaminated food (Fo, Hy)	
		Staphylococci	1–6 hours
		Bacillus cereus	1–12 hours
		Clostridium perfringens	12–24 hours
		Vibrio parahaemolyticus	12–48 hours
Fort Sherman virus	Fever (A)	Culicine mosquito (Vc)	–
Gan Gan virus	Fever, arthritis (A)	Culicine mosquito (Vc)	–
Gastrodiscoides	Diarrhoea (H)	Raw vegetables and water plants (Fo)	–
Gastroenteritis	Diarrhoea (B, V)	Faecal–oral, food, water and milk (Fo, Hy, Im, Sa, Wa)	12–72 hours
Germiston virus	Fever, rash (A)	Culicine mosquitoes (Vc)	5–15 days
Giardia	Diarrhoea, bloating (P)	Faecal–oral, water and food (Fo, Hy, Sa, Wa)	3–25 days
Glanders	Multiple abscesses (B)	From horses (An)	–
Glomerulonephritis	Oedema and haematuria (B)	Airborne or direct (Ch, Hy)	1–3 weeks

Continued

Continued

Disease/causative organism	Clinical features (agent)	Means of transmission (control method)	Incubation period
Gnathostoma	Systemic abscess (N)	Uncooked fish or poultry (Fo)	–
Gonorrhoea	Urethral discharge (B)	Sexual contact (Ch, Xe)	2–7 days
Granuloma inguinale	Anogenital ulcers (B)	Sexual contact (Ch, Xe)	1–16 weeks
Guama fever	Fever (A)	Culicine mosquito (Vc)	5–15 days
Guanarito haemorrhagic fever	Haemorrhagic fever (V)	Inhalation or swallowing of cane rat excreta (Hy, Ra)	7–16 days
Guaroa fever	Fever (A)	Culicine mosquito (Vc)	5–15 days
Guinea worm disease	Leg worm (N)	Water (swallowing infected copepods) (Wa)	1 year
Haemorrhagic fever with renal syndrome	Fever, haemorrhage, shock, oliguria (V)	Aerosol transmission from rodent urine, faeces and saliva (Ra)	2–4 weeks
Hand, foot and mouth disease	Stomatitis and skin lesions (V)	Direct contact with mouth lesions, airborne and faecal–oral (Hy)	3–5 days
Hantavirus pulmonary syndrome	Fever, myalgia, respiratory distress and shock (V)	Aerosol transmission from rodent (deer mouse, pack rats, chipmunks) excreta (Ra)	1–6 weeks
Hanzalova virus	Fever (A)	*Ixodes* ticks (Vc)	–
Helicobacter pylori	Gastritis, ulcer and adenocarcinoma (B)	Faecal–oral or oral–oral (Ch, Hy)	5–10 days
Hendra	Encephalitis (V)	Contact with horses; reservoir in fruit bats (An)	4–18 days
Hepatitis A (HAV)	Jaundice (V)	Faecal–oral, water or food (Fo, Hy, Im, Wa)	15–50 days
Hepatitis B (HBV)	Jaundice (V)	Inoculation, blood transfusion, sexual contact, perinatal (Bl, Im, Ne, Xe)	6 weeks–6 months
Hepatitis C (HCV)	Jaundice, chronic active hepatitis (V)	Inoculation, blood transfusion, sexual contact (Bl, Ne, Xe)	2 weeks–6 months
Hepatitis delta (HDV)	Jaundice, associated with HBV (V)	Inoculation, sexual contact (Im – HBV vaccine, Ne, Xe)	2–8 weeks
Hepatitis E (HEV)	Jaundice, mortality in pregnancy (V)	Water-borne; pig reservoir (An, Hy, Wa)	3–9 weeks
Herpangina	Pharyngitis (V)	Contact with nose and throat discharges, faecal–oral and airborne (Hy, Wa)	3–5 days
Herpes genitalis	Genital sores, in infants encephalitis (V)	Sexual, oral and perinatal contact (Xe)	2–12 days
Herpes simplex	Cold sores or systemic lesions in infants (V)	Contact with saliva or lesions, perinatal (Hy)	2–12 days
Heterophyes	Enteritis (H)	Uncooked freshwater fish (Fo)	–
Histoplasmosis	Pulmonary and systemic lesions (F)	Inhalation of spores from soil (decrease dust)	3–17 days
Hookworm	Anaemia (N)	Larvae penetrate skin (Ch, Hy, Sa, Wa, footwear)	8–10 weeks
Human immunodeficiency virus (HIV)	Fever, diarrhoea, weight loss, opportunistic infection (V)	Sexual contact, blood transfusion, needle–transfer, perinatal (Bl, Ne, Xe)	1–18 years
Human papilloma virus (HPV)	Genital warts, cervical cancer (V)	Sexual or direct contact (Xe)	1–3 months
Hymenolepis	Enteritis (H)	Faecal–oral, food or water (Fo, Hy, Sa, Wa)	1–2 weeks
Ilesha virus	Fever and rash (A)	Vector (unknown)	3–12 days

Continued

Disease/causative organism	Clinical features (agent)	Means of transmission (control method)	Incubation period
Ilheus virus	Encephalitis (A)	Culicine mosquito (Vc)	5–15 days
Impetigo	Crusted spots (B)	Direct contact/airborne (Hy)	4–10 days
Infectious mononucleosis	Glandular fever (V)	Swallowing saliva directly or on toys, etc. (Hy)	4–6 weeks
Influenza	Respiratory infection (V)	Airborne droplets inhaled, swallowed or direct contact with mucous (Hy, Im)	1–5 days
Inkoo virus	Fever (A)	Culicine mosquitoes (Vc)	5–15 days
Isospora	Diarrhoea (P)	Faecal–oral and from dogs and cats (An, Hy, Sa, Wa)	–
Issyk-Kul fever	Fever (A)	Tick vector (Vc)	4–5 days
Itaqui virus	Fever (A)	Culicine mosquito; rodent reservoir (Vc)	3–12 days
Jamestown canyon virus	Encephalitis (A)	Culicine mosquito (Vc)	5–15 days
Japanese encephalitis	Encephalitis (A)	*Culex* mosquito; reservoir in birds and pigs (Im, Vc)	4–14 days
Junin haemorrhagic fever	Haemorrhagic fever (V)	Aerosol or contact with rodent excreta (Im, Ra)	7–16 days
Jurona virus	Fever (A)	Culicine mosquito (Vc)	–
Kaposi's sarcoma	Vascular neoplasia (V)	Sexual contact, associated with HIV infection (Xe)	–
Karshi virus	Fever, encephalitis (A)	Tick vector (Vc)	–
Kasokero virus	Fever (A)	Vector, unknown	5–15 days
Kawasaki syndrome	Fever and rash in children (T)	Unknown, probably airborne	–
Kemerovo virus	Fever (A)	Tick vector (Vc)	4–5 days
Kokobera fever	Fever, arthritis (A)	Culicine mosquito (Vc)	5–15 days
Koutango virus	Fever and rash (A)	Culicine mosquito (Vc)	5–15 days
Kumlinge disease	Fever (A)	*Ixodes* tick; reservoir in rodents and birds (Vc)	–
Kunjin fever	Encephalitis (A)	Culicine mosquito (Vc)	5–15 days
Kuru	Cerebella ataxia (O)	Eating human brain	4–20 years
Kyasanur Forest disease	Haemorrhagic fever and encephalitis (A)	*Haemaphysalis* tick; reservoir in rodents and monkeys (Vc)	3–8 days
La Crosse encephalitis	Encephalitis (A)	*Aedes* mosquito; reservoir in *Aedes* eggs, birds, pigs (Vc)	5–15 days
Larva migrans	Creeping eruptions (N)	Larva penetrates skin (Ch, Hy, Sa, Wa, footwear)	8–10 weeks
Lassa fever	Haemorrhagic fever (V)	*Mastomys* excreta, human blood and excretions, sexual (Hy, Ne, Ra, barrier nurse)	6–21 days
Le Dantec virus	Encephalitis (A)	Vector, unknown	3–12 days
Legionellosis	Pneumonia (B)	Airborne aerosol of water	2–10 days
Leishmaniasis	Cutaneous, mucocutaneous and visceral lesions (P)	*Phlebotomus* and *Lutzomyia* sandflies; mammalian reservoir specific to locality; blood transfusion and needles (An, Bl, Ne, Vc)	2 weeks–6 months
Leprosy	Skin and nerve lesions (B)	Respiratory and close personal contact (Ch, Hy, Im)	1–20 years
Leptospirosis	Fever and jaundice (S)	Contact with rat, pig, cow or dog urine or in water (An, Ra)	4–19 days
Linguatula disease	Nasopharyngitis (E)	Eating raw liver of sheep, goats and cows (Fo)	–

Continued

Continued

Disease/causative organism	Clinical features (agent)	Means of transmission (control method)	Incubation period
Lipovnik virus	Meningitis (A)	Tick vector (Vc)	4–5 days
Listeriosis	Meningoencephalitis in adults and neonates (B)	Eating milk and cheese, contact with animals and perinatal (An, Fo, Hy)	3–70 days
Loiasis	Calabar swelling (N)	*Chrysops* fly (Ch, Vc)	Years
Louping ill	Encephalitis (A)	*Ixodes* tick (Vc)	7–14 days
Lyme disease	Erythematous migrans, meningitis (S)	*Ixodes* tick, reservoir in ticks and mammals (An, Im, Vc)	3–32 days
Lymphocytic choriomeningitis	Choriomeningitis (V)	Excretions of mice in food, contact or aerosol (Fo, Hy, Ra)	8–13 days
Lymphogranuloma venereum	Anovaginal lesions (B)	Sexual and direct contact with lesions (Ch, Xe)	3–30 days
Lymphonodular pharyngitis, acute	Lymphonodular lesions in pharynx (V)	Direct contact with nose, throat discharges and faeces or by aerosol (Hy)	5 days
Machupo haemorrhagic fever	Haemorrhagic fever (V)	*Calomys* rodent urine in dust or through skin (Ra)	7–16 days
Madrid virus	Fever (A)	*Aedes* and *Culex* mosquitoes; rodent reservoir (Vc)	3–32 days
Malaria	Fever (P)	*Anopheles* mosquito (Vc)	9–17 to 18–40 days[b]
		Blood transfusion (Bl, Ne)	2–4 days
Manangle virus	Fever and rash (V)	Close contact with pig fluids and tissues (An, Hy)	14–18 days
Mansonella	Fever, joint pain (N)	*Culicoides* and *Simulium* (Ch)	–
Marburg disease	Haemorrhagic fever (V)	Contact with blood and body fluids (barrier nurse)	2–21 days
Marituba fever	Fever (A)	*Aedes* and *Culex* mosquitoes, rodent reservoir (Vc)	3–12 days
Mayaro fever	Fever, rash, arthritis (A)	*Mansonia* and *Haemagogus* mosquitoes (Vc)	3–11 days
Measles	Fever and rash (V)	Airborne or contact with nose or throat secretions (Im)	10–14 days
Melioidosis	Pulmonary consolidation (B)	Ingestion, inhalation or contact of broken skin with soil	Months–years
Meningitis, *Haemophilus*	Fever and meningitis (B)	Airborne or contact with nose and throat secretions (Ch, Im)	2–4 days
Meningitis, meningococcal	Fever and meningitis (B)	Airborne or contact with nose and throat secretions (Ch, Im)	2–10 days
Meningitis, pneumococcal	Fever and meningitis (B)	Airborne or contact with nose and throat secretions (Ch, Im)	1–3 days
Meningitis, viral	Fever and meningitis (V)	Airborne or contact with nose and throat secretions (Hy, Im)	Depends on organism
Metagonimus	Diarrhoea (H)	Uncooked fish (Fo)	–
Microsporidiosis	Diarrhoea (P)	Ingestion, inhalation? (Hy)	–
Mokola virus	Rabies-like illness (V)	Animal saliva or bite (An)	–
Molluscum contagiosum	Skin papules (V)	Direct contact with lesions, sexual contact (Hy, Xe)	19–50 days
Monkeypox	Pox rash (V)	Close contact with animal or person to person (An, Im)	–
Morumbi virus	Fever (A)	Culicine mosquito (Vc)	–
Mucambo virus	Fever (A)	Vector, unknown	3–11 days

Continued

Disease/causative organism	Clinical features (agent)	Means of transmission (control method)	Incubation period
Mucormycosis	Thrombosis and infarction (F)	Inhalation, ingestion or inoculation of spores (Ne)	–
Mumps	Parotitis (V)	Airborne and contact with saliva (Im)	14–24 days
Murray Valley encephalitis	Encephalitis (A)	*Culex* mosquito, reservoir in birds (Vc)	5–15 days
Murutucu virus	Fever (A)	Culicine mosquito, rodent reservoir (Vc)	3–12 days
Mycetoma	Localised induration and sinuses (B, F)	Inoculation from soil or wood splinters or thorns (footwear)	Months
Mycoplasma	Pneumonia	Airborne droplets or direct contact with secretions (Hy)	6–32 days
Myiasis	Furuncle, wound or various sites (E)	Fly larvae (Vc)	–
Naegleriasis	Meningoencephalitis (P)	Stagnant water in nasal passages, e.g. swimming	3–7 days
Nairobi sheep disease	Fever (A)	Tick vector (Vc)	4–5 days
Nasopharyngeal cancer	Obstruction of nasopharynx (V)	Epstein–Barr virus (EBV) from saliva exchange	Years
Negishi virus	Encephalitis (A)	Vector, unknown	5–15 days
Nepuyo virus	Fever (A)	Culicine mosquito; rodent reservoir (Vc)	3–12 days
Nipah	Encephalitis (V)	Close contact with pig fluids and tissues (An, Hy)	4–45 days
Nocardiosis	Systemic abscesses (B)	Inhalation of soil dust	Weeks
Noma ulcer	Mouth ulcer (B)	Contact with lesions (Hy)	–
Non-gonococcal urethritis	Urethritis and discharge (B)	Sexual contact (Xe)	1–2 weeks
Non-Hodgkin's lymphoma	Lymphoma (V)	Reactivated EBV infection due to immunodeficiency	–
Norwalk or Norovirus	Diarrhoea (V)	Faecal–oral, airborne or via food and water (Fo, Hy, Wa)	1–2 days
Nyando virus	Fever (A)	Culicine mosquito (Vc)	3–12 days
Ockelbo	Arthralgia, rash (A)	*Aedes* and *Culex* mosquitoes (Vc)	–
Omsk haemorrhagic fever	Haemorrhagic fever (A)	*Dermacentor* tick or contact with muskrat (Im, Vc)	3–8 days
Onchocerciasis	Blindness and skin damage (N)	*Simulium* fly (Vc)	1 year
O'nyong-nyong fever	Arthralgia (A)	*Anopheles* mosquito (Vc)	3–12 days
Ophthalmia neonatorum	Conjunctivitis in newborn (B)	Genital secretions of mother to infant (Ch, Hy, Xe)	2–7 days[c] 7–14 days[d]
Opisthorcis	Liver damage (H)	Uncooked freshwater fish (Fo)	4 weeks
Orf virus	Maculopapular lesions (V)	Contact with mucous membranes of infected sheep and goats (An, Hy)	3–6 days
Oriboca virus	Fever (A)	*Aedes* and *Culex* mosquitoes (Vc)	3–12 days
Oropouche fever	Fever and meningitis (A)	Culicine mosquito; reservoir in monkeys, sloths, birds (Vc)	3–12 days
Orungo fever	Fever (A)	*Aedes* and *Anopheles* mosquitoes (Vc)	3–12 days
Ossa virus	Fever (A)	Culicine mosquito; rodent reservoir (Vc)	3–12 days
Osteomyelitis	Bone abscess (B)	Blood or wound infection (Ch)	4–10 days
Otitis media	Ear infection (B)	Secondary to respiratory or throat infection (Ch, Hy, Im)	1–4 days

Continued

Chapter 20

Disease/causative organism	Clinical features (agent)	Means of transmission (control method)	Incubation period
Paracoccidioidomycosis	Mycosis of respiratory tract and skin (F)	Airborne soil dust	Months–years
Paragonimus	Lung damage (H)	Freshwater crabs/crayfish (Fo)	6–10 weeks
Parainfluenza	Croup, pneumonia (V)	Respiratory or contact (Hy)	1–10 days
Paratyphoid	Diarrhoea and rash (B)	Faecal contamination of food and water (Fo, Hy, Im, Sa, Wa)	1–10 days
Pasteurellosis	Cellulitis (B)	Cat scratch or dog bite (An)	12–24 hours
Pediculosis	Urticaria (E)	From infested person (Hy, Vc)	10–14 days
Pertussis	Whooping cough (B)	Airborne droplets (Im)	7–10 days
Pinta	Maculopapular rash (S)	Contact with lesions or by flies (Ch, Hy, Sa, Wa)	1–3 weeks
Piry virus	Fever (A)	Vector, unknown	3–12 days
Plague	Bubonic (B)	*Xenopsylla* fleas (Ra, Vc)	2–6 days
	Pneumonic (B)	Airborne (barrier nurse)	1–4 days
Pneumococcal pneumonia	Pneumonia (B)	Airborne droplets or direct contact with discharges (Im)	1–3 days
Pneumocystis	Pneumonia (P/F)	Airborne or reactivated infection (Ch)	1–2 months
Pneumonia, chlamydial	Pneumonia in neonates and adults	To infant during birth; adult by direct contact (Hy)	1–12 weeks
Poliomyelitis	Paralysis (V)	Faecal–oral or respiratory (Im)	5–30 days
Pongola virus	Fever, arthritis (A)	Culicine mosquito (Vc)	3–12 days
Powassan virus	Encephalitis (A)	Tick vector (Vc)	7–14 days
Psittacosis	Pneumonia (B)	Inhale bird droppings (An, Hy)	5–15 days
Puerperal fever	Genital tract infection following delivery (B)	Droplets, hands or faecal contamination (Ch, Hy)	1–3 days
Punta Toro virus	Fever (A)	*Phlebotomus* sandfly (Vc)	3–6 days
Pyelonephritis	Pain passing urine, fever (B)	Contamination during pregnancy, catheter, etc.	6–8 days
Q fever	Fever, endocarditis (R)	Direct from animal fluids, airborne or milk (An, Fo, Hy)	2–3 weeks
Quaranfil virus	Fever (A)	Tick vector (Vc)	4–5 days
Rabies	Encephalomyelitis (V)	Animal saliva via bite or abrasion, also bats (An, Im)	2–12 weeks
Rat-bite fever	Fever and rash (B, S)	Rat bite, also secretions (Ra)	1–3 weeks
Relapsing fever	Periodic fever, mainly children (S)	*Pediculus* louse (Hy, Vc) or	5–15 days
		Ornithodorus tick (Ra, Vc)	3–10 days
Respiratory syncytial virus	Fever, rhinitis, pneumonia (V)	Respiratory, contact or swallowed (Hy)	2–8 days
Restan virus	Fever (A)	Culicine mosquito; rodent reservoir (Vc)	3–12 days
Rheumatic fever	Cardiac damage (B)	Secondary to sore throat from respiratory (droplet) (Ch)	1–3 days[e] 19 days[f]
Rhinosporidiosis	Growth in nose (B)	Stagnant fresh water, swimming	–
Rickettsial pox	Fever and rash (R)	Mite vector; rodent reservoir (Vc)	3–13 days
Rift Valley fever	Haemorrhagic fever (A)	*Culex* mosquito, contact with animal tissues (An, Vc)	3–12 days
Rio Bravo virus	Encephalitis (A)	Vector (unknown)	5–15 days
Rocio encephalitis	Encephalitis (A)	*Culex* mosquito (Vc)	5–15 days
Rocky mountain spotted fever	Fever and rash (R)	*Amblyomma* and *Dermacentor* ticks (An, Vc)	3–14 days

Continued

Continued

Disease/causative organism	Clinical features (agent)	Means of transmission (control method)	Incubation period
Ross River fever	Arthritis (A)	*Aedes* and *Culex* mosquitoes (Vc)	3–11 days
Rotavirus	Diarrhoea (V)	Faecal–oral, respiratory, direct or water (Im, Hy, Wa)	1–3 days
Rubella, congenital rubella syndrome (CRS)	Rash in adults, neonatal lesions (V)	Respiratory or direct to congenital (Im)	15–20 days
Sabia haemorrhagic fever	Haemorrhagic fever (V)	Inhaled rodent excreta (Ra)	7–16 days
St Louis encephalitis	Encephalitis (A)	*Culex* mosquito (Vc)	5–15 days
Salmonellosis	Diarrhoea (B)	Meat, milk, eggs, faecal–oral and water (Fo, Hy, Wa)	12–36 hours
Sandfly fever	Fever (A)	*Phlebotomus* and *Lutzomyia* sandflies (Vc)	3–6 days
Sarcocystis	Diarrhoea (P)	Uncooked meat (Fo)	–
Scabies	Urticaria (C)	Direct contact (Ch, Hy, Wa)	2–6 weeks
Scarlet fever	Rash (B)	Respiratory (Ch, Hy, Wa)	1–3 days
Schistosomiasis	Liver or bladder damage (H)	Water contact (Ch, Hy, Sa, Wa, decrease water contact)	2–6 weeks
Semliki Forest virus	Encephalitis (A)	Culicine mosquito (Vc)	3–12 days
Sepik virus	Fever (A)	Culicine mosquito (Vc)	5–15 days
Serra Norte virus	Fever (A)	Vector (unknown)	–
Severe acute respiratory syndrome	Cough, pneumonia, difficult breathing (V)	Respiratory, close contact, faecal–oral? (Hy)	1–14 days
Shingles	Vesicular rash (V)	Reactivated chickenpox	2–3 weeks
Shokwe virus	Fever (A)	Culicine mosquito (Vc)	3–12 days
Shuni virus	Fever (A)	Mosquito, *Culicoides* (Vc)	3–12 days
Simian B virus	Meningoencephalitis (V)	Monkey bite or contact with saliva (An, Hy)	3 days–3 weeks
Sindbis virus	Arthritis, rash (A)	*Culex* mosquito; reservoir in birds (Vc)	3–12 days
Sleeping sickness	Fever, headache, somnolence (P)	*Glossina* tsetse fly (An, Ch, Vc)	Weeks–months
Smallpox	Pox rash (V)	Respiratory, skin contact (Im)	7–19 days
Snowshoe hare virus	Encephalitis (A)	Culicine mosquito (Vc)	3–12 days
Sparganosis	Subcutaneous nodules (H)	Water, or eating frogs and other amphibians (Fo, Wa)	–
Spondweni virus	Fever (A)	Culicine mosquito (Vc)	3–12 days
Sporotrichosis	Skin nodules (F)	Percutaneous, inhalation from wood or sphagnum moss	1 week–3 months
Staphylococcus	Skin, wound, bone or organ infections (B)	Autoinfection, contact with lesions or flies (Ch, Hy, Wa)	5–10 days
Streptococcal sepsis of the newborn	Pneumonia and meningitis (B)	Perinatal from genital tract infection (Ch, Hy)	1–7 days
Streptococcal sore throat	Inflamed throat and tonsils (B)	Respiratory or ingestion of food or milk (Ch, Fo, Hy)	1–3 days
Strongyloides	Creeping eruption (N)	Larvae penetrate skin, oral or autoinfection (Hy, Sa)	2–4 weeks
Syphilis, endemic	Skin and bone lesions (S)	Shared drinking vessels and direct contact (Ch, Hy, Wa)	2 weeks–3 months
Syphilis, venereal	Skin, heart and CNS lesions (S)	Sexual or direct contact, via blood or congenital (Bl, Ch, Xe)	9–90 days
T-cell leukaemia	Sarcoma, lymphoma or leukaemia (V)	Breast milk, blood, needles or sexual contact (Bl, Ne, Xe)	–
Tacaiuma virus	Fever (A)	*Anopheles* mosquito (Vc)	3–12 days
Taenia saginata	Tapeworm (H)	Eating uncooked beef (An, Fo)	10–14 weeks

Continued

Continued

Disease/causative organism	Clinical features (agent)	Means of transmission (control method)	Incubation period
Taenia solium	Tapeworm and cysticercosis (H)	Uncooked pork, autoinfection, swallowing eggs (An, Fo)	8–12 weeks
Tahyna virus	Fever (A)	Culicine mosquito (Vc)	–
Tamdy virus	Fever (A)	Tick vector (Vc)	4–5 days
Tataguine virus	Fever and rash (A)	Culicine mosquito (Vc)	5–15 days
Tensaw virus	Encephalitis (A)	Culicine mosquito (Vc)	3–12 days
Tetanus (and neonatal tetanus)	Muscular contractions and rigidity (B, T)	Contamination of abraded skin or umbilicus (Hy, Im)	4–21 days
Thogoto virus	Meningitis (A)	Tick vector (Vc)	4–5 days
Tick-borne encephalitis	Encephalitis (A)	Tick vector (Vc)	7–14 days
Tick typhus	Fever (R)	Dog tick vector and reservoir (An, Vc)	1–15 days
Tinea	Fungal skin and nail disease (F)	Direct skin contact, also animals (An, Hy, Wa)	4–14 days
Tonate virus	Fever (A)	Culicine mosquito (Vc)	3–12 days
Toscana virus	Meningitis (A)	*Phlebotomus* sandfly (Vc)	3–6 days
Toxic shock syndrome	Fever and shock (B)	Frequently associated with use of absorbent tampons and contraceptive devices in women (Ch)	4–10 days[g] 1–3 days[h]
Toxocara	Fever, cough, rash, liver enlargement, blindness (H)	Ingestion of earth or food contaminated with dog and cat faeces (An, Fo, Hy)	Weeks–months
Toxoplasmosis	Often asymptomatic in adult, but brain damage to neonate (P)	Eating uncooked meat, earth contaminated with cat faeces or direct from cat (An, Fo, Hy)	10–20 days
Trachoma	Red eye, blindness (B)	Contact with eye discharges from fingers, wipes and clothing. Flies (Ch, Hy, Sa, Wa)	5–12 days
Trench fever	Fever, endocarditis (B)	*Pediculus* louse (Hy, Vc)	7–30 days
Trichinosis	Fever and systemic cysts (N)	Uncooked pork and other meat (An, Fo, Ra)	8–15 days
Trichomonas	Vaginitis (P)	Sexual contact (Ch, Xe)	5–20 days
Trichuris	Diarrhoea, debility in children (N)	Ingestion of soil and soil on vegetables (Fo, Hy, Sa, Wa)	2–3 months
Trivittatus virus	Fever (A)	Culicine mosquito (Vc)	–
Tropical spastic paresis	Myelopathy and spasticity (V)	Blood or sexual contact (Bl, Xe)	–
Tropical ulcer	Skin ulcer with tissue loss (B)	Contamination of abraded skin, flies (Hy, Sa, Wa)	2–7 days
Trubanaman virus	Fever, arthritis (A)	Culicine mosquito (Vc)	–
Tuberculosis (TB)	Cough, weight loss and anaemia (B)	Respiratory, spitting, unpasteurized milk (Ch, Hy, Im)	4–12 weeks
Tucunduba virus	Encephalitis (A)	Culicine mosquito (Vc)	–
Tularaemia	Lymphadenopathy, systemic lesions (B)	Tick, *Chrysops*, *Aedes*, animal bite, water and meat or inhalation (An, Fo, Hy, Vc)	1–14 days
Tunga	Foot furuncles (E)	Invasive flea (footwear)	–
Typhoid	Fever and bowl ulceration (B)	Faecal contamination of food, water. Flies (Fo, Hy, Im, Sa, Wa)	3–30 days
Typhus, epidemic	Fever, prostration and rash (B)	*Pediculus* faeces scratched in or inhaled (Hy, Im, Vc)	1–2 weeks
Typhus, murine	Fever and rash, mild (B)	*Xenopsylla* flea faeces inhaled (Hy, Ra, Vc)	1–2 weeks

Continued

Disease/causative organism	Clinical features (agent)	Means of transmission (control method)	Incubation period
Typhus, scrub	Fever, eschar and rash, mild–severe (B)	*Leptotrombidium* mite, reservoir in small mammals (Vc)	1–3 weeks
Usutu virus	Fever, rash (A)	Culicine mosquito (Vc)	3–12 days
Venezuelan equine encephalitis	Fever and encephalitis (A)	Culicine mosquito; reservoir in rodents and horses (Im, Vc)	2–6 days
Vesicular stomatitis	Fever, pharyngitis (A)	*Lutzomyia* sandfly (Vc)	–
Wanowrie virus	Fever and bleeding (A)	Tick vector (Vc)	4–5 days
Warts	Skin growths (V)	Direct contact, inoculation or indirect (e.g. floors) (Hy)	2–3 months
Wesselsbron disease	Fever (A)	Culicine mosquito (Vc)	3–12 days
Western equine encephalitis	Encephalitis (A)	*Culex* mosquito (Vc)	5–15 days
West Nile fever	Fever (A)	*Culex* mosquito; reservoir in birds (Vc)	3–12 days
Wyeomyia fever	Fever (A)	Culicine mosquito (Vc)	3–12 days
Xingu virus	Fever, hepatitis (A)	Vector, unknown	–
Yaws	Skin and bone lesions (S)	Contact with lesions and exudates, flies (Ch, Hy, Sa, Wa)	2–8 weeks
Yellow fever	Haemorrhagic fever (A)	*Aedes* mosquito; reservoir in monkeys (Im, Vc)	3–6 days
Yersiniosis	Fever and diarrhoea (B)	Faecal–oral, contaminated food and water; pig reservoir (An, Fo, Hy, Sa, Wa)	3–7 days
Zika virus	Fever (A)	Culicine mosquito (Vc)	5–15 days

[a]CNS, central nervous system.
[b]Incubation period depends on *Plasmodium* spp.
[c]Gonococcal ophthalmic neonatorum.
[d]Chlamydial ophthalmic neonatorum.
[e]Initial streptococcal infection.
[f]Time to development of acute rheumatic fever.
[g]Staphyloccal infection.
[h]Streptococcal infection.

Index

Diseases are listed by the name most commonly used, such as whooping cough rather than pertussis, but leptospirosis rather than Weil's disease. Cross-references are given to all other names of each disease. Countries where relevant are listed, except for European countries where they are all under the single heading of Europe. Page numbers in **bold** refer to figures and tables.

insecticides *see* vector control
interstitial plasma-cell pneumonia *see* pneumocystis
intestinal fluke *see* Fasciolopsis
Iran 117, 140, 239, 260
    see also Asia
Iraq 138, 260
    see also Asia
Isospora sp. **263**, 306
Israel 158, 198
Israeli tick typhus *see* tick typhus fever
Issyk-Kul fever **256**, 306
itaqui virus 306
Ixodes spp., disease transmission **256**, **257**, 301, 304,
    305, **306**, 307
      I. holocyclus 257
      I. ricinus 19, 258
      I. scapularis 258
Ixodidae 255

jackals, diseases association 123, **239**, 264, 266
Jamestown Canyon virus 306
    see also encephalitis
Japan 117, 119, 120, 138, 140, **197**, 200, 251, **256**,
    259, 272, 275, 293
    see also Asia
Japanese encephalitis (JE) 14, 36–**37**, **53**, 119–120, 198,
    259, 260, **271**, 306
Junin haemorrhagic fever 306
jurona virus **306**

kala-azar *see* leishmaniasis, visceral
Kaposi's sarcoma 2, 158, 184, 281, 291, **306**
karelian fever *see* sindbis
karshi virus **256**, 306
kasokero virus 306
Kawasaki syndrome 306
Kemerovo virus **256**, 306
Kenya 19, 54, **74**, **157**, 183, 193, 210, 214,
    227, **239**, 266
    see also Africa
Kenya tick typhus *see* tick typhus
keratoconjunctivitis 78, 83, 87–88, 304
    see also epidemic keratoconjunctivitis
kerion *see* tinea
Klebsiella granulomatis 180
kokobera fever **306**
Korea 117, 119, 200, 293
    see also Asia
Korean haemorrhagic fever *see* haemorrhagic fever with
    renal syndrome
koutango virus 306
kumlinge disease **256**, 306
kunjin fever **306**
kuru 9, 292, **306**
Kyasanur Forest disease 198, 199, 260, **306**

La Crosse encephalitis **271**, 306
Laos 117, 119, 138, 200, 293
    see also Asia
larva currens 130
larva migrans 129, **263**, 268–269, 306
larvicides *see* vector control
laryngitis *see* acute respiratory infections
Lassa fever 10, 32, 57, 193–194, 275–276,
    283, 291, **306**
latency 3, 4, 143, 168, 238
latent period 4, 23, 176, 177, 281
Le Dantec virus **306**
legionellosis **306**
Leishmania spp. 19, 237, **238**, **239**, **240**
leishmaniasis 19, **53**, 185, 237–241, **263**, 281, **306**
leprosy 9, **43**, **45**, 63, 69, 72, **73**, 150–153, 183,
    278, **279**, 306
    see also BCG; *Mycobacterium leprae*
Leptospira interrogans 168, **271**, 274
leptospirosis 19, **43**, **44**, **45**, 57, **73**, **104**, 274–275, **306**
Liberia 74, 203, 276
    see also Africa
lice 8, **53**, 56, 57, 76, 78, 79–80, 143, 195, 242
Linguatula 264, **271**, 306
Lipovnik virus **265**, 307
listeriosis **279**, 284–285, **307**
liver cancer *see* hepatocellular cancer
Loa loa 218, 222, 225, 227
lockjaw *see* tetanus
loiasis 227–228, **307**
louping ill **256**, 307
lues *see* syphilis, venereal
lung fluke *see* Paragonimus westermani
Lutzomyia spp. 238, **239**, 302, **306**, 310, **312**
lyme disease 19, 20, **168**, **256**, 258–259, **271**, 307
lymphatic filariasis *see* filariasis, lymphatic
lymphocytic choriomeningitis virus 168, **307**
lymphogranuloma venereum *see* inguinale
lymphonodular pharyngitis, acute **307**
lyssa *see* rabies
lyssavirus 262

Machupo haemorrhagic fever **307**
Madagascar **74**, 143, 164, 198, **219**, 246, 295, 296
    see also Africa
Madrid virus **307**
Madura foot *see* mycetoma
malaria
    forest fringe 13, 14
    life cycle **206**, 210–211, **212**
    mathematical models 26, 210–212
    see also Anopheles spp.; *Plasmodium* spp.
malaria risk map for Africa (MARA) 157
Malawi 225, 281
    see also Africa
Malayan filariasis *see* filariasis, lymphatic

necrotizing ulcerative stomatitis *see* noma ulcer

negishi virus **308**

neonatal inclusion blennorrhoea *see* ophthalmia neonatorum

Nepal **55**, 152, 162, 169, 200, **209**, 239, 278
  see also Asia

nephropathia epidemica *see* haemorrhagic fever with renal syndrome

nepuyo virus **308**

New Guinea Island 109, 141, 197, 200, 205, 214, 215, **219**

New World spotted fever *see* Rocky Mountain spotted fever

New Zealand **197**

Niger 106, 170
  see also Africa

Nigeria **74**, 85, 92, 106, **157**, 203, 227, 272, 276
  see also Africa

Nipah virus **263**, **271**, 295, **308**

njovera *see* syphilis

nocardiosis **308**

noma ulcer **308**

nomads/pastoralists 13, 273, 274

non-A non-B hepatitis *see* hepatitis C; hepatitis E

non-gonococcal urethritis (NGU) 87, 177, 178, 179–180, **308**

non-Hodgkin's lymphoma 2, 185, **308**

non-venereal syphilis *see* syphilis, endemic

norovirus *see* Norwalk

North American tick typhus *see* Rocky Mountain spotted fever

North Asian tick fever *see* tick typhus

Norwalk **308**

notification of diseases **33**, 52, 59, 60, 72–74, 98, 157, **159**
  England and Wales 73
  WHO 72, 73, 97, 105, 112, 144, 200, 247, 252, 265, 276

nyando virus **308**

occupational diseases 28, 139, 190, 232, 260, 274
  see also anthrax; arbovirus infections; hepatitis, B; schistosomiasis; sleeping sickness

ockelbo *see* sindbis

Ohara disease *see* tularaemia

Omsk haemorrhagic fever **256**, 260, **308**

Onchocerca volvulus **218**, 223

onchocerciasis 79, 130, 220, 222, 223–227
  vectors 14, **42**, **45**, 223, **224**, **225**, **308**

onychomycosis *see* tinea

o'nyong-nyong virus 197, **308**

ophthalmia neonatorum 73, 78, 87, 179, **279**, 280, 288, 290, **308**
  see also eye diseases

Opisthorchis sp. 2, 102, 117, **118**, **263**, **271**, 303, **308**

opossum, diseases association 235, 249, 275

oral rehydration solution (ORS) 89, **91**, 96, 108

orf virus **308**

organophosphates 55–56

oriboca virus **308**

oriental sore *see* leishmaniasis

Orientia sp. 247, 249

Ornithodorus spp. **253**, 254, **256**, 288, **309**

ornithosis *see* psittacosis

oropouche fever 197–198, **308**

Oroya fever *see* bartonellosis

ORS (oral rehydration solution) 89, **91**, 96, 108

orungo fever 197–198, **308**

ossa virus **308**

osteomyelitis 170, **308**
  see also staphylococcus infection; streptococcal infections

otitis media 35, 75, 145, 149, 164, 170, 171, 172–173, 174, 184, **308**
  see also staphylococcal infections; streptococcal infections

outbreak, investigation 28

oxyuriasis *see* *Enterobius*

Pacific Islands 57, 80, 81, 86, 95, 109, 112, 152, 158, 169, 172, 174, 192, **197**, 202, 214, 215, 217

Pakistan 92, 106, 140, **157**, 185, 251, 260
  see also Asia

Panama 74, **204**, 258
  see also America, Central

Panstrongylus sp. 235, 236

papatasi fever *see* sandfly fever

Papua New Guinea 2, 9, 19, 131, 171, 181, 185, **219**, 292, 295

paracoccidioidomycosis **309**

Paragonimus spp. 6, **42**, **44**, **49**, **115**, 118, 119, **263**, **271**, **309**

Paraguay 74, 236
  see also America, South

parainfluenza virus 161, **162**, 163, **309**

paramyxoviridae 144, 148

parapertussis *see* whooping cough

paratrachoma *see* opthalmia neonatorum

paratyphoid 73, 103, **309**
  see also typhoid

parotitis *see* mumps

parrot fever *see* psittacosis

Parvovirus B19 **279**, 285, 289
  see also erythema infectiosum

passive case detection *see* surveillance, passive

pasteurellosis **263**, **309**

pasteurization, milk 102, 109, 113, 158, 259, 260, 270, 272, 284, 285, **311**

pastoralists/nomads 13, 273, 274

pediculosis *see* lice

period of communicability, *definition* 23

persistence, pathogens 4, 5, 93, 95, 102, 273, 274

shigellosis **84**, 97–98
  see also Shigella sp.
shingles 10, 143–144, **310**
  see also chickenpox
shipyard eye *see* epidemic keratoconjunctivitis
shokwe virus **310**
shuni virus **310**
Siberian tick typhus *see* tick typhus
Sierra Leone 74, 203, 276
  see also Africa
simian B virus **310**
Simulium spp. 14, **42**, 223, **224**, **225**, 227, 241, **307**, **308**
sindbis virus **310**
Singapore 292
sixth disease *see* exanthem subitum
skin infections **76**, 83, 87, 143–163, 182, **304**
skunk, diseases association 249, 264, 275
slave trade, disease dissemination 130, 138
sleeping sickness
  African 8, 64, 228–233
  American *see* Chagas' disease
  Gambian 13, 230–232
  Rhodesian 9, 232–233
  vectors 9, 14, 228, **229**, 231, 234, **271**, **310**
small round structured virus (SRSV) *see* Norwalk
smallpox 11, 26, 64, **73**, 143, 144, 291, 294, 295, 298, **310**
snail, as intermediate host
  food-borne diseases 114, **116**, 117, **118**, 119
  helminths **42**
  meningitis cause **168**, **301**
  schistosomiasis 6, 8, 14, 30, 31
  water contact diseases 136, 138, 139, 141, 142
snowshoe hare virus **310**
sodoku *see* rat-bite fever
soft chancre *see* chancroid
soil contact diseases **76**, 77, 87, 124, 125–134
soil eating *see* pica
solar water disinfection (SODIS) 47, 95
Solomon Islands 19, **63**, 205
  see also Pacific Islands
South Africa **157**, 162, 174, 185, 186, 281
South American blastomycosis *see* paracoccidioidomycosis
sparganosis **310**
spirillosis *see* rat-bite fever
spondweni virus **310**
sporotrichosis **310**
Sri Lanka 209, 219, 221
  see also Asia
Staphylococcus aureus **162**, 164, 172, 297
staphylococcus infection 109, **310**
  see also food, poisoning; otitis media
streptobacillary fever *see* rat-bite fever
streptococcal infections 23, 87, 173, 174, **271**
  newborn sepsis **310**
  skin infections **76**, 83, 87, 149–150, 182, **304**

sore throat **162**, 162, 166, 172, 174, 192, 262, 275, 293, 295, **309**, **310**
  see also impetigo; rheumatic fever; scarlet fever
Streptococcus pneumoniae 161, **162**, 164, **168**, 171, 172, 173, 297
  vaccination 297
Strongyloides spp. 4, **42**, 49, 124, 130–132, 185, **263**, **310**
subacute spongiform encephalopathy
  see Creutzfeldt–Jakob disease
subclinical transmission 8–9, 167
Sudan 74, 85, 106, 140, 192, 193, **225**, **239**, 272
  see also Africa
surveillance 62, 63–64, 73, 79, 80, 86
  active 59, 62–63, 68, 69
  emergency 63
  passive 62, 67, 68
  routine 62
  sentinel 63
Swaziland 281
  see also Africa
swineherd disease *see* leptospirosis
syphilis
  congenital **279**
  during pregnancy 280–281
  endemic 7, 78, 81, 83, **310**
  meningitis cause **168**
  venereal 81, 176–177, **310**

T-cell leukaemia/lymphosarcoma **310**
tacaiuma virus **310**
Taenia spp. 5, **42**, 43, **44**, 49, **115**, 122
  T. saginata 6, 120, **122**, **271**, **310**
  T. solium 6, **122**, **271**, **311**
tahyna virus **311**
Taiwan 114, 117, 119, 138
  see also Asia
tamdy virus **311**
Tanzania 5, **18**, **19**, 68, 74, 147, 152, **157**, 197, 214, **225**, 230, 231, 246
  see also Africa
tapeworm
  beef 6, 120, **122**, **271**, **310**
  fish 6, 119–120, **121**
  pig 6, **122**, **271**, **311**
  see also Diphyllobothrium spp.; *Dipylidium* spp.; *Hymenolepis* spp.; *Taenia* spp.
tataguine virus **311**
TB *see* tuberculosis
temephos (Abate) 54, 56, 204, 224, 251
  see also insecticides; larvicides
temperature 5, 14–15, 19, 20, 37, 38, 39, 43, 81, 93, 100, 101, 109, 112, 113, 122, 123, 126, 136, 203, 207, 210, 215, 223, 229, 238, 243, 247, 250, 259, 262, 270, 272, 299
tensaw virus **311**